MY LABORATORY   MY PR

AUTHOR SIGNATURE FORM

Name of book	How to be a Lab Director 2020 edition		
Author of Book	Philip A. Dauterman, MD PMB 276 P.O. Box 10001 Saipan, MP 96950 E-mail: drp_dauterman@yahoo.com	Board Certified in Anatomic Pathology and Clinical Pathology	Since 1996
Mandatory Comment Field	In my Pathology training days, the program strongly favored Anatomic Pathology. The Clinical Pathology training was the minimum number of months to be eligible for boards, and all classroom work. There was not even a single "hands on" course that involved on-the-job training in a real life setting. After graduation, I had a great deal of classroom knowledge, but did not know how to deal with real-life situations in real labs. I learned that on the fly and on the job. America's Pathology training programs still strongly emphasize Anatomic Pathology at the expense of Clinical Pathology. To date, there has not been an educational book written about how to be a hospital Lab Director. This book is intended to fill that void.		
Optional comment field			
Owner of book		Note: if the book ownership changes, strike the former book owner's name and affiliation with a single line and write in the new book owner's name and affiliation. All changes must be signed and dated. Use of white-out is prohibited.	
Affiliation of owner of book			
Author signature	*Philip A. Dauterman, M.D.*	**Seventh edition published Jan. 1, 2020**	

How to be a Lab Director 2020 edition by Philip A. Dauterman, MD
with graphs by Steven Matthew R. Dauterman
Table of Contents

Chapter 1 – Intro to the Clinical Lab

Chapter 2 – Things you probably don't need to know as a Lab Director
    A. The color on the top of the drawing tubes.
    B. Diagnostic precision and accuracy
    C. Sensitivity and specificity
    D. Limit of detection and limit of quantitation

Chapter 3 – How to read a Levey-Jennings chart

Chapter 4 – Pick your Westgard rules carefully

Chapter 5 – Proficiency testing and corrective actions

Chapter 6 – What to do if one analyte fails two or more proficiency testing events in one year

Chapter 7 – How to put a new analyzer into service
    A. Pick which equipment you want to buy
    B. Decide to rent, buy or lease the equipment
    C. The new analyzer and the Service Rep arrive
    D. Check correlation
    E. Do calibration, verification of calibration and check linearity
    F. Set the Analytical Measurement Range (AMR), Reference Range and Critical Values
    G. Write the procedures for the new equipment
    H. Controls, final preparations, going live with the new analyzer and retiring the old analyzer

Chapter 8 – How to put a new test onto an existing analyzer

Chapter 9 – How to deal with analyzer breakdowns

Chapter 10 – How to read a linearity proficiency test report

Chapter 11 – How to write a policy and/or procedure

Chapter 12 – Quality Assurance, complaints, incident reports and root cause analysis

Chapter 13 – How to deal with personnel problems
    A. How to spot a potentially homicidal employee
    B. How to spot a potentially suicidal employee
    C. How to deal with two lab employees that do not get along
    D. How to deal with a disagreement between employees inside and outside lab
    E. How to deal with the chronically late to work employee
    F. How to deal with an employee with performance and/or behavioral issues

Chapter 14 – Physician and administrator demands on lab and physician ordering practices

Chapter 15 – Professional relations. Making sure you are not a problem employee
    A. What to wear to work
    B. Always know your relationship to your employer
    C. Avoid conflicts of interest

Chapter 16 – Lab tech hiring, orientation, competency testing, promotion, retention and discipline

Chapter 17 – Administration, management, planning and deciding which tests to do in-house

Chapter 18 – Other duties delegated to the Lab Director

Chapter 19 – How to be a Lab Supervisor

Chapter 20 - Section supervisor qualifications, duties, responsibilities, promotion and retention

Chapter 21 – Pathologist hiring, orientation, competency testing, promotion, retention and retirement

Chapter 22 – How to go through the inspection process
    A. How to pick an inspecting agency and prepare for the inspection
    B. The day of the inspection
    C. How to fill out CMS form 2567 and write a Plan of Correction
    D. Testing your abilities to make a Plan of Correction

Chapter 23 – Regulatory scrutiny syndrome

Chapter 24 – How to avoid HIPAA pitfalls

Chapter 25 – How to interact with the legal profession

Chapter 26 – How to be a waived test Lab Director and a PPM Lab Director

Chapter 27 – How to start a new lab from nothing

Chapter 28 – Lab Director ethics

Chapter 29 – Lab Director leadership skills and how to deal with conflict in the clinical laboratory

Chapter 30 – How to chair a meeting

Chapter 31 – Lab Director hiring, orientation, competency testing, promotion, retention and retirement

Chapter 32 – Advanced topics in Lab Directorship
    Topic #1 - How to handle certificates and PT when patient testing is spread across multiple sites
    Topic #2 - How to perform verification for a non-waived qualitative analyzer
    Topic #3 - How to perform "off label" test verification
    Topic #4 - How to make an Individualized Quality Control Plan (IQCP)
    Topic #5 - Public relations. Lab Director as Public Information Officer (PIO)
    Topic #6 - Lab Director liability (malpractice) insurance
    Topic #7 - Laboratory Information Technology (IT) and Laboratory Information Systems (LIS)
    Topic #8 - The End. How to perform voluntary closure of a laboratory

Chapter 1 – Intro To the Clinical Lab

In the US almost all lab testing is governed by a Federal law called the Clinical Laboratory Improvement Amendments of 1988 (known in the business as "CLIA"). There are a few exceptions, such as pre-employment drug screening. However, every lab in the US that does patient testing (i.e. clinical labs) must follow the CLIA regulations. As a Lab Director a good part of your time will be spent ensuring that your lab complies with all CLIA regulations.

Some states set higher requirements for clinical laboratories than is mandated by the federal CLIA law. For example CLIA only requires retention for 2 years for most clinical lab test records whereas the State of Idaho requires retention of these records for at least 5 years from the date of the test. The reference is Idaho Code Ann. § 39-1394. In this situation, you must follow the more stringent requirements of the State in which your lab is located. In Idaho, you must retain all test records for at least 5 years, but in most other states you can dispose of most lab records after 2 years.

Some municipalities have municipal regulations that affect clinical labs. This is typically limited to waste disposal. For the remainder of this book, I will only be covering the federal CLIA requirements and not giving a State by State or municipal breakdown of clinical lab requirements. In order to be effective as a Lab Director you will need to know not only the CLIA requirements but also all State and municipal regulations affecting clinical labs in your locale.

Under CLIA there are three levels of complexity for lab testing: waived, moderate and high complexity. There is a separate entity called Provider Performed Microscopy (PPM). PPM is largely limited to outpatient clinics where the providers do their own microscopic work such as wet mounts and fern tests. In the typical hospital lab this is limited to urine microscopy, KOH prep, fern tests and wet mounts. This is an insignificant part of the typical hospital lab's workload. For this reason, I will not refer to PPM in this book again, except for Chapter 26 which deals with outpatient testing.

That being said, any given lab test is assigned to one of the three levels of complexity (waived, moderate or high complexity) based on the difficulty of doing the test. Given the way the regulations are set up, the director of a lab doing any moderate and/or high complexity testing is almost always a pathologist. Anyone can be the lab director of a lab doing only waived testing.

While reading this entire book, unless stated otherwise and with the exception of Chapter 26, one can assume that the information given refers to moderate and/or high complexity testing. Chapter 26 deals with waived testing and the outpatient setting.

The typical hospital lab is divided into several sections – Hematology, Blood Bank, Chemistry, Microbiology, Urinalysis, Send-out testing, and Anatomic Pathology. The Receptionist's Office will be at the front of the lab. Immediately behind the Receptionist's Office is the drawing area.

In the typical small to midsize hospital lab the Lab Secretary's, Lab Director's and Lab Supervisor's Offices are in an office area at the back of the Lab. The chemistry, hematology, send-out and urinalysis sections are in a large open area at the center of the lab. Blood Bank, Microbiology and Anatomic Pathology each have their own separate side rooms adjoining the main part of lab. There is considerable variation in floor plan from one lab to another.

The Lab Director is the immediate supervisor to the pathologists and the Lab Supervisor. The Lab Supervisor is immediate supervisor to the section supervisors. The section supervisors are immediate supervisors to the bench level lab techs. The Lab Director answers to the hospital Medical Director who in turn answers to the Hospital Administrator. The typical chain of command chart is as follows:

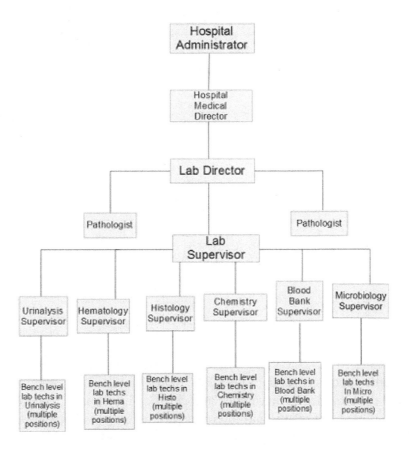

There is some variation in terminology from lab to lab. In some labs the position termed "Lab Supervisor" above is called "Lab Manager" or something similar.

The lab's day is divided into three shifts which typically run as follows: day shift 7AM to 3PM, evening (swing) shift 3PM to 11PM and overnight (graveyard) shift 11PM to 7AM. A lab tech working the day shift will typically work in one section only.

The term "floating" is used when a lab tech works in more than one section of lab during the same 8 hour shift. For example, if a lab tech scheduled to work in chemistry section is called upon to do Blood Bank work, the person is said to "float" to Blood Bank. The ability to work in more than one section of lab is considered a desirable quality. Not all lab techs can do this.

At some labs the evening shift and overnight shift are considered to be separate sections of lab. In this case the evening shift supervisor and overnight shift supervisor are equal in status to section supervisors. The typical small hospital lab has minimal staffing on these shifts (i.e. a "skeleton crew"). The lab techs on these shifts must work in most or all sections of lab. There is typically a pay differential for the evening and overnight shifts since these are considered undesirable shifts, and require the lab techs to "float" to most or all sections of lab.

Next I will go into filling out CMS form 209 Laboratory Personnel Report. This is required prior to all CMS inspections, and helps illustrate the relationships of the parties involved.

Here is what CMS form 209 Laboratory Personnel Report looks like:

DEPARTMENT OF HEALTH AND HUMAN SERVICES
CENTERS FOR MEDICARE & MEDICAID SERVICES

Form Approved
OMB No. 0938-0151

LABORATORY PERSONNEL REPORT (CLIA)
(For moderate and high complexity testing)

1. LABORATORY NAME	2. CLIA IDENTIFICATION NUMBER

3. LABORATORY ADDRESS *(NUMBER AND STREET)*	CITY	STATE	ZIP CODE

4. Instructions:
a. List below all technical personnel, by name, who are employed by the laboratory. Check (✓) the appropriate column for each position held. For TC and TS follow instructions on reverse.
b. Indicate whether shift worked is (1) day, (2) evening or (3) night.
c. Indicate highest level of testing for which personnel are qualified: Use (M) for moderate and (H) for high complexity.
d. Indicate whether position held is full (F) or part-time (P).

Positions:
D - Director
CC - Clinical Consultant
TC - Technical Consultant
TS - Technical Supervisor
GS - General Supervisor
TP - Testing Personnel
CT/GS - Cytology General Supervisor
CT - Cytotechnologist

5. TELEPHONE *(INCLUDE AREA CODE)*

FOR OFFICIAL USE ONLY
(NOT TO BE COMPLETED BY LABORATORY)
QUALIFIES ACCORDING TO SUBPART M

DATE OF SURVEY _____

EMPLOYEE NAMES			a. POSITION HELD								b. SHIFT 1 2 3	c. M OR H	d. F OR P	
LAST NAME	FIRST NAME	MI	D	CC	TC	TS	GS	TP	CT/GS	CT				

For the purposes of CMS form 209, the Lab Director is the same as the Clinical Consultant. The Lab Director provides overall supervision to the Lab. CLIA states that the Lab Director must have an MD, DO, DPM or an earned doctoral degree in science and certified by a board. The Clinical Consultant ensures the quality of reported test results and interprets test results. In all states, the interpretation of test results requires an MD, DO or possibly a DPM degree. The work of the Lab Director and Clinical Consultant typically only justifies one full time equivalent; hence one person typically fills both roles. In my experience the minimum qualifications are an MD or DO degree plus state licensure and Pathology board certification.

Next down the totem pole is the "Technical Consultant" in a moderate complexity testing lab. This is essentially identical to the "Technical Supervisor" in a high complexity testing lab. These positions are effectively the same as the "Lab Supervisor" position in the lab chain of command diagram above. This position deals with quality control of all areas of Lab, proficiency testing, competency testing of all personnel in lab, etc.

The "General Supervisor" in a high complexity testing lab is more or less the same as a section supervisor in the above chain of command diagram. This position is responsible for the quality control of one section of Lab. This person should be able to do corrective actions and troubleshoot any problems (equipment breakdowns, controls not in, etc.) in their own section of Lab, but not necessarily for Lab as a whole.

The "Testing Personnel" are the people doing the day-to-day hands on work of Lab testing. Their job is to do the testing, document and maintain records of their work as necessary, follow the laboratory's procedure manual and quality control policies, identify and correct problems that may adversely affect testing and follow instructions from their supervisors.

The check boxes for "CT/GS" and "CT" are used for the cytotech supervisor and cytotech respectively. There are also check boxes for shift worked, highest level complexity testing that person is allowed to perform and for part time/full time status.

If your lab is doing both moderate and high complexity testing (i.e. the typical hospital lab), you must have at least one person designated as Laboratory Director, Clinical Consultant, Technical Supervisor, Technical Consultant, General Supervisor and Testing Personnel. One person can occupy multiple of these positions in which case multiple boxes are checked off for that person in the form above.

If your lab is only doing moderate complexity testing (i.e. most respiratory labs since arterial blood gas testing is typically moderate complexity) you don't need a General Supervisor or a Technical Supervisor designated in the form above. You only need a Lab Director, Clinical Consultant (almost always the same person as the Lab Director), Technical Consultant and Testing Personnel. One person can occupy multiple of these positions in which case multiple boxes are checked off for that person on CMS form 209.

For the Technical Supervisor and Technical Consultant positions, specialties should be indicated by numbers. See the CMS form 209 instructions as to which numbers correspond to which specialties. Here is an example of what it looks like when you are done:

EMPLOYEE NAMES			POSITION HELD							S/H/1/F/3	M or H	F or P	
LAST NAME	FIRST NAME	MI	D	CC	TC	TS	GS	TP	CTGS	CT			
Dauterman	Philip	A	X	X							1	H	F
Doe	John				7,8	1,9	X	X			1,2,3	H	F
Doe	Jane				12,35	12,35		X			1,2,3	H	F
Washington	George						X	X			1,2,3	H	P
Jefferson	Thomas							X			1	M	F
Adams	John								X	X	1	H	F

Only the positions listed above go on CMS form 209. Below the bench level lab techs there are phlebotomists, secretaries, billing specialists, etc. None of these lower ranking positions are listed on CMS form 209. The janitorial, security, maintenance and repair positions typically come under the main hospital, not the Lab, such that Lab is not responsible for overseeing those positions. None of these positions go on CMS form 209 either.

The CLIA educational, training and competency testing requirements only apply to the positions on CMS form 209. These CLIA requirements do not apply to the lower ranking positions that do not appear on CMS form 209. In other words, the lab does not need to perform competency testing on the phlebotomists, secretaries and janitors. My advice is that it is in your best interest to competency test the phlebotomists, since the entire testing process depends on specimens they have drawn.

After CMS form 209 is filled out you will sign it as Lab Director. Make sure to read the fine print:

READ THE FOLLOWING CAREFULLY BEFORE SIGNING

Statement or Entities Generally: Whoever, in any manner within the jurisdiction of any department or agency of the United States knowingly and willfully falsifies, conceals or covers up by any trick, scheme, or device a material fact, or makes false, fictitious or fraudulent statements or representations, or makes or uses any false writing or document knowing the same to contain any false, fictitious or fraudulent statements or entry, shall be fined not more than $10,000 or imprisoned not more than five years, or both. (U.S. Code, Title 18, Sec. 1001)

CERTIFICATION: I CERTIFY THAT ALL OF THE INDIVIDUALS LISTED ABOVE QUALIFY, TO FUNCTION IN THE POSITION INDICATED, ACCORDING TO THE PERSONNEL REGULATIONS OF 42 CFR PART 493 SUBPART M.

6. SIGNATURE OF LABORATORY DIRECTOR	7. DATE

FORM CMS-209 (09/92)   IF CONTINUATION SHEET PAGE ___ OF ___

As with most documents you will send in to the CMS, there are severe penalties for falsification. Before you sign this form, make sure the information is as accurate as possible. If you are new to that lab and have not seen the lab techs' credentials previously, double-check the credential folders for the lab techs to make sure that all the documentation is in place.

Lab tests can be ordered as STAT, ASAP, routine or timed depending on when and how quickly the results are needed. Turnaround time is the duration from ordering the test to results sign-out in the computer (or manual sign-out of results) by the Lab.

Lab tests are only supposed to be ordered STAT in true emergencies. Ordering a lab test as a STAT causes the lab techs to stop whatever they are doing (routine tests) and concentrate on the STAT specimen. Tests should only be ordered STAT when absolutely necessary. Unnecessary STAT ordering will delay other patient's routine tests. STAT lab tests are typically allowed a turnaround time of 1 hour.

STAT test ordering tends to be abused by Physicians with a tendency to indiscriminate STAT ordering. If STAT ordering becomes a problem (most tests ordered STAT) it may help to put in place criteria as to what really does constitute a medical emergency requiring a STAT test.

Lab tests ordered ASAP (As Soon As Possible) are not as urgent as a STAT but higher priority than routine. A test ordered ASAP will not cause the lab techs to stop whatever they are doing to concentrate on this test. Instead, the ASAP test is prioritized ahead of all the routine work. Allowable turnaround time of a test ordered ASAP is typically up to 3 hours.

Lab tests ordered as routine are collected and tested only after the above more urgent tests are dealt with. Routine tests can be batched, in other words saved up in order to be tested with multiple other specimens. Routine lab tests are typically allowed a turnaround time of 24 hours.

Lab tests ordered as timed are collected at the time requested, usually in the early morning hours so that the results are ready for the Physician's morning rounds. These tests are typically batched and analyzed with the next routine batch.

Chapter 2 – Things you probably don't need to know as a Lab Director

    A. The color on the top of the drawing tubes.

While I was in medical school, The first 2 years were pure classroom work. In the third year, I did very limited drawing of patient lab specimens then went on to electives in the fourth year that involved no drawing. During Pathology residency, none of the residents did any drawing of lab specimens. From talking with other Pathologists, my education is typical of the US Pathology training system.

When I graduated from training in 1996 and took my first job, I did not know which color top tube corresponds to which lab test and vice versa. The phlebotomists and technologists considered this basic, first day on the job knowledge. The initial impression of the lab staff working under me was that my training was not very good. I had to memorize the following very quickly:

Light blue top tubes
 -Contains sodium citrate which anticoagulates by forming insoluble complexes with calcium
 -Used for testing coagulation (PT, PTT, INR, etc.)

Red/Black (tiger top) tubes
-No anticoagulant. Allows blood to clot. Gel acts as a barrier to separate serum and cells.
-Used primarily for chemistry panels

Red top Tubes
-No anticoagulant. Allows blood to clot. No gel present
-Used primarily for Blood Bank procedures and some drug testing

Green top tubes:
-Lithium heparin (light green top) or sodium heparin (dark green top) which anticoagulates by neutralizing thromboplastin and thrombin
-Used primarily for electrolytes and STAT chemistry panels

Lavender (purple) top tubes
-Potassium ethylenediaminetetraacetate (EDTA) anticoagulates by binding calcium
-Used primarily for Complete Blood Counts (CBCs)

Gray Top Tubes
-Potassium oxalate (anticoagulates by binding calcium) and sodium fluoride (preservative)
-Used for glucose testing and some chemistry tests

Yellow Top Tubes
-Acid-citrate-dextrose (ACD) inactivates complement. Citrate anticoagulates by binding calcium
-Used for HLA typing, paternity testing and DNA studies

Orange Top Tubes
-Contains thrombin which acts as a procoagulant.
-Used for STAT serum chemistries

Dark blue (royal blue) top tubes
-Sodium heparin with or without EDTA additive
-This tube is specifically designed to be devoid of metals.
-Used for trace element testing (zinc, copper, lead, mercury) and toxicology

Black top tubes
-Contains buffered sodium citrate which anticoagulates by binding calcium
-Used for Westergren sedimentation rate

Pink top tubes
-Potassium EDTA anticoagulates by binding calcium
-Used primarily for Blood Bank

There are a variety of special tubes on the market each with a different color on top. In general these are used for esoteric testing that you don't have to worry about.

Plasma is the acellular, liquid part of blood with the clotting factors still in it. This is what you get in a tube with anticoagulant when the anticoagulant is mixed properly with the blood. Serum is the acellular, liquid part of blood without the clotting factors. This is what you get in a tube without anticoagulant or in an improperly collected anticoagulant tube in which the blood has clotted due to improper mixing of blood and anticoagulant.

B. Diagnostic precision and accuracy

The terms precision and accuracy appear frequently in the literature. The analogy I will give here is shooting at a target. Accuracy means having the average of your shots correspond exactly to the center of the target (i.e. "true" value). Precision is how tightly clustered your shots are relative to each other. For clinical lab testing, the "true" value you are aiming for is typically the peer mean on a Proficiency Test (PT) or the known mean of a control substance.

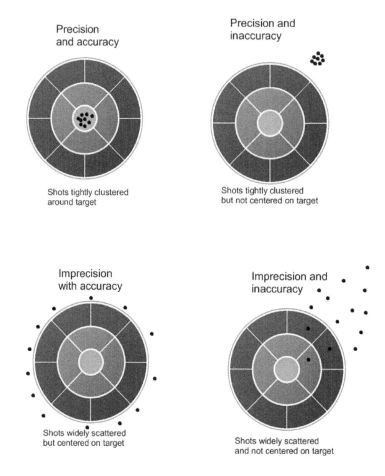

In diagnostic testing, you want to have both accuracy and precision. The main point of quality control is to make sure that testing is both accurate and precise.

Inaccuracy implies measurement bias. Bias is the difference between the average of your measurements and the target. Bias in turn implies systematic error. Systematic error does not occur by chance but instead results from a consistent, reproducible error in the measurements. Imprecision implies random error. Random error occurs by pure chance.

Measurement error is the difference between the measured value and the "true" value. Measurement error can result from systematic error or random error or both.

Outside the US, the ISO nomenclature and regulations are used. The ISO terminology equates accuracy with the absence of bias and absence of imprecision. This is different from the American CLIA definition which equates accuracy with absence of bias (but not necessarily absence of imprecision). I will be using American terminology throughout this book and will not refer further to international ISO terminology. It is my understanding that the international ISO regulations governing laboratories are generally similar to the CLIA regulations, but they not exactly identical.

C. Sensitivity and specificity

The terms sensitivity and specificity are heavily used in the Lab literature. When calculating sensitivity and specificity, it is assumed that the world is binary. There are only positive and negative tests, and no such thing as an equivocal or borderline test. It is assumed that the patient does or does not have a fully developed disease, and there is no such thing as a "form fruste", early stage of disease, etc.

Thus sensitivity and specificity assume a perfect binary world. In the real world, these calculations may have some value, but are overrated in my opinion. Here's the simplest way of looking at it:

	Patient has disease	Patient without disease
Test positive	True positive	False positive
Test negative	False negative	True negative

Sensitivity = number of true positive tests divided by number of patients with disease

Specificity = number of true negative tests divided by number of patients without disease

Positive predictive value = number of true positives divided by the total number of positive tests

Negative predictive value = number of true negatives divided by the total number of negative tests

Prevalence = number of patients with disease divided by total number of patients

As an example I will use the fictitious test serum radon levels. At present there is no such test, it doesn't exist. I will use serum radon levels throughout this book as an example of a generic, garden variety test and will further assume that this nonexistent test is strongly associated with lung cancer as shown below:

	lung cancer	no lung cancer	totals
serum radon positive	99	10	109
serum radon negative	1	890	891
totals	100	900	1000

Sensitivity = 99 ÷ 100 = 99.0%   Specificity = 890 ÷ 900 = 98.9%

Positive predictive value = 99 ÷ 109 = 90.8%   Negative predictive value = 890 ÷ 891 = 99.9%

Prevalence = 100 ÷ 1000 = 10.0%

For any given test, the sensitivity and specificity depend on the cutoff used. For example, screening for prostate cancer in asymptomatic elderly men using PSA. If the cutoff is set very low (PSA of 2 is positive) you will have large numbers of positive tests and few of them will be true positive (prostate cancer). The sensitivity will be increased but the specificity will be reduced compared to using a middling cutoff number.

If the cutoff is set very high (PSA of 7 is positive), there will be very few positive tests, but a larger percent of those positives will be true positive (prostate cancer). The sensitivity is reduced but the specificity is increased compared to using a middling cutoff number.

In general for population screening, you want to have the highest sensitivity that is practicable. In the example above, you don't want to miss anyone with prostate cancer, and it doesn't matter much if you do a large number of prostate biopsies. Hence, the cutoff is set relatively low for this type of testing. For diagnostic testing, the cutoff is set higher.

D. Limit of detection and limit of quantitation

The limit of detection (LoD), also known as the detection limit or lower limit of detection, is the amount of an analyte that can be distinguished from zero with reasonable certainty. This is the smallest amount of analyte that can be detected, but this does not necessarily mean you can quantify it.

The limit of quantitation (LoQ) is the amount of analyte that can be quantitatively measured with acceptable precision and accuracy.

In this setting false positive is determining that an analyte is present when it really isn't. False negative is determining that an analyte is absent when it really is present.

If you test a sample with no analyte, most analyzers will give a minimal signal that is slightly greater than zero. This minimal signal is referred to as "noise". The negative sample used in this setting is typically saline and is referred to as a "blank". If you repeatedly run blank specimens the results can be used to calculate the mean of blanks (i.e. the "noise" level) and the standard deviation (SD) of the blanks. If you repeatedly run weakly positive specimens you can determine a mean and SD for the weakly positive specimens.

The blanks and the weakly positive specimens will have a roughly Gaussian distribution. The mean for these two populations will be very close together, such that the distributions overlap:

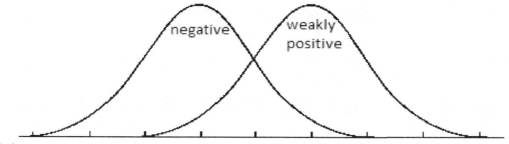

There is little agreement in the literature on how to calculate the LoD and LoQ. I have seen the LoD defined as the mean of blanks plus 1.645 or 2 or 3 times the blank SD. The LoD has also been defined as 3 or 5 times the mean of blanks (i.e. signal to noise ratio of 3 or 5).

The LoQ can be equal to the LoD or higher, but cannot be below the LoD. The LoQ is most frequently defined as the mean of blanks plus 10 times the blank SD. I have also seen it defined as 10 times the mean of blanks (i.e. signal to noise ratio of 10) and defined as the lower limit of linearity.

The higher you set the LoD, the less risk there is of a false positive with a truly negative specimen. However, setting the LoD higher means there is more risk of a false negative when testing a truly positive specimen containing trace amounts of the analyte. This results in reduced sensitivity but increased specificity compared to a lower LoD situation. Here is what happens if you set a high LoD:

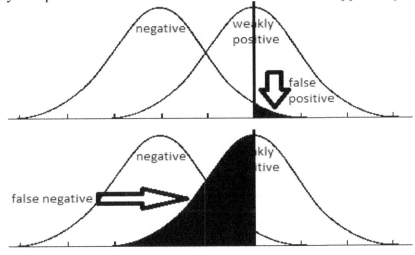

If you set a low LoD there is more risk of a false positive and less risk of a false negative. This results in increased sensitivity but reduced specificity compared to the high LoD situation described above. Here is what happens if you set a low LoD:

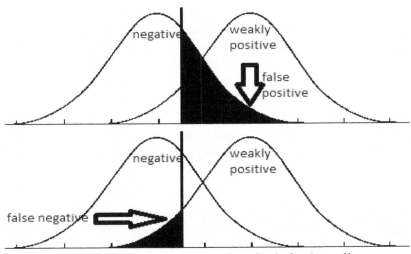

Deciding where to set the LoD is very important in testing for infectious diseases such as nucleic acid testing for Hepatitis C Virus (HCV). In this setting any detectable amount at all represents a positive test for HCV. For general patient testing, you want to avoid false positives for HCV (i.e. you want high specificity but don't care as much about the sensitivity), so you set the LoD high enough that any equivocal results are reported as negative. However, setting the LoD this high will result in false negatives in patients with minimal, barely detectable viral nucleic acid loads.

For blood donor testing, you want to avoid false negatives (i.e. you want high sensitivity but don't care as much about the specificity), so you set the LoD much lower. The lower LoD means you will almost never give out a false negative. However, equivocal results will be reported as positive and you will have more false positives.

For any given test methodology the sensitivity and specificity are always a trade-off. One must decrease as the other increases. The only possible way to increase both the sensitivity and the specificity at the same time is to change the test methodology.

Chapter 3 – How to read a Levey-Jennings chart

A Levey-Jennings chart displays data points in chronological order from left to right (x axis). Typically it represents one or two month's worth of controls. The y-axis is measured in standard deviations. A point one standard deviation above the mean indicates that test resulted one standard deviation above the known mean of the control substance, and so on. The chart starts the month blank, as follows:

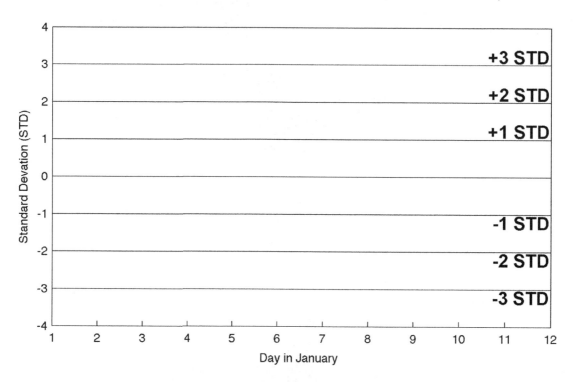

The chart is then filled in one day at a time. On January 7 it looks like the following:

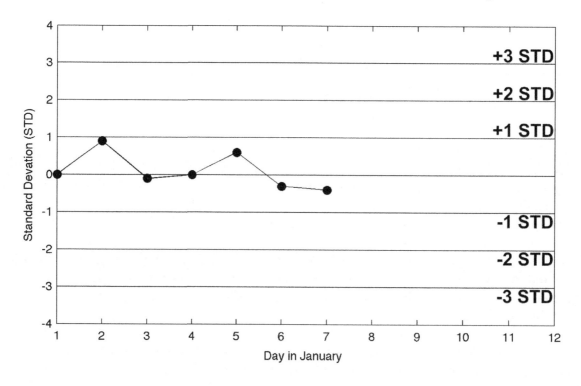

Eventually the chart is completely filled in

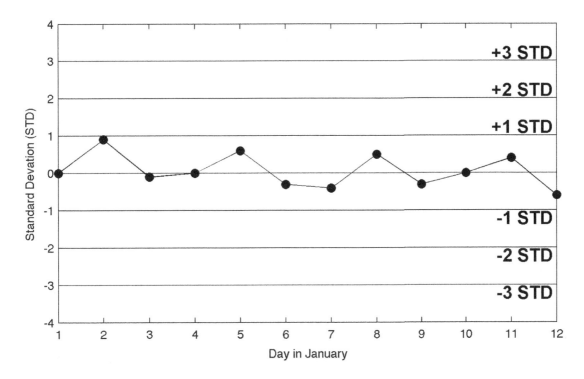

In this example, the chart only runs 12 days. That is all the time we will need to demonstrate the Westgard rules (see next chapter). In reality the typical Levey-Jennings chart runs for one or two months. After one Levey-Jennings chart is filled the next chart should start contiguously. For the above example, the next Levey-Jennings chart should start no later than January 13. If it were to start later, it would imply there were days when controls were not tested. This would result in an inspection citation.

The Levey-Jennings chart in the example above passes all the Westgard rules given in the next chapter. The data points are clustered close to the mean, and randomly scattered above, below and on the mean. There are roughly equal numbers of data points above the mean and below the mean.

For clinical lab testing, the "true" mean you are aiming for is typically the peer mean on a Proficiency Test (PT) or the known mean of a control substance. Controls typically come from the manufacturer with the mean and SD already determined. Each time you test a control, you are comparing your test results against the expected outcome.

In the above Levey-Jennings chart the mean of your results is extremely close to the "true" mean (i.e. your results are accurate). For clinical lab testing, your mean does not have to exactly match the true mean, it just has to be reasonably close. In the above Levey-Jennings chart the clustering of data points close to the mean indicates your SD is not any larger than it should be (i.e. your results are precise). Similar to the accuracy, the precision does not need to be perfect but does need to be reasonably good.

The next chapter will deal with the rules used to determine if your control test results are close enough to the expected outcome (i.e. there are no problems with your testing) or too far away from the expected outcome (i.e. something is wrong with your testing).

Chapter 4 – Pick your Westgard rules carefully

In the last chapter we covered the basics of Levey-Jennings charts. In order to review these charts for quality control (QC) purposes, one must have a set of rules to determine if the chart passes or fails the rules. Multi-rule QC is called Westgard rules after the inventor. The reference is:

Westgard JO, Barry PL, Hunt MR, Groth T. A multi-rule Shewhart chart for quality control in clinical chemistry. Clin Chem 1981;27:493-501.

Extensive description of Westgard rules can be found at the Westgard website www.westgard.com. Examples of Westgard rules are as follows:

1-3S – any one point falls outside of 3 standard deviations (SD) from the mean. In the following graph the offending data point is circled:

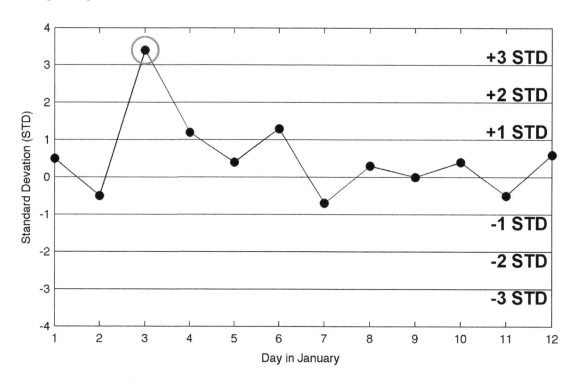

Assuming a Gaussian distribution, the probability of any given point falling more than 3SD from the mean is 0.3%. For 31 consecutive random points (a month's worth of data) the chance that any one of these 31 data points will randomly fall outside 3SD is 0.3% times 31 equals 9.3%.

8x – any 8 consecutive points are on the same side of the mean. In the example below, there are 8 consecutive points above the mean, and the offending area of the graph is circled:

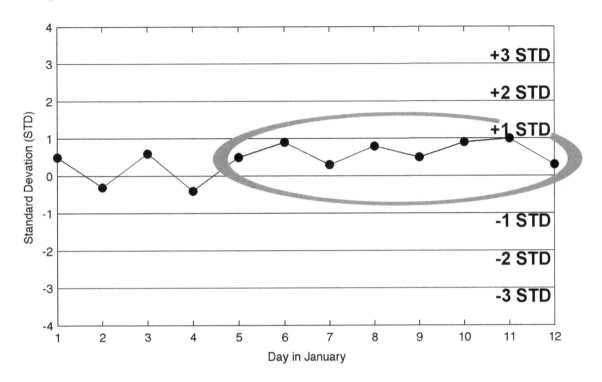

For any given number the probability of the next number being on the same side of the mean is 50%. The other 50% will be on the other side of the mean. For the purpose of this calculation we are excluding numbers on the mean. The numbers are random and discrete. This is just like a coin toss, which can be either heads or tails.

Let's say that the coin toss on day one is heads. The probability that the next seven coin tosses are heads is 0.5 x 0.5 x 0.5 x 0.5 x 0.5 x 0.5 x 0.5 = 0.78%. In the chart above the first day's data point is above the mean. The probability of the following 7 being above the mean is 1 in 2 to the seventh power, about 0.78%. Day one has a 0.78% chance of the following 7 days coming out the same. Day two also has a 0.78% chance of the following 7 days coming out the same. This continues up until day 25 at which point there are only 6 days left in the month, not enough for seven more tries. The cumulative probability over those 25 days is 0.78% times 25 equals 19.5% In the course of a 31 day month that comes out to 19.5% probability of eight consecutive data points above or below the mean by chance alone.

10x – any 10 consecutive points are on the same side of the mean. In the example below, there are 10 consecutive points above the mean, and the offending area of the graph is circled:

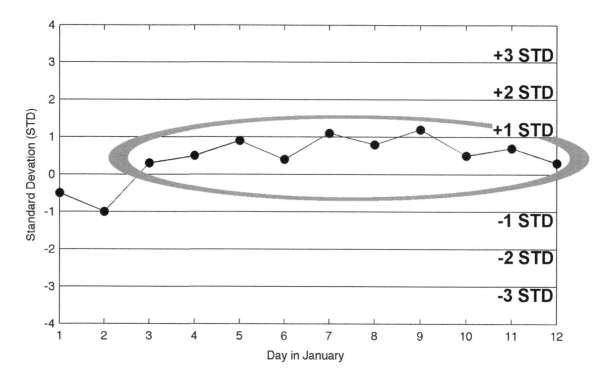

For any given number the probability of the next number being on the same side of the mean is 50%. The other 50% will be on the other side of the mean. For the purpose of this calculation we are excluding numbers on the mean. The numbers are random and discrete. This is just like a coin toss, which can be either heads or tails.

Let's say that the coin toss on day one is heads. The probability that the next nine coin tosses are heads is 0.5 x 0.5 x 0.5 x 0.5 x 0.5 x 0.5 x 0.5 x 0.5 x 0.5 = 0.19%. In the chart above the first day's data point is below the mean. The probability of the following 9 being below the mean is 1 in 2 to the ninth power, about 0.19%. Day one has a 0.19% chance of the following 9 days coming out the same. Day two also has a 0.19% chance of the following 9 days coming out the same. This continues up until day 23 at which point there are only 8 days left in the month, not enough for nine more tries. The cumulative probability over those 23 days is 0.19% times 23 equals 4.5% In the course of a 31 day month that comes out to 4.5% probability of ten consecutive data points above or below the mean by chance alone.

12x – any 12 consecutive points are on the same side of the mean. In the example below, every data point is above the mean.

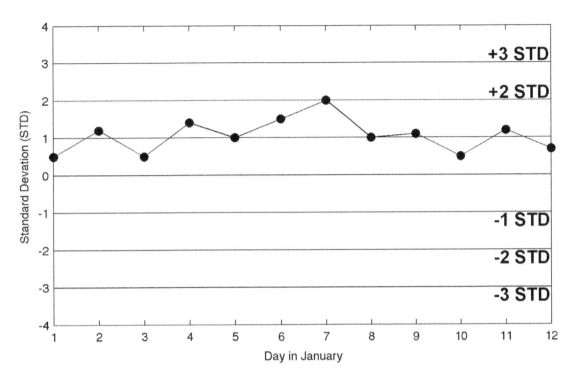

For any given number the probability of the next number being on the same side of the mean is 50%. The other 50% will be on the other side of the mean. For the purpose of this calculation we are excluding numbers on the mean. The numbers are random and discrete. This is just like a coin toss, which can be either heads or tails.

Let's say that the coin toss on day one is heads. The probability that the next eleven coin tosses are heads is 0.5 x 0.5 x 0.5 x 0.5 x 0.5 x 0.5 x 0.5 x 0.5 x 0.5 x 0.5 x 0.5 = 0.049%. In the chart above the first day's data point is above the mean. The probability of the following 11 being above the mean is 1 in 2 to the eleventh power, about 0.049%. Day one has a 0.049% chance of the following 11 days coming out the same. Day two also has a 0.049% chance of the following 11 days coming out the same. This continues up until day 21 at which point there are only 10 days left in the month, not enough for eleven more tries. The cumulative probability over those 21 days is 0.049% times 21 equals 1.1% In the course of a 31 day month that comes out to 1.1% probability of twelve consecutive data points above or below the mean by chance alone.

7t – seven consecutive data points all trending in the same direction:

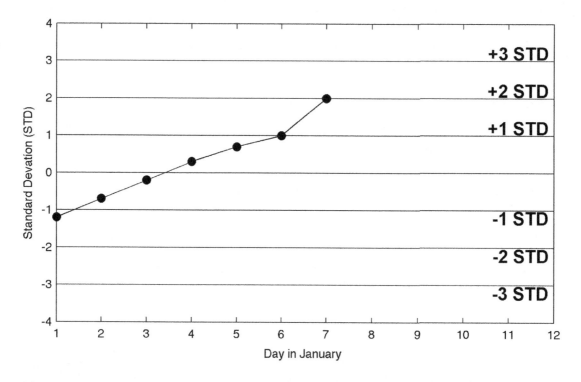

For any given number, I am making the assumption that the probability of the next number going further in the same direction is roughly 50%. This is not entirely correct since the distribution is Gaussian, but this is a rough guesstimate. Using these assumptions, this is just like a coin toss, which can be either heads or tails.

The probability that the next six coin tosses are heads is 0.5 x 0.5 x 0.5 x 0.5 x 0.5 x 0.5 = 1.5%. The probability of the following 6 data points trending is 1 in 2 to the sixth power, about 1.5%. Day one has a 1.5% chance of the following 6 days trending. Day two also has a 1.5% chance of the following 6 days trending. This continues up until day 26 at which point there are only 5 days left in the month, not enough for six more tries. The cumulative probability over those 26 days is 1.5% times 26 equals 40.6% In the course of a 31 day month that comes out to 40.6% probability of seven data points trending by chance alone.

10t – ten consecutive data points all trending in the same direction:

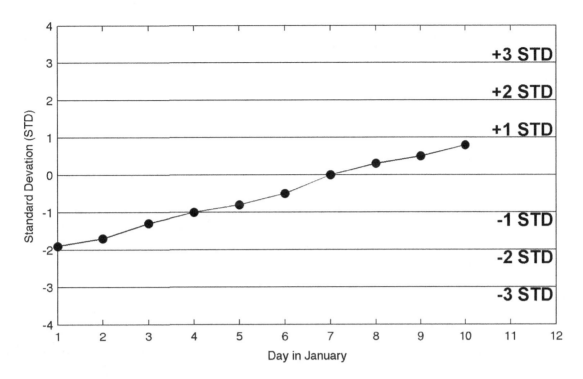

For any given number, I am making the assumption that the probability of the next number going further in the same direction is roughly 50%. This is not entirely correct since the distribution is Gaussian, but this is a rough guesstimate. Using these assumptions, this is just like a coin toss, which can be either heads or tails.

The probability that the next nine coin tosses are heads is 0.5 x 0.5 x 0.5 x 0.5 x 0.5 x 0.5 x 0.5 x 0.5 x 0.5 = 0.19%. The probability of the following 9 data points trending is 1 in 2 to the ninth power, about 0.19%. Day one has a 0.19% chance of the following 9 days trending. Day two also has a 0.19% chance of the following 9 days trending. This continues up until day 23 at which point there are only 8 days left in the month, not enough for nine more tries. The cumulative probability over those 23 days is 0.19% times 23 equals 4.5%. In the course of a 31 day month that comes out to 4.5% probability of ten data points trending by chance alone.

4-1S – any 4 consecutive points are more than one SD from the mean on the same side of the mean. In the example below, there are 4 consecutive points more than one SD above the mean, and the offending area of the graph is circled:

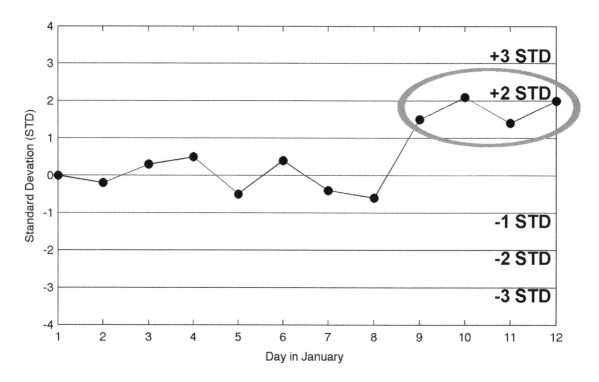

Assuming a Gaussian distribution, the probability of any given point falling more than 1SD from the mean is 32%. That comes out to 16% for each side of the mean. The probability that one data point is more than one SD from the mean and the subsequent 3 are more than 1 SD from the mean on the same side is 0.32 x 0.16 x 0.16 x 0.16 = 0.13%. Day one has a 0.13% chance of this happening. Day two also has a 0.13% chance of this happening. This continues up until day 29 at which point there are only 2 days left in the month, not enough for three more data points. The cumulative probability over those 29 days is 0.13% times 29 equals 3.8%. In the course of a 31 day month that comes out to 3.8% probability of one point more than 1 SD from the mean followed by three consecutive points more than 1 SD from the mean on the same side.

There are only two ways for a test to go out of control, a shift or a trend. A shift is a sudden, abrupt change in the mean of the data points. A trend is a slow gradual change in the mean over time. The rule 4-1S relates to shifts. In the above example the shift occurred sometime on January 8 or 9. The mean for the data points shifted by at least one SD higher. This is in contradistinction to the rules 7t and 10t which deal with trends.

In my experience as a Lab Director, most of the Westgard rule violations I have seen on the analyzers in my lab have been "false alarms". Thus I have made a point of calculating the false positive rates for each of the tests above. In all fairness, I need to point out that the Westgard rules are very sensitive for picking up errors. In other words, if you are starting to have a problem with a test, the Westgard rules should quickly detect that there is a problem developing.

Notice that I used the monthly rate when calculating "false alarms". As a Lab Director you will review the Levey-Jennings charts, typically on a monthly basis. The lab tech running the equipment should be reviewing the Levey-Jennings charts daily, and if there is a problem should refer the charts to you immediately, not waiting for the next monthly cycle of chart reviews. Most modern day lab instruments can be programmed with whatever Westgard rules you want, and will flag you immediately when they begin to fail the Westgard rules they are programmed with. Keep in mind that the point of doing QC is to catch a problem as soon as possible, before it can cause any real damage.

Under CLIA, you can pick whichever Westgard rules you want. You are not obligated to pick any rule over the others. I prefer to keep it simple – three rules only: 10t, 12x and 1-3S. The theoretical probability of a false positive is 4.5% plus 1.1% plus 9.3% per month, around 14.9% per month.

Try to avoid 7t or 8x as your rules. If you pick 7t or 8x you will be forever chasing down random data points. You will spend a great deal of time and effort doing corrective actions for data points that fall by random chance in an order that fails your rules.

An analyzer typically comes from the manufacturer pre-programmed with its Westgard rules, but the lab can change these if it wants to. I have seen some labs change the Westgard rules before setting an analyzer into service. To the best of my knowledge no lab has ever changed the Westgard rules on an analyzer already in service. Although there is nothing in CLIA that would prevent you from changing Westgard rules on-the-fly, it would complicate your evaluation of the QC.

In order to pass QC a Levey-Jennings chart cannot violate any of the Westgard rules you have chosen. If your Levey-Jennings chart passes the rules, it implies your mean is reasonably close to the "true" mean, your SD is acceptable and you don't need to take any further action. A Levey-Jennings chart that violates one or more of the Westgard rules is said to fail that rule or those rules. If your Levey-Jennings chart fails any rule, it implies your mean is unacceptably far from the "true" mean and/or your SD is too large such that you need to take action.

Theoretically, by using the 1-3S rule, there is a 9.3% chance per month you are going to be chasing down a ghost, a point that falls outside of 3SD by random chance. In reality, what will happen is that the lab tech who is running QC the day of the more than 3SD outlier will re-run the control, and on the second attempt is likely to get a result within 3SD of the mean. The second attempt will be recorded as the relevant data point for the purpose of the Levey-Jennings chart.

In a perfect world, every control that falls beyond 3SD from the mean would get a corrective action. In the real world, most hospital labs are short of staff and many are very short. There isn't enough manpower to generate large numbers of corrective actions, so everybody looks the other way, and lets the tech repeat a greater than 3SD outlier once or twice.

If the repeat control results continue to fall outside 3SD of the mean, you really do have a problem. Your analyzer has failed Westgard rule 1-3S. It needs a corrective action. Do not allow the tech to keep repeating the control over and over, until a number is obtained that is within 3SD. If you repeat the controls until such time as you get the desired result, it will reduce your ability to detect a real shift or trend. Set a limit that the tech can repeat an outlier only once or twice.

If the control is still outside of 3SD after the second repeat, the analyzer is assumed to be out of control. You can skip ahead to the chapter on what to do when you have failed proficiency testing, since failing QC is essentially the same thing, caught at an earlier stage. The tech cannot perform patient testing on the analyzer and has to inform the section supervisor and/or Lab Supervisor that the analyzer is out of control. A corrective action must be completed. It must be documented that this analyzer is in control before it can be put back into service for patient testing.

The same applies for all the other Westgard rules you have chosen. If your Westgard rules involve 12x or 10t and your analyzer fails 12x or 10t, the tech can repeat the offending control only twice. If the results for that control still fail any Westgard rule after the second repeat, the analyzer is taken out of commission until such time as a corrective action can be completed. The instrument can only be brought back online for patient testing when it is documented that it is in control.

There have been instances where the tech fails to realize that a Westgard rule has been violated, such as a quality control data point falls outside of 3SD above or below the mean. In this situation the tech will record the data point and move on as if nothing is wrong. If this happens, and you catch it at the end of the month reviewing the Levey-Jennings charts, you need to make a corrective action. If you miss this as well, and the inspector catches it, you will get a citation on the inspection. No matter how this mistake is caught, it needs a corrective action. See the subsequent chapter on proficiency testing and corrective actions.

Here is a Westgard rule **test**. Look at the following and determine if it passes Westgard rules:

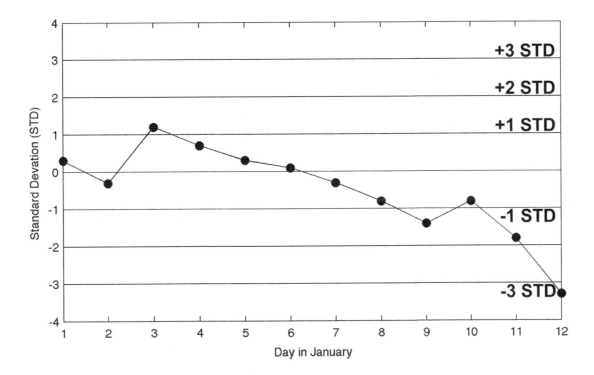

I'll give you some help on this. When looking at charts, there is a tendency to look at the middle of the chart, and miss things happening at one end or the other. This happens not only with Levey-Jennings charts, but with everything that people look at. If you take a dollar bill out of your pocket, the first thing you are going to look at is the picture of President Washington, not the numbers in the corners. You recognize this piece of paper as a dollar bill more by the picture in the middle than the numbers in the corners.

My advice: when looking at a Levey-Jennings chart, you have to look at the whole chart. Start at the left end and work your way right. Do this for each rule. Start with 1-3S. Look at every data point one at a time. Does the first data point fall outside of 3SD from the mean? Look at the second data point. Does the second data point fall outside of 3SD from the mean? Continue until you get to the last data point.

Then go from left to right on the same chart using your next Westgard rule, 7t. Look at the first data point. Do the next six points all trend in the same direction? Look at the second data point. Do the next six data points trend in the same direction? Continue until you get to the last data point.

Do this for every rule that you are using. If the chart has not failed any rules it is a passing Levey-Jennings chart. Most modern day lab analyzers can be programmed with whatever Westgard rules you want and then will automatically tell you if you are failing those Westgard rules.

I trained many years ago at a time when most analyzers wouldn't automatically flag Westgard rule failures. At that time, the evaluation of the Levey-Jennings charts were done by looking at them. The first few times you do this, it is tedious work. As you become more proficient, you will be able to do this quickly and accurately.

ANSWER: It fails both 7t and 1-3S

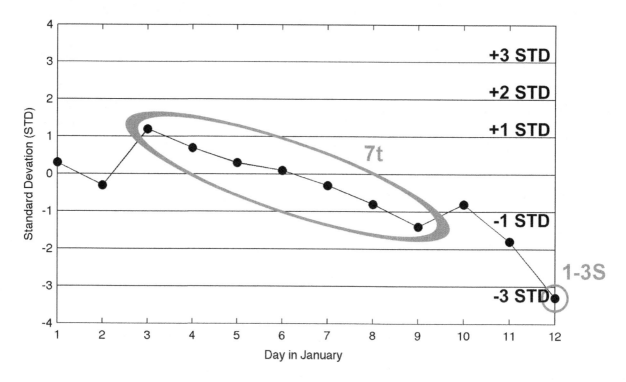

There are a number of take-home points in this graph. The first point is that the chart fails two rules at the same time. This is typical of a test that is having problems, it will fail multiple rules not just one. The analyte is having a downward trend, which results in one outlier more than 3SD below the mean. The outlier is the last data point on the chart as would be expected for a trend.

The second take-home point is to always look at the chart from end to end. If you had looked at the middle of the chart only, you would have missed the outlier more than 3SD below the mean because it is at the back end of the chart.

The above graph is a classic example of a trend. This involves a gradual drift in the mean in which the mean is slowly changing over time. The date the problem started cannot be pinpointed. This is in contradistinction to a shift in which the change in mean is sudden, abrupt and can usually be pinpointed to within a day or two.

Here is another Westgard rule **test**. Look at the following and determine if it passes all Westgard rules:

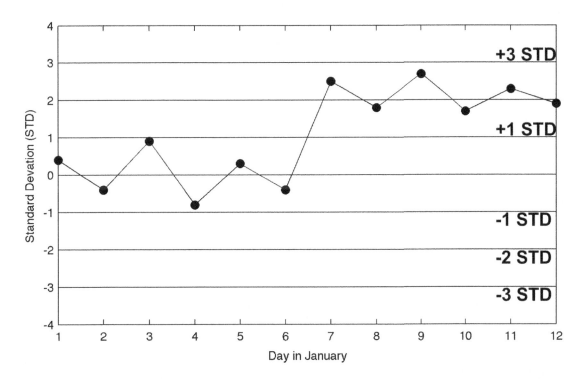

The same advice applies here as for the prior Westgard rule test. When looking at a Levey-Jennings chart, you have to look at the whole chart. Start at the left end and work your way right. Do this for each rule. Start with 1-3S. Look at every data point one at a time. Does the first data point fall outside of 3SD from the mean? Look at the second data point. Does the second data point fall outside of 3SD from the mean? Continue until you get to the last data point.

Then go from left to right on the same chart using your next Westgard rule, 7t. Look at the first data point. Do the next six points all trend in the same direction? Look at the second data point. Do the next six data points trend in the same direction? Continue until you get to the last data point.

Do this for every rule you are using. If the chart has not failed any rules it is a passing Levey-Jennings chart. Most modern day lab analyzers can be programmed with whatever Westgard rules you want and then will automatically tell you if you are failing those Westgard rules.

I trained many years ago at a time when most analyzers wouldn't automatically flag Westgard rule failures. At that time, the evaluation of the Levey-Jennings charts were done by looking at them. The first few times you do this, it is tedious work. As you become more proficient, you will be able to do this quickly and accurately.

ANSWER: It fails 4-1S

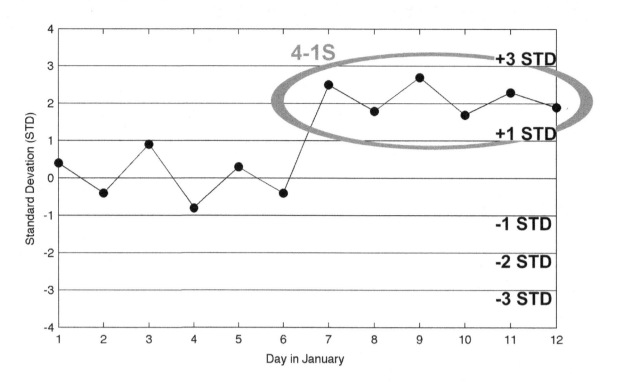

The above failure of the 4-1S rule is a classic example of a shift. Sometime on January 6 or 7 the mean abruptly shifted upward by about 2 SD, and this upward shift persisted intact for the remainder of the time represented in the graph. This is in contradistinction to the gradual drift in mean seen with the violation of rule 7t representing a trend in the prior Westgard rule test.

The date the problem started can be pinpointed with a shift, but not with a trend. For the example 4-1S rule violation given above, check to see what happened on January 6 or 7. Was a new lot put into place? If so was the analyzer correctly programmed with the new lot number, new lot mean, etc.?

Chapter 5 – Proficiency testing and corrective actions

CLIA requires proficiency testing (PT) for a subset of moderate and high complexity testing analytes referred to as the "regulated analytes". CLIA does not require PT for the non-regulated analytes, waived testing analytes, calculated values, etc. However, CAP requires PT for all tests in your lab. This is why I strongly prefer CMS inspection over CAP inspection, not that the inspection is easier to pass, but in between the inspections you will be doing a whole lot less work. I generally don't PT the waived testing analytes, nor do I perform PT on the calculated values like anion gap and calculated LDL.

Proficiency testing must be done three times per year for each regulated analyte. The exception is mycobacteriology (AFB smear, mycobacterial culture and sensitivity) where PT only needs to be done twice a year. Each round of PT testing is referred to as a PT "event".

For each PT event, passing is 80% or more for all parts of lab except for ABO grouping, Rh (D) typing and compatibility testing. Passing is 100% for ABO grouping, Rh (D) typing and compatibility testing. CLIA requires a minimum of 5 specimens per PT event for the regulated analytes.

In order to pass each PT event, the Blood Bank has to get 5 out of 5 right on ABO grouping, Rh (D) typing and compatibility testing. All other parts of Lab only have to get 4 out of 5 right. Successful PT performance is defined as passing at least two of the three PT events per year. The reference for the above is 42 CFR part 493, Subpart I.

Only one failed PT event is allowed per year for each analyte. If you fail two or more PT events in one year for any given analyte, in theory you have to stop testing in-house for that analyte and start sending the testing out. I will go into more detail on repeat PT failure in the next chapter.

For analytes that are not regulated the laboratory must verify the accuracy of the test twice annually. The reference is 42 CFR § 493.1236. CLIA does not specifically require PT testing of the non-regulated analytes, and other methods could be used to verify the accuracy of the testing. Although it is possible to separate out the non-regulated analytes and verify the accuracy of their testing by some method other than PT testing, this would be too cumbersome and time consuming. It is easier to test all the regulated and non-regulated analytes together at the same PT events. As mentioned above I generally don't PT the waived testing analytes or calculated values (calculated LDL, anion gap, etc.).

For the non-regulated analytes, there is a tendency to take the PT less seriously. Failure does not have the consequences of a PT testing failure on a regulated analyte. In theory you cannot receive a cease testing letter or regulatory closure for failing PT on a non-regulated analyte. Even the PT providers take non-regulated analyte PT less seriously. For regulated analytes all PT providers I am aware of will only send PT events as sets of 5 specimens. You cannot order a regulated analyte PT event with 4 specimens or 6 specimens because none of the PT providers would fulfill such a request. For non-regulated analytes, some PT providers will send you only one PT specimen per analyte per event.

In my opinion all PT testing should be taken seriously. My advice is if you fail PT on a non-regulated analyte you should make a corrective action as outlined below. You should correct the problem, or else you should send out the testing for that non-regulated analyte, the same as you would for a regulated analyte.

CLIA requires that the PT specimens must come from a CMS approved PT provider. CLIA mandates that the testing for PT specimens must be done the same way and by the same personnel as the patient testing. The way most people interpret this is that if you have multiple lab techs testing an analyte you can pick whichever tech you want from the list of techs testing that analyte to test the PT specimens. You cannot pick a tech that does not ordinarily test that analyte.

The assignment of the PT testing is typically rotated among all the lab techs who perform the test. This way, the PT testing acts as an unofficial competency test. On a rotating basis you are checking each tech's ability to perform the PT testing.

If you are testing by multiple methodologies you have to test the PT specimen by the "primary system" meaning the methodology most commonly used for patient testing. If you have multiple analyzers, CLIA only requires you to PT the "primary" analyzer meaning the analyzer most commonly used for patient testing.

The big sin to avoid is referral of PT specimens to an outside lab, or asking another lab what their results were, until such time as you have returned your results to the PT provider. If you get caught referring PT specimens your lab will be in deep trouble.

The PT specimens must be treated the same as patient specimens. If you test patient specimens one time each by one methodology, you are only allowed to test the PT specimens one time each by one methodology before reporting the PT results. If you test patient specimens in duplicate, you must test the PT specimens in duplicate, etc. You are not allowed to recalibrate and/or change reagents before each PT run unless you do so before each patient run. The reference for the above is 42 CFR § 493.801. If you break these rules, it will be considered "cheating" on your PT and your lab will be in deep trouble.

In the typical lab, most analytes are tested once before reporting. Given the above rules, the PT material can only be used to PT one analyzer per PT event. However, after the due date of the PT event you are allowed to use the same PT material to QC the other analyzers. If you have multiple analyzers, wait until after the PT due date has passed to run the PT material on the other analyzers. The other analyzers should report results within the acceptable limits for that PT event. Any analyzer reporting unacceptable results should be taken out of commission until a corrective action can be completed. This should be done as internal QC within the lab and should not be reported to any PT provider. The same data points generated by testing the PT material on multiple analyzers can also be used to correlate the analyzers against each other. This correlation of the analyzers against each other is required by CLIA twice per year; the reference is 42 CFR § 493.1281(a). Thus, the same PT material can be put to multiple uses, so as to reduce expenses.

If you have multiple analyzers, my advice is not to order multiple PT events from multiple different vendors so as to PT each analyzer individually. This would be more expensive and creates issues of its own, namely which of the PT events is the "primary" PT event that counts towards passing or failing PT. If you have five analyzers and one fails PT, does it put all five analyzers in jeopardy for the next two PT events? This approach clouds the issue unnecessarily and should be avoided.

CLIA requires that the PT specimens must be tested with the laboratory's regular patient workload. The strictest reading of the regulations would require that all PT specimens be integrated with a routine run of patient specimens. At most labs I am familiar with the PT specimens are run separately from the patient specimens, but on the same day of testing. I am not aware of any CMS inspector giving a citation for running the PT specimens as a separate run from patient specimens, but it would be possible to cite this if the regulations are read in the strictest sense.

Many of the PT specimens you receive will be lyophilized (freeze dried) and have to be reconstituted. This step is not done with routine patient testing and many problems can occur at this step (incorrect amount of diluent and/or wrong diluent used to reconstitute the PT sample).

PT specimens tend to decay in transit, which is a bigger problem the farther away you are from the PT manufacturer. It should be made clear to all lab techs that they should immediately open all parcels received from the PT manufacturer and check the condition of the PT material. If a PT specimen is received warm, hemolyzed or otherwise deteriorated that specimen should not be tested. Instead your lab should immediately call the PT provider's customer service number and request a replacement for the PT specimen. In my experience the PT providers will typically tell your lab to test any specimens received warm as long as there are no visible signs of deterioration (hemolysis, etc.). In this situation it is important to document the compromised condition of the PT material used for testing. Your lab may be performing corrective action after the PT event is over. In this case use the documentation of the compromised PT material as part of the corrective action. In the remote areas I have worked, deteriorated PT specimens are the most common cause of PT failure.

I have seen instances when the PT material was received obviously deteriorated (very hemolyzed) and the PT provider could not produce more PT material. In this situation, the PT provider has always given us a "pass" on the PT event in question and told us to verify the accuracy of the test by some other method. This outcome is better than testing an obviously deteriorated PT specimen. A badly hemolyzed specimen is bound to produce a "fail" on a PT event.

After testing the PT specimen the results have to be transcribed onto a form, or typed into a computer to report the results back to the PT provider. This transcription step is not done with routine patient testing, and is another big source of error, in this case clerical error in data entry.

Every PT event has an attestation page which must be signed by the testing personnel and the Lab Director. After all signatures are completed this attestation page is filed in the PT binder along with a printout of the reported results. The PT evaluation report will be filed in this same binder when it returns, typically several weeks after you submit the results. The documentation for any corrective actions should be filed in this same binder. The inspector will want to look at all these documents at the same time, so it is best to keep them all in the same binder.

Each PT event will have a due date. Be very careful to return results by the due date. If you are one day late this counts as a PT failure. In my experience, this is one of the most common causes of PT failure. It is not uncommon to have one tech or even a few techs procrastinate with the PT specimens. The PT specimens can be seen as less important than the routine patient testing, and tend to be left for last, or not tested at all. In most labs it is the Lab Supervisor's responsibility to ensure that all steps in the PT process are completed in a timely manner.

After the results are reported for the PT event, the PT specimens are typically frozen and stored indefinitely. If there are any failures on the PT event, you will need to retrieve the PT specimens and retest them. If there are no failures, the PT specimens can be used in any situation where you need a specimen with known quantity of analyte (e.g. making a correlation, performing verification of calibration, etc.).

Every year your lab will need to renew its PT subscription. PT subscriptions typically run for one calendar year and do not automatically renew. Each year your lab must submit additional paperwork for renewal. Most PT providers will send a bill and an enrollment form during the third quarter of each year for the next year's PT subscription. It is imperative to pay this bill and submit the enrollment form on time. If submission is late, your lab may not receive the first PT events after the start of the new year. For regulated analytes, failure to enroll in PT is considered equivalent to failing the PT events in question.

When renewing the PT each year, if you are CAP inspected make sure PT is ordered for every analyte tested in-house. If you are CMS inspected make sure PT is ordered for all regulated analytes tested in-house. If CMS inspected, you don't need to PT the non-regulated analytes including the waived testing analytes and calculated values (calculated LDL, anion gap, etc.). As mentioned above, for regulated analytes, failure to enroll in PT for that analyte is considered equivalent to failing PT for that analyte.

After receiving your payment and renewal paperwork the PT provider will send you a confirmation letter listing the specialties and analytes to be tested, scheduled shipping dates, etc. Check this confirmation letter to ensure you will be receiving the PT you ordered then file the confirmation letter in the PT binder. If any PT event is not received within a few days of the scheduled ship date, call or E-mail the PT provider to check the status of the shipment. Ask for a replacement for any shipments lost in transit. As mentioned above, failure to participate in a PT event is considered equivalent to failing that PT event.

Here is what a passing proficiency test result looks like:

Bilirubin, direct mg/dL											
	CHM-01	2.1	2.13	0.09	836	-0.3	1.7	2.6	Acceptable	C-A 2014	
	CHM-02	1.3	1.24	0.07	831	+0.8	0.8	1.7	Acceptable	C-C 2013	
	CHM-03	0.9	0.90	0.07	842	0.0	0.4	1.3	Acceptable	C-B 2013	
	CHM-04	0.1	0.05	0.05	664	+0.9	0.0	0.5	Acceptable		
	CHM-05	1.2	1.23	0.08	838	-0.3	0.8	1.7	Acceptable		-100 -80 -60 -40 -20 0 20 40 60 80 100

The report comes back with several columns of data. For each analyte you are measured against your peer group, meaning all other labs using the same instruments and methodology that you are using. From left to right, the data represents your result, the peer mean result, the peer standard deviation (SD), the number of peer labs reporting, your SD from the peer mean (for most analytes you must be within 3SD of the peer mean to pass), the lower limit of acceptability, the upper limit of acceptability, and your grade for each test. Your results are graded as "acceptable" which means passing or "unacceptable" which means failing. The graphs on the far right represent your performance for the most recent three proficiency testing events, and are expressed in percent of allowable error.

The example above is about as good as PT results can be. All results are within 1 SD from the peer mean, and are randomly distributed around the peer mean with roughly equal numbers of data points above and below the peer mean. When you get results this close to the peer mean, it indicates your testing has excellent accuracy. The clustering of your results close to the peer mean indicates your SD is not any larger than it should be (i.e. your results are precise). When you get results this good, all you have to do is sign the PT report and file it. No further action is needed.

If all results had been above or below the peer mean, you would have to worry about a high or low bias, respectively. You should also get worried if any data point is more than 2.5 SD from the peer mean, as you are getting close to having an outlier.

Some of the proficiency testing results may come back not graded because they are an "educational challenge" or have "no consensus" among respondents. Here are examples:

LDL Cholesterol, calc	CHM-11	30.00	34.134	8.682	3053	-0.5	[26]
mg/dL	CHM-12	105.80	98.302	19.574	3128	+0.4	[26]
CHOL - HDL - (TRIG/5)	CHM-13	61.80	62.767	15.084	3123	-0.1	[26]
	CHM-14	102.60	98.453	19.769	3130	+0.2	[26]
	CHM-15	53.40	55.666	10.815	3121	-0.2	[26]

BLOOD CELL IDENTIFICATION

Analyte / Method	Sample	Reported Result	Expected Result	Grade
Blood Cell ID (Educational)	BCI-06	Hairy cell	See commentary	Not Graded
	BCI-07	Monocyte	See commentary	Not Graded[6]
Blood Cell Identification **	BCI-01	Neutrophil, segmented (poly)	Neutrophil, segmented (poly)	Acceptable
	BCI-02	Myelocyte	Myelocyte	Not Graded[2]
	BCI-03	Eosinophil, all stages	Eosinophil, all stages	Acceptable
	BCI-04	Lymph, reactive(atyp, variant)	Lymph, reactive(atyp, variant) Lymphoma cell (malignant)	Not Graded[2]
	BCI-05	Lymphocyte, normal	Lymphocyte, normal See commentary	Acceptable

In this case, you have to compare your response to the majority response or peer mean. The accompanying booklet will contain this information. Write the majority response or your difference from the peer mean on the PT results printout. If your lab gave the majority response or was within 3SD of the peer mean, document this as a handwritten note on the PT results form indicating that your results are acceptable. If you were in the minority or missed by more than 3SD on an "educational challenge" or "no consensus" specimen, you should indicate this on the PT results form and make a corrective action as outlined below for a failed PT. Here's what it looks like when you are done:

LDL Cholesterol, calc	CHM-11	30.00	34.134	8.682	3053	-0.5	Within -1SD Acceptable	[26]
mg/dL	CHM-12	105.80	98.302	19.574	3128	+0.4	Within +1SD Acceptable	[26]
CHOL - HDL - (TRIG/5)	CHM-13	61.80	62.767	15.084	3123	-0.1	Within -1SD Acceptable	[26]
	CHM-14	102.60	98.453	19.769	3130	+0.2	Within +1SD Acceptable	[26]
	CHM-15	53.40	55.666	10.815	3121	-0.2	Within -1SD Acceptable	[26]

BLOOD CELL IDENTIFICATION

Analyte / Method	Sample	Reported Result	Expected Result	Grade
Blood Cell ID (Educational)	BCI-06	Hairy cell 51% hairy cell	See commentary acceptable	Not Graded
	BCI-07	Monocyte 62% monocyte	See commentary acceptable	Not Graded[6]
Blood Cell Identification **	BCI-01	Neutrophil, segmented (poly)	Neutrophil, segmented (poly)	Acceptable
	BCI-02	Myelocyte	Myelocyte acceptable	Not Graded[2]
	BCI-03	Eosinophil, all stages	Eosinophil, all stages	Acceptable
	BCI-04	Lymph, reactive(atyp, variant)	Lymph, reactive(atyp, variant) acceptable Lymphoma cell (malignant)	Not Graded[2]
	BCI-05	Lymphocyte, normal	Lymphocyte, normal See commentary	Acceptable

All CMS inspectors like to see these types of handwritten notes in your PT results forms, it indicates you are paying attention to your PT. Some inspectors consider these notes to be mandatory and will give you a citation if you don't make such notes. Most will not cite you for failure to do this, however.

You are required to make a corrective action for each instance your results for an analyte are outside the expected range. For the remainder of this chapter I will refer to this situation as "failed PT". In reality, if you get 4 out of 5 right on a chemistry analyte, your overall performance is successful, but you still have to make a corrective action for the one erroneous result out of five. In effect that one erroneous result is treated as a failure even though your overall result (4 out of 5 correct) is successful.

Here is an example of a PT event where one of five failed, but the overall is passing:

T3 Uptake Percent uptake (%)	CHM-11	46.00	44.376	2.130	165	+0.8	37.98	50.77	Acceptable
	CHM-12	50.00	45.262	2.088	166	+2.3	38.99	51.53	Acceptable
	CHM-13	49.00	46.954	2.420	167	+0.8	39.69	54.22	Acceptable
	CHM-14	49.00	45.226	2.010	167	+1.9	39.19	51.26	Acceptable
	CHM-15	61.00	44.753	2.101	167	+7.7	38.45	51.06	Unacceptable

x: Result is outside the acceptable limits

Your lab should begin working on the corrective action immediately upon notification of the PT failure. Some of the corrective action steps are time sensitive such as retesting the PT specimen. The stored specimen tends to decay over time making retesting more problematic as time goes on. Other steps in the corrective action process can become more difficult if done well after the fact.

The lab management's response to having a failed PT varies from lab to lab. In some labs, the failed PTs occur relatively commonly, and everybody knows how to handle them. You make the corrective action and you move on.

In one lab I worked at, failed PT was essentially unheard of. In the year I was there, it happened one time. The Lab Director called in the Lab Supervisor, the section supervisor and the lab tech who did the testing into one room for a very nervous finger pointing session as to how this happened.

The corrective action is typically delegated to the section supervisor of the area where the failure occurred. Most laboratories have a corrective action form that is used in this situation. The form is filled out and signed by the section supervisor, advanced to the Lab Supervisor to review and sign, and then advanced to the Lab Director to sign off on. The corrective action form on the next page corresponds to the failed PT event given above.

My advice to the tech handed this task is that if you fail PT, take a deep breath and try to stay calm. Stay focused on filling out the corrective action form, as it will guide you in what to look for and what could have gone wrong in the PT testing.

MY LABORATORY -- PROFICIENCY TESTING CORRECTIVE ACTION/INVESTIGATION

Name of Survey	Chemistry 3rd event 2013				Date Originally Tested	10/12/13
Lab Section	Chemistry				Reconst. By	N/A
Analyte	T3 Uptake				Date Review Initiated	12/10/13
Specimen No.	CHM-15				Repeated Result	Repeated X1
Intended Result	38.4-51.0				Review Performed By	P. Dauterman, MD
Reported Result	61.00				Init / Date Completed	12/12/13
Analyte Grading	Unaccep					

SAMPLE	YES	NO	N/A	COMMENTS
Reconstituted Correctly			X	
Correct Sample Tested	X			
Correct Results Reported	X			
Correct Dilution Calc.			X	
Other				CHM-15 repeat T3 Uptake test result 45
PROCEDURE/INSTR.				
Specify Instr				Siemens Dimension
Report Correct Meth/Instr				
P.M. Current	X			
Calibrations Done When				Most recent prior calibration 8/19/13
Calibration Since PT				Subsequent calibration 10/16/13
Reagent Problems		X		
Procedure Verified			X	
Problems on Run		X		
QUALITY CONTROL				
Within Limits	X			
Shifts Noted		X		
Trends Noted		X		
Other				
WORKSHEET				
Any Problems with PT Tests				
Any Patients Repeated				
Trend with Patients				
Other				
PREVIOUS PT FAILURE				
		X		

Final Conclusion of Above Investigation: There was no problem with controls, linearity, etc. for this analyte. The repeat test was within the expected range for this proficiency testing event. The original unacceptably high result is an unexplainable, random error.

Corrective Action to Prevent Re-Occurrence:

Evidence of Successful Corrective Action: Subsequent PT testing.

Reviewed By: Signature   Date   Comments

Lab Supervisor/Lab Director

Assuming a Gaussian distribution, the probability of a test result falling more than 3SD from the mean is 0.3%. Most analytes do not have a perfectly Gaussian distribution, but for the most part it is still assumed that 0.3% of results will fall more than 3SD from the mean by random chance. A proficiency testing event involves testing 5 tubes of blood for maybe 30 to 50 analytes each. Just by random chance, you might have one or two results outside of 3SD from the mean per PT event. This is referred to as "inexplicable, random error" in the form above.

In order to make this assumption, you have to exclude more sinister causes for failed PT. This requires you to review the entire process of quality control for the analyte involved. This includes reviewing the controls, calibration, linearity, etc. In general the process for corrective action is:

1. Compare the original analyzer tape to the reported results to make sure there are no transcription errors.
2. Check for evidence of a specimen switch (low PT specimen had high results, high PT specimen had low results, etc.)
3. For PT specimens received lyophilized (freeze dried), make sure the reconstitution was done with correct diluent, correct amount of diluent, etc.
4. Rerun the failed PT specimens x 2 each if there is enough remaining specimen to test. Record the rerun results on the corrective action form.
5. Document that all controls are in and were in for this analyte at the time of PT testing, the analyzer is passing all Westgard rules and passed all Westgard rules for this analyte at the time of PT testing, testing for this analyte passed linearity, the analyzer's preventive maintenance and calibration are current, there were no problems with the most recent calibration, etc.
6. Document if the PT specimen was received warm, delayed transit, arrived hemolyzed or deteriorated, delayed testing after arrival, improper storage after arrival, the correct procedure was followed when testing the PT specimen, etc.
7. Make a notation that patient testing was not affected.
8. Sign the corrective action form and file it in the same binder with the paperwork for the PT event. A copy of the corrective action form goes in the folder for the Quality Assurance Committee.

Most failed PT is a "false alarm" as described above in which case no further action is needed. In my experience it is very rare that a failed PT really does indicate there is a problem with the underlying test. Any problem with the test should have been caught well before it resulted in failed PT. If you are having major problems with a test, the controls should be out for that test. This would be caught the next time the controls are run, typically once per day of testing or once per 8 hour shift depending on the test.

If you find that there really is a problem with the test you have to get the test back into control. Take the easiest steps first, such as changing pipettes, cuvettes and/or other disposables. Make sure all reagents, controls and calibrators are in-date and not expired, the analyzer's preventive maintenance is current, etc. You can try recalibration, ordering new controls, new reagents and/or new calibrators, sending an aliquot of your existing controls and/or calibrators to an outside lab for testing to see if your controls and/or calibrators have deteriorated, calling the analyzer manufacturer's headquarters, calling the Service Representative (known in the business as a "Service Rep") for the analyzer and ask for maintenance on the instrument and for the Service Rep to help with getting the instrument back in control, etc. All actions taken must be documented in writing.

Once you get the test back in control, retest any remaining patient specimens from the time the test was out of control. If you have to turn out corrected reports for those tests, the providers who submitted the test requests must be notified of the corrected results.

You will not be very popular with any providers receiving corrected results. Even if it is a relatively minor change, for example correcting a serum sodium level from 140 to 142, it will cause your providers to distrust you, distrust your lab, and distrust your lab results. Thus, it is imperative to make sure that all tests are in control on all days of testing, so that you don't ever find yourself in the position of turning out large numbers of corrected results. It should be made very clear to all lab techs that they are not to release test results unless their daily controls are in.

You need to document that there was no patient harm from the testing that was out of control. If there was any patient harm you have to mitigate it to the extent possible. You will also need to put in place measures to prevent the same problem from recurring, and a way of monitoring this potential problem to ensure the problem does not recur. After you are done, sign the corrective action form and file it in the same binder with the paperwork for the PT event. A copy goes in the folder for the Quality Assurance Committee.

Chapter 6 – What to do if one analyte fails two or more proficiency testing events in one year

Per CLIA, for each analyte you need 80% or more correct to pass a PT event for all parts of lab except Blood Bank where passing is 100% correct for ABO grouping, Rh (D) typing and compatibility testing. For the purpose of this chapter, when I refer to "failed PT" I am referring to the situation where the lab had less than 80% correct (i.e. less than 4 out of 5 correct) for the main lab or less than 100% correct (i.e. 5 out of 5 correct) for Blood Bank on any analyte on a PT event. This is more correctly referred to as "unsatisfactory current PT event performance" for that analyte. Here is what a failed PT looks like:

Sodium, serum mmol/L	CHM-06	131	137.9	1.6	222	-4.3	133	142	Unacceptable
	CHM-07	137	142.9	1.6	222	-3.6	138	147	Unacceptable
	CHM-08	131	137.7	1.6	225	-4.1	133	142	Unacceptable
	CHM-09	144	150.8	1.9	223	-3.7	146	155	Unacceptable
	CHM-10	114	118.9	1.3	221	-3.7	114	123	Acceptable

x: Result is outside the acceptable limits

Every time you fail a PT, you must make a corrective action. See the prior chapter on how to make a corrective action. For the remainder of this chapter, when I go through the steps of mitigating multiple failed PT, I am assuming that you have made a corrective action for each failed PT.

For any given analyte, if you have not failed any other PT event in the last year the corrective action process given in Chapter 5 is sufficient to meet regulatory requirements. File the corrective action form in the same binder as the PT results form. Your inspector should accept this as being sufficient to remediate the failure. The situation becomes more complicated when you have failed more than one PT event for any given analyte in the last year.

I will use as an example a test that doesn't exist – serum radon levels. Let's say that you had a transcription error earlier in the year, you switched the transcription on the high and low PT specimens, and failed your first proficiency testing event of the year. You passed the second PT event of the year. Then on the third PT event, you incorrectly reconstituted the specimen, and failed on all 5 PT specimens for this serum radon level PT event.

Right now the last three proficiency testing events in chronological order are FAIL-PASS-FAIL. The term "initial unsuccessful participation" in proficiency testing is used to describe any situation in which the last two out of three PT events are failures. The easiest thing to do at this point is to discontinue in-house testing for serum radon levels and send the test out. In some circumstances and for some analytes, the test is life or death, and you can't wait for send-out testing to come back.

Here is what you do for analytes that can't be sent out:

1. Get the test back into control and/or fix the underlying problem as soon as possible. This should be considered urgent, and given priority over other work in the lab. Do not perform any PT or patient testing while the test is out of control as this would only make the situation worse.
2. After the test is back in control order a new, unscheduled PT event from any vendor that is willing to send it immediately. This should be in addition to your regularly scheduled PT events. Have the new PT event sent as soon as possible.
3. Do everything you can to pass the new PT event. Assign the best tech to do the testing, have a second person double-check the reconstitution of the PT specimens, double-check the transcription, etc.
4. If you pass the new PT event you will then be PASS-FAIL-PASS for the 3 most recent PT events. When the new, passing PT event is added to your tally, the first failed PT event will be "pushed off the back" of the list of your three most recent PT events. You will receive a new PT report indicating "successful" performance since the last two of three PT events are passing. The "successful" PT report is filed in the PT binder along with all the corrective action paperwork.
5. For PT purposes, you are allowed to define the year as starting on any day you want. Define the start of the PT testing year as starting somewhere in the time interval between the two failures. Thus, the two failures fall in different PT testing years.
6. Be extremely careful to pass all subsequent PT for this analyte. As discussed below, repeat unsuccessful PT participation is defined as failing three or more out of the last six PT events. In other words, once you have gotten yourself into the situation of initial unsuccessful PT participation, the last six PT events are held against you, not just the last three PT events. If you fail another PT on this analyte within the next three PT events, skip ahead to the section on repeat unsuccessful PT participation.

As a caveat, the CAP will not allow unscheduled PT events. However, unscheduled PT events are allowed by the API, the MLE, the AAFP-PT and the AAB. If you want to use the "pushing of the back" strategy, you might have to switch your inspecting agency and/or primary PT provider (i.e. the PT provider keeping track of your scores).

In my 29 years in Pathology and Lab Medicine I have had two instances of an analyte in the FAIL-PASS-FAIL situation. In both instances the above steps were taken. The Lab passed the additional proficiency testing event. The CMS inspectors were satisfied with the results, or at least gave us a pass at the subsequent CMS inspection. The CMS inspectors have the ability to give citations and/or sanctions (fines) and they do not automatically pass everything.

Let's say your lab has failed the last two consecutive PT events for one analyte such that the last three PT events are FAIL-FAIL-PASS. Similar to the situation described above, this counts as "initial unsuccessful participation" in proficiency testing because the last two of three PT events are failures. This is worse than the situation described above, and will require more work to remediate, since the failures are back to back. As above, the easiest thing to do is discontinue in-house testing and send the test out. For an essential test that can't be sent out, there are still a few desperate last-ditch maneuvers you could try:

1. Get the test back into control and/or fix the underlying problem as soon as possible. Do not perform any PT or patient testing while the test is out of control as this would only make the situation worse. After the problem is fixed, order and run unscheduled PT events in rapid succession, until such time as two of the most recent three PT events are passing. You are attempting to "push off the back" one of the two failing PT events.
2. After the problem is fixed, begin ordering PT material from a new PT provider. Do not discontinue the standing orders for PT material from your old PT provider. When you are enrolled in PT from 2 different providers for the same analyte, you must designate one of the 2 PT providers as the "primary" PT provider. Only the results from the primary PT provider count towards passing for CLIA purposes. Order three PT events from your new provider and run them in rapid succession. Once you have successfully completed three passing PT events with your new PT provider, designate that PT provider as your primary PT provider. You are attempting to invalidate the failing PT from the PT provider you have replaced as your primary PT provider. The caveat here is that if you switch primary PT providers, you are required to keep the new PT provider as your primary provider for at least one year. This option will not work if you have already switched primary PT providers within the last year.
3. Put a new analyzer into place that employs a different methodology to test the same analyte.
4. If waived testing is available for this analyte, change to waived testing.

In my 29 years in Pathology and Lab Medicine I have only once headed a Lab that had an analyte in the FAIL-FAIL-PASS situation. In August, 2013 I was hired to "turnaround" a Lab with problems. When I started work there I found that one of the problems was the sodium test results were coming out too low. The above failed sodium PT evaluation report is from this lab. By the time I took the helm of this lab, it had already failed two out of the last three PT events for sodium. This is an essential analyte and send-out is not an option. Here is the actual proficiency testing performance summary showing that the sodium has failed the last two out of three PT events.

CMS Peformance Summary for Analytes Regulated Under the Clinical Laboratory Improvement Amendments of 1988

CLIA ID #: _____ Subspecialty: Routine Chemistry

Regulated Analyte	Proficiency Event 2012 3			Proficiency Event 2013 1			Proficiency Event 2013 2			Current Event Performance Interpretation	Cumulative CLIA '88 Performance Interpretation
	Test Event	Score	%	Test Event	Score	%	Test Event	Score	%		
ALT	C-C	5/5	100	C-A	5/5	100	C-B	5/5	100	Satisfactory	Successful
Albumin	C-C	5/5	100	C-A	5/5	100	C-B	5/5	100	Satisfactory	Successful
Alkaline Phosphatase	C-C	5/5	100	C-A	5/5	100	C-B	5/5	100	Satisfactory	Successful
Amylase	C-C	5/5	100	C-A	5/5	100	C-B	5/5	100	Satisfactory	Successful
AST	C-C	5/5	100	C-A	5/5	100	C-B	5/5	100	Satisfactory	Successful
Bilirubin, Total	C-C	5/5	100	C-A	5/5	100	C-B	5/5	100	Satisfactory	Successful
Calcium, Total	C-C	5/5	100	C-A	5/5	100	C-B	5/5	100	Satisfactory	Successful
Chloride	C-C	5/5	100	C-A	5/5	100	C-B	5/5	100	Satisfactory	Successful
Cholesterol, Total	C-C	5/5	100	C-A	5/5	100	C-B	5/5	100	Satisfactory	Successful
Cholesterol, HDL	C-C	5/5	100	C-A	5/5	100	C-B	5/5	100	Satisfactory	Successful
Creatine Kinase	C-C	5/5	100	C-A	5/5	100	C-B	5/5	100	Satisfactory	Successful
Creatinine	C-C	5/5	100	C-A	5/5	100	C-B	5/5	100	Satisfactory	Successful
Glucose	C-C	5/5	100	C-A	5/5	100	C-B	5/5	100	Satisfactory	Successful
Iron, Total	C-C	5/5	100	C-A	5/5	100	C-B	5/5	100	Satisfactory	Successful
LD	C-C	5/5	100	C-A	5/5	100	C-B	5/5	100	Satisfactory	Successful
Magnesium	C-C	5/5	100	C-A	5/5	100	C-B	5/5	100	Satisfactory	Successful
Potassium	C-C	5/5	100	C-A	5/5	100	C-B	5/5	100	Satisfactory	Successful
Sodium	C-C	5/5	100	C-A	3/5	60	C-B	1/5	20	Unsatisfactory	Unsuccessful <3>

The Lab took option #3 from the list of possible remediations given above, putting a new chemistry instrument into service that replaced an excessively old, worn out piece of equipment. At the subsequent CMS inspection in December, 2013, the CMS inspector gave the lab a pass without any sanctions (fines), and no citations directly related to the sodium testing, new chemistry equipment, etc.

This was a judgment call on the part of the inspector. The strictest reading of the regulations would require that this lab cease sodium testing for 6 months, correct the problem, pass two sodium PT events (called "reinstatement PT events") and then reapply to CMS for sodium testing. This was a small hospital lab in the middle of nowhere, hours away from the next nearest hospital or clinic lab able to test sodium. If this lab was not able to test sodium, there would have been severe consequences to medical care in this small town. Hence, the inspector "bent the rules" for this lab by interpreting the regulations in the most lenient manner possible.

The CLIA reference is given at 42 CFR § 493.803 and states that for a lab with initial unsuccessful participation in PT the CMS may direct the laboratory to undertake training of its personnel or to obtain technical assistance, or both, rather than imposing sanctions such as a cease testing letter. There are a few exceptions, such as poor compliance history (i.e. you have repeatedly promised the CMS inspectors to fix problems then failed to do so). Thus, at this stage of the game the decision to issue or not issue a cease testing letter is largely a judgment call on the part of the CMS inspectors. In all situations I am aware of, the CMS inspectors made the judgment call to allow the lab to keep testing, based on a promise to fix the problem. If you make this promise and are allowed to keep testing, it is imperative to keep your promise and fix the problem as quickly as you can. The CMS inspectors will expect to see a "full court press" (i.e. 100% effort) to get the problem fixed.

I will give the subsequent PT results for this analyte as an example of the process of "pushing off the back" prior PT failures. In this particular case, the lab put a new analyzer into service using a different methodology. The PT prior to the installation of the new analyzer does not apply to the new analyzer. The new analyzer was passing all along, even though the PT results given here indicate unsuccessful performance for sodium. The sodium failures occurred on the 2013 first and second events. After the 2013 second event, the most recent three sodium PT events are FAIL-FAIL-PASS and the cumulative performance is unsuccessful. The new analyzer went live shortly before the 2013 third event. The 2013 third event results are given below:

CMS Peformance Summary for Analytes Regulated Under the Clinical Laboratory Improvement Amendments of 1988

	CLIA ID #:			Subspecialty:	Routine Chemistry					
	Proficiency Event 2013 1			Proficiency Event 2013 2			Proficiency Event 2013 3			Current Event Performance Interpretation	Cumulative CLIA '88 Performance Interpretation
Regulated Analyte	Test Event	Score	%	Test Event	Score	%	Test Event	Score	%		
ALT	C-A	5/5	100	C-B	5/5	100	C-C	5/5	100	Satisfactory	Successful
Albumin	C-A	5/5	100	C-B	5/5	100	C-C	5/5	100	Satisfactory	Successful
Alkaline Phosphatase	C-A	5/5	100	C-B	5/5	100	C-C	5/5	100	Satisfactory	Successful
Amylase	C-A	5/5	100	C-B	5/5	100	C-C	5/5	100	Satisfactory	Successful
AST	C-A	5/5	100	C-B	5/5	100	C-C	5/5	100	Satisfactory	Successful
Bilirubin, Total	C-A	5/5	100	C-B	5/5	100	C-C	5/5	100	Satisfactory	Successful
Calcium, Total	C-A	5/5	100	C-B	5/5	100	C-C	5/5	100	Satisfactory	Successful
Chloride	C-A	5/5	100	C-B	5/5	100	C-C	5/5	100	Satisfactory	Successful
Cholesterol, Total	C-A	5/5	100	C-B	5/5	100	C-C	5/5	100	Satisfactory	Successful
Cholesterol, HDL	C-A	5/5	100	C-B	5/5	100	C-C	5/5	100	Satisfactory	Successful
Creatine Kinase	C-A	5/5	100	C-B	5/5	100	C-C	5/5	100	Satisfactory	Successful
Creatinine	C-A	5/5	100	C-B	5/5	100	C-C	5/5	100	Satisfactory	Successful
Glucose	C-A	5/5	100	C-B	5/5	100	C-C	5/5	100	Satisfactory	Successful
Iron, Total	C-A	5/5	100	C-B	5/5	100	C-C	5/5	100	Satisfactory	Successful
LD	C-A	5/5	100	C-B	5/5	100	C-C	5/5	100	Satisfactory	Successful
Magnesium	C-A	5/5	100	C-B	5/5	100	C-C	5/5	100	Satisfactory	Successful
Potassium	C-A	5/5	100	C-B	5/5	100	C-C	5/5	100	Satisfactory	Successful
Sodium	C-A	3/5	60	C-B	1/5	20	C-C	5/5	100	Satisfactory	Unsuccessful <3>

The sodium has passed the 2013 third PT event. A passing PT event has been "pushed off the back" of the most recent three PT events. The three most recent PT events are now PASS-FAIL-FAIL. The cumulative performance for sodium is still showing as unsuccessful, since two of the three most recent PT events are failing. Here are the 2014 first event results:

CMS Peformance Summary for Analytes Regulated Under the Clinical Laboratory Improvement Amendments of 1988

CLIA ID #: ▇▇▇▇▇▇▇   Subspecialty: Routine Chemistry

Regulated Analyte	Proficiency Event 2013 2			Proficiency Event 2013 3			Proficiency Event 2014 1			Current Event Performance Interpretation	Cumulative CLIA '88 Performance Interpretation
	Test Event	Score	%	Test Event	Score	%	Test Event	Score	%		
ALT	C-B	5/5	100	C-C	5/5	100	C-A	4/5	80	Satisfactory	Successful
Albumin	C-B	5/5	100	C-C	5/5	100	C-A	5/5	100	Satisfactory	Successful
Alkaline Phosphatase	C-B	5/5	100	C-C	5/5	100	C-A	5/5	100	Satisfactory	Successful
Amylase	C-B	5/5	100	C-C	5/5	100	C-A	5/5	100	Satisfactory	Successful
AST	C-B	5/5	100	C-C	5/5	100	C-A	5/5	100	Satisfactory	Successful
Bilirubin, Total	C-B	5/5	100	C-C	5/5	100	C-A	5/5	100	Satisfactory	Successful
Calcium, Total	C-B	5/5	100	C-C	5/5	100	C-A	5/5	100	Satisfactory	Successful
Chloride	C-B	5/5	100	C-C	5/5	100	C-A	5/5	100	Satisfactory	Successful
Cholesterol, Total	C-B	5/5	100	C-C	5/5	100	C-A	5/5	100	Satisfactory	Successful
Cholesterol, HDL	C-B	5/5	100	C-C	5/5	100	C-A	5/5	100	Satisfactory	Successful
Creatine Kinase	C-B	5/5	100	C-C	5/5	100	C-A	5/5	100	Satisfactory	Successful
Creatinine	C-B	5/5	100	C-C	5/5	100	C-A	4/5	80	Satisfactory	Successful
Glucose	C-B	5/5	100	C-C	5/5	100	C-A	5/5	100	Satisfactory	Successful
Iron, Total	C-B	5/5	100	C-C	5/5	100	C-A	5/5	100	Satisfactory	Successful
LD	C-B	5/5	100	C-C	5/5	100	C-A	5/5	100	Satisfactory	Successful
Magnesium	C-B	5/5	100	C-C	5/5	100	C-A	5/5	100	Satisfactory	Successful
Potassium	C-B	5/5	100	C-C	5/5	100	C-A	5/5	100	Satisfactory	Successful
Sodium	C-B	1/5	20	C-C	5/5	100	C-A	5/5	100	Satisfactory	Successful

The sodium has passed the 2014 first PT event. A failing PT event has been "pushed off the back" of the most recent three PT events. The three most recent PT events are now PASS-PASS-FAIL. The cumulative performance for sodium is now showing as successful, since two of the three most recent PT events are passing.

As mentioned above, this lab had put a new analyzer into service. If the lab had not put in a new analyzer, there would be some urgency in getting the failing PT events remediated. As described above, my advice is to fix the underlying problem as quickly as possible and then order multiple unscheduled PT events. Do not wait for the routine scheduled PT events which only occur three times per year.

I have never had an analyte in the situation in which the last three PT events are FAIL-FAIL-FAIL. This situation would be referred to as "repeat unsuccessful participation" in proficiency testing. Repeat unsuccessful participation is defined in different ways by the various regulatory agencies. For the purpose of this book, I will assume repeat unsuccessful participation is defined as three or more PT failures out of the last six PT events.

I am only aware of one lab getting itself into this situation. At all other labs having PT problems in-house testing was discontinued and the analyte was sent out after the second failed PT event and/or the underlying problem was fixed before it came to this. In the event of repeat unsuccessful PT participation my advice is to discontinue in-house testing and send out the test if you can. If you can't send the test out, you should try the remediation steps given above over and over until you are successful or until regulatory intervention is imminent. As mentioned above, in this situation the last six PT events are held against you. You will be desperately ordering and running multiple unscheduled PT events until there is no more than one failure in the last six PT events.

As your PT situation worsens, your lab will come under increasing regulatory scrutiny. This is discussed in more detail in the chapter on Regulatory Scrutiny Syndrome later in this book. After being hired in August, 2013 to "turnaround" the lab referenced above, I was in nearly constant contact with the team of CMS inspectors assigned to that lab. There was nearly daily E-mail and weekly teleconferences with the CMS inspectors as the lab struggled to right itself. The CMS inspectors provided helpful input and useful suggestions on how to remediate problems. At the next CMS inspection in December, 2013 this lab was found to have all prior citations corrected. After this inspection, the contact with the team of CMS inspectors dropped to occasional E-mail as needed.

At some point the regulators may tell you that the next failed PT will result in a "cease testing" letter. In this situation my advice is that you should voluntarily discontinue in-house testing for that analyte and send the test out rather than risk a "cease testing" letter. A "cease testing" letter typically comes with sanctions including loss of your ability to bill Medicare or Medicaid for 6 months.

My advice is to always do exactly as the regulators tell you. If they send you a "cease testing" letter you must immediately stop testing that analyte at all labs covered under the CLIA number referenced. You could try switching the testing to a waived test if possible. Put the waived test in a separate room and on a separate CMS certificate (i.e. a Certificate of Waiver) from the rest of the lab. In theory, the CMS cannot routinely inspect a waived testing lab and can only inspect when there has been a complaint against that lab. If that doesn't work you would then be sending out an essential analyte, but you would have no other choice, you have run out of options.

At some point the regulators may tell you that the next failed PT will result in revocation of your CMS certificate (i.e. regulatory closure of your lab). In this situation my advice is that you should voluntarily shut down that part, or all, of your lab rather than risk regulatory closure. The effects of regulatory closure are devastating and should be avoided at all cost.

There is a saying that an ounce of prevention is worth a pound of cure. It is your responsibility as Lab Director to ensure that all tests are in control on all days of testing. If your tests are in control, you should not have recurrent failure on PT testing.

Like all government regulations, the rules related to PT are subject to change. On February 4, 2019 the CMS made known its intention to narrow the acceptability limits for proficiency testing, add many more analytes to the list of regulated analytes, and make various other changes to the PT rules spelled out in this chapter. The reference is the Federal Register Vol. 84, No. 23, pages 1536 to 1567. The current CLIA law was passed in 1988 but could not be fully implemented until 2003. Given past experience the proposed rule changes will likely take several years to finalize and more than a decade to fully implement. Thus, the PT rules stated in this chapter will likely remain in effect for the foreseeable future.

Chapter 7 – How to put a new analyzer into service

In this chapter, I will go through the steps of setting a Food and Drug Administration (FDA) cleared or approved non-waived quantitative analyzer into service. This is the typical type of analyzer for all sections of lab except microbiology. For verification of an FDA approved or cleared non-waived qualitative analyzer (i.e. the typical microbiology analyzer) see Chapter 32, Topic #2. For verification of a test that is not FDA cleared or approved see Chapter 32, Topic #3.

The Food, Drug and Cosmetic Act refers to all lab testing instruments and systems as "in vitro diagnostic products" and defines them as a "device". The reference is 21 CFR § 809.3. Based on this definition, the FDA has regulatory authority over the manufacture of all lab testing equipment in the

US. In order to sell an analyzer in the US, the manufacturer has to get FDA clearance or approval. I will briefly discuss the manufacturer's requirements for getting FDA clearance or approval since this is relevant to your subsequent installation of the same equipment into your lab.

According to the FDA, validation of an analytic procedure is determining it is fit for the intended use. Typical validation characteristics which should be considered are: accuracy, precision, specificity, detection limit, limit of quantitation, linearity, range and ruggedness. Ruggedness is also called robustness and refers to a test's ability to remain unaffected by small variations in test methods and test conditions. If all the quality objectives are met, the method is considered as validated.

The manufacturer of lab testing equipment must validate the equipment, unless the equipment uses standard methods. Standard methods are those published by international, regional or national standards-writing bodies, by reputable technical organizations and FDA published methods.

Verification of an analytical procedure is demonstrating that the test replicates with an acceptable level of performance a standard method. Verification ensures that the laboratory is capable of performing the analysis. This is required for the first use of a new method within a laboratory. The reference for the above is FDA's Office Of Regulatory Affairs (ORA) Laboratory Manual Volume I - 5.4 Test Methods and Method Validation and Volume II - 5.4.5 Methods, Method Verification and Validation.

Given the above information, validation and verification are different. The manufacturer has already done the validation in order to make the analyzer available for sale. You can assume that any lab testing equipment being sold in the US meets the minimum standards for clinical lab testing. All you have to do is verification, which is proving that the analyzer you received performs as well as the manufacturer claims it should while in use in your lab by your lab's testing personnel. You must also meet all other regulatory requirements (enroll in proficiency testing, have a procedure manual for the analyzer, etc.).

Although validation and verification are different, there is a tendency for these terms to be used interchangeably. All the activities described in this chapter represent verification, not validation. A small hospital lab typically does not have the resources to make its own tests from nothing and generally doesn't have the volume of testing to make it worthwhile. Thus a small hospital lab will essentially never do validation, only verification.

A test that is not FDA approved or cleared is referred to as a laboratory developed test (LDT) or "off label" test. Such a test can only be performed in-house. The testing equipment cannot be sold to or used in another lab without FDA clearance or approval. However, other labs can send you specimens for "off label" testing.

The typical situation where a lab makes a test in-house involves molecular testing for infectious agents. Labs doing this type of testing usually have a long list of infectious organisms they can test for. Each of these tests typically involves a different Analyte Specific Reagent (ASR). As the name suggests, an ASR is a reagent used to identify an individual chemical or ligand in the specimen. An ASR is specific for one test (e.g. mumps virus) and cannot be used for a different test (e.g. measles virus).

When a lab makes an in-house test involving an ASR the following statement must appear on the test report: "This test was developed and its performance characteristics determined by (Laboratory Name). It has not been cleared or approved by the U.S. Food and Drug Administration". The reference is 21 CFR § 809.30. The CAP recommends additional verbiage at the end of this statement to indicate that

FDA approval or clearance is not necessary for this type of test.

I have only seen the above disclaimer on test reports coming from large university hospital labs and reference labs and have never seen such disclaimers on test reports coming from a small hospital lab. As mentioned above, a small hospital lab typically does not have the resources to make a test in-house, and generally doesn't have the volume of testing to make it worthwhile.

Per CLIA each laboratory that introduces an unmodified, FDA-cleared or approved test system before reporting patient test results must demonstrate that it can obtain performance specifications comparable to those established by the manufacturer for the following performance characteristics: accuracy, precision and reportable range of test results. The lab must verify that the manufacturer's reference intervals (normal values) are appropriate for the laboratory's patient population. The laboratory must determine the test system's calibration procedures and control procedures based upon the performance specifications it has established. The laboratory must document all these activities.

If you modify a test you would additionally need to establish the following: analytical sensitivity, analytical specificity to include interfering substances, reference intervals (normal values) and any other performance characteristic required for test performance. The reference for the above is 42 CFR § 493.1253.

In my 29 years experience in Pathology and Lab Medicine I have never once needed to modify a test into something that was different from the manufacturer's instructions. To the best of my knowledge, test modification is only done at large university hospital labs and reference labs. In some instances, the reason for wanting to modify the test was petty - wanting to use a collection device different from the manufacturer's instructions or wanting to use a less expensive reagent for the test. These large labs routinely make their own molecular tests from nothing, and have extensive experience doing all the additional work required (making an in-house reference range, in-house reportable range, etc.).

My advice is that if you are working in a community hospital lab, never modify a test. It is much easier to put an unmodified test into place. There are other reasons not to modify a test. For example for most analyzers, if you do anything to the analyzer that the manufacturer does not approve of this will void the warranty. For the remainder of this chapter, when I go through the steps of putting a new analyzer into service, I am referring to an analyzer which has not been modified in any way from the manufacturer's instructions.

A. Pick which equipment you want to buy

Lab equipment has a usable life span and depreciates over that life span. Lab equipment wears out and needs to be replaced at regular intervals. The usable life span of a lab testing instrument is around 5 to 10 years depending on the equipment.

As the equipment gets older, it will have more breakdowns. At some point it will be more expensive to continue repairing the old equipment than to buy new equipment. This is the typical point at which the decision to purchase is made.

You will need approval from the hospital's administration to buy new equipment. It tends to be very expensive, such that the decision to buy or not to buy can be very difficult. Once the old equipment has gone beyond the typical lifespan of lab testing instruments and is having frequent breakdowns, purchasing a new instrument is usually not a "hard sell" with the hospital's administration.

If the old equipment breaks down, and can't be repaired, you will be making the purchase as an emergency procurement. If you can't do basic testing like CBCs or Chem-12s and end up sending them out for testing, the medical staff will be very upset with the turnaround time. In this situation the hospital's administration will be signing all the equipment procurement paperwork you bring them and worrying about the cost later.

For most types of equipment (chemistry, hematology, etc.) there are multiple manufacturers to choose from. Typically the decision as to which one to buy from is made based on economics – pick the cheapest vendor. Sometimes the decision is made based on convenience – if every other lab in your community uses one vendor, you should as well so that you are able to share reagents with the surrounding labs.

CLIA makes the Lab Director responsible for "appropriate test method selection". In my experience the equipment is usually selected based on which manufacturer is the cheapest to deal with. As far as I am concerned as a Lab Director the instrument's methodology, radioimmunoassay (RIA) versus enzyme linked immunosorbent assay (ELISA) versus other methodology, doesn't really matter. I really only care that the testing has precision and accuracy.

The big caveat here is to make sure that the new piece of equipment does not have special requirements that exceed the specifications of your existing facility. Is the new piece of equipment too large to fit in the existing space? Does it have requirements for a special type of water, narrow temperature and/or humidity requirements? Will it need special ducting for contaminated exhaust air? You don't want to buy a piece of equipment only to find that you have to move your whole lab into a larger space to accommodate the new equipment, ducting for the new equipment, etc.

All essential equipment (e.g. hematology analyzers, chemistry analyzers, etc.) are typically bought as a set of two identical instruments (i.e. same manufacturer and preferably the same model). You need to have two instruments so that one can serve as the backup in case the other goes down. There are several good reasons for having identical instruments. If you have two or more analyzers performing the same tests, CLIA requires that you correlate the two instruments against each other once every 6 months. If you have identical instruments you will likely have a near perfect correlation. Furthermore, both instruments will have the same reference range, specimen requirements, critical values, supplies/reagents, etc.

If you were to have two instruments from different manufacturers (i.e. you replace one analyzer but not the other with a newer instrument) this would cause a whole series of problems. You would likely have a poor correlation between the two instruments since you are comparing different analyzers. Each instrument would likely have its own reference range. The two instruments could have different specimen requirements, critical values, etc. You would be dealing with two different vendors, different supplies/reagents, different preventive maintenance schedules for the two analyzers, etc. You would have to maintain inventory for both analyzers and you would likely have more expired reagents. This would be prohibitively expensive and creates so many problems that it should be avoided if at all possible.

The only instance I have ever seen a hospital consider replacing one analyzer but not the other that hospital was desperately short of cash with two old hematology analyzers both breaking down at the same time. That hospital opted instead for a reagent rental agreement with zero up front cost. Thus, I am not familiar with even one instance of a hospital having two different hematology or chemistry analyzers from two different manufacturers.

        B. Decide to rent, buy or lease the equipment

It is possible to buy, rent or lease lab equipment. This is just like any other piece of capital equipment, such as a car.

For lab equipment, lease arrangements are the most common in my experience. Leasing has many advantages over buying. Leasing has less up-front costs compared to buying. If the equipment breaks down, the leasing company has to repair it. At the end of the lease term, typically 5 years, you can trade in the old instrument for a brand new instrument while making a new lease. Alternatively, the lease can be set up so that you can buy the equipment at the end of the 5 years and obtain outright ownership of the equipment after the lease is over.

The main disadvantage to leases is that the interest rate is typically variable. If interest rates go up, you will be paying more for the lease. However, if interest rates go down, you will be paying less for the lease. In the business world uncertainty is unnerving. It is hard to budget for a lease if you don't know how much next year's payments will be.

Another disadvantage of a lease is that you are legally committed to the deal for the term of the lease, which is typically five years. It is possible for a test or technology to become obsolete in less time. If you had leased equipment to do CK-MBs at the same time your competitor down the street got troponins going on their equipment, you would have been out of luck, stuck with obsolete, unused equipment for the remainder of the lease.

Reagent rental is another option. In this option you pay per test. There is usually a minimum payment based on the minimum number of tests that will be done. This option is best for reference labs doing a large volume of testing. Even if you don't meet the minimum number of tests you will still have to pay the minimum payment, in effect paying for tests that are not done.

After making the decision to buy, rent or lease, the next step is to negotiate the price and other terms with the vendor. After reaching agreement on all terms, the hospital and vendor sign an acquisition contract. Most hospitals have a Materials Management or Procurement Office that will handle most of the purchase paperwork. After the paperwork is executed, the vendor will send the equipment. Usually the hospital pays for the transport of the equipment. The vendor should supply you with a "starter kit" of reagents and supplies to be used training the staff and verifying the analyzer. I have only seen one instance where the "starter kit" ran out before the verification was complete. In this case we informed the vendor we needed more supplies to complete the verification of the analyzer, and they sent us the needed supplies.

If the deal is executed with a new vendor, you should receive a "hello" letter or E-mail from that vendor informing you of all relevant contact information for that company – corporate headquarters address and phone number, phone number for troubleshooting technical problem calls, names and phone numbers of your sales representative and service representative, etc. This information is important, so file the "hello" letter in a secure location.

Someone from the equipment manufacturer should contact you to discuss the upcoming installation of the new analyzer. They should inform you of the requirements for the analyzer – space needed, electric requirements, type of internet connection needed, biohazard waste containers, etc. If necessary, make a work order for the preparation of the area where the analyzer will be situated. It is best to complete these preparations before the analyzer arrives. The installer is going to be on a tight schedule. If there are any delays the installer may have to leave before all the installation work is complete, leaving some of this work for your lab staff to finish.

C. The new analyzer and the Service Rep arrive

The new analyzer will arrive a few days to weeks after the acquisition contract is signed. In general most of the work of putting a new analyzer into service will be done by the Service Representative (known in the business as a "Service Rep"). The Service Rep is a traveling representative of the company that made the analyzer.

The Service Rep tends to be more of a hardware person than a quality control person. As such, the Service Rep typically has technologists available for phone consultations from the company headquarters. These techs know more about quality control, but they rarely leave the corporate headquarters and you will likely never meet them in person. You are allowed to call these techs directly without needing to have the Service Rep on the line.

If the analyzer has quality control problems (fails controls) that you can't mitigate internally, call the company headquarters first. If the analyzer has an issue that is obviously a hardware problem call the Service Rep first.

Almost all analyzer acquisition contracts state that the company must approve of any and all changes to the analyzer or else these changes will void the warranty and servicing agreement. The Service Rep is your point of contact for the company that made that analyzer. As such the Service Rep has the authority to decide what changes the company will or will not allow to the analyzer.

The Service Rep will also do all the preventive maintenance for that analyzer, flying in a few times a year to do this work. The Service Rep can be called in on an unscheduled basis if there is a major problem with the analyzer such as the analyzer goes down and can't be brought back up again.

As soon as the analyzer arrives on site the Service Rep should fly in to do the calibration, correlation, linearity, etc. Your staff should not have to do the majority of this work. Validation only needs to be done once before you put a new analyzer into service and does not need to be repeated during the life of the analyzer. The documentation of this work should be kept for the life of the analyzer and should be easily retrievable. This is usually accomplished by keeping the documentation in a three ring binder stored in the same place as the procedure manuals for the analyzer. At the next CMS or CAP inspection, the inspector will almost certainly ask to review this documentation.

CLIA lists the verification work that is necessary, but does not specifically require the Lab Director to sign off on this work. The CAP requires the Lab Director to sign off on new methods and recommends a statement to the effect the Lab Director has reviewed the verification work and determined the performance of the method is acceptable for patient testing. See the reference, CAP checklist item COM.40000, for the exact verbatim to put down when signing off on the verification.

D. Check correlation

Correlation is tested by selecting 20 or more random patient specimens, splitting the specimens and running one split of each on the old instrument and the new instrument. The minimum of 20 is recommended, but not a regulatory requirement. If you don't have enough patient specimens, you are allowed to use controls, calibrators and/or proficiency testing specimens to reach the minimum number needed for a correlation. Even so, there should be some patient specimens included, not all controls, calibrators and proficiency testing specimens. The results are used to calculate the correlation of the new instrument to the old instrument. If there is no old instrument (i.e. you are adding a new type of testing) you will need to send a split of the specimens to an outside lab and correlate against their test results.

The testing for the correlation should reflect patient testing to the extent possible. Assign some of the correlation testing to each of the lab techs who will be doing the patient testing. Do not assign all the correlation testing to one lab tech unless that lab tech will be doing all the patient testing.

Usually the Service Rep calculates the correlation, but this calculation can also be done by the Lab Supervisor. Alternatively, the raw data can be E-mailed to the analyzer manufacturer's corporate headquarters for them to do the calculation. The results are usually expressed as correlation coefficient (R). The correlation testing is usually reviewed by the Service Rep and Lab Supervisor for their approval and then brought to the Lab Director to sign off on.

R can range from -1 (perfect negative correlation) through zero (no correlation) to +1 (perfect positive correlation). In my experience the typical R obtained when comparing one analyzer to another is at least 0.98. For setting a new analyzer into service, most people in the profession, myself included, prefer an R of 0.95 or higher.

Here is an example of a correlation that was used to put a new piece of equipment into service:

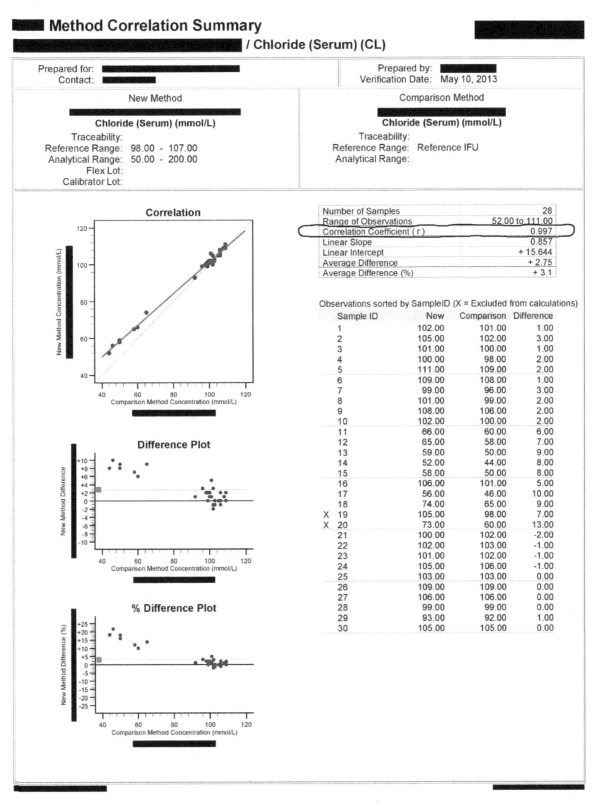

This correlation came out to 0.997 which is near perfect. Perfect positive correlation is 1.000. When you see a correlation this good you don't have any hesitation on accepting it. Just sign it and move on. If the correlation comes out to less than 0.95 that is when I start getting worried that something is wrong.

Here is the worst correlation I have ever seen:

MPV

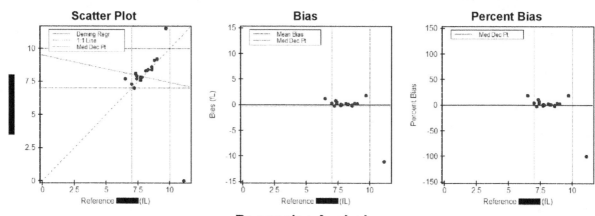

This is a correlation of Mean Platelet Volume (MPV) from an old instrument to a new instrument. The correlation coefficient came out to -0.3257. Quite frankly, I did not think it was possible for a correlation coefficient to come out negative in actual clinical practice until it happened. This is the only negative correlation I have ever seen in my 29 years in Pathology and Lab Medicine.

When you get a correlation this bad, you should check the precision for both the old and new analyzer. Aside from imprecision, such poor correlation could also result from exceeding the Analytical Measurement Range (AMR) of one or both analyzers while doing this testing, deteriorated specimens used for testing, miscalculating the dilution on one analyzer, interfering substances affecting one but not the other analyzer, etc. Compare the original analyzer tapes to the data used for the calculations to make sure there are no clerical errors in transcription. Check the math manually on a calculator.

The test in question is only MPV, which is not that significant. Even so, I would not accept this analyzer without further work to improve the MPV correlation.

The corrective action was carried out for the above MPV correlation. The correlation was made with only 19 data points which is less than the recommended 20 data points minimum. Of those 19 data points, 5 were found to have transcription error. After correction of the 5 data points with transcription error, and running ten more specimens, the above correlation was repeated. Here are the repeat results:

Supporting Statistics

Corr Coef (R) 0.9076	Y Mean ± SD 8.25 ± 0.59	Points (Plotted/Total) 27/29
Bias 0.14 (1.68 %)	Std Dev Diffs 0.30	Outliers None
X Mean ± SD 8.11 ± 0.70	SubRange Bounds None	Scatter Plot Bounds None

The correlation has improved to 0.9076. This is not a great correlation; I prefer 0.95 or higher. However, it is better than having a negative correlation. It is possible to do additional work on this correlation, by running additional specimens.

CLIA does not set a minimum for correlation. If the correlation comes out below 0.95 you can accept that if you want. If the correlation comes out below your expectation, you can improve it by running some more samples. Use a few very low (or negative) samples and a few very high samples.

The very high samples should be just below the cutoff of the AMR. Do not exceed the AMR on either instrument. Exceeding the AMR typically worsens the correlation and will only make the situation worse.

You will find that adding in a few very low and very high samples will drive the correlation coefficient up to nearly +1, near perfect positive correlation. I have heard of some Clinical Chemistry people referring to this technique as "cheating". Keep in mind that CLIA does not specifically forbid this technique. It's a free country, you can do whatever you want unless there's a law or regulation against it. There is no law or regulation to stop you from running very high and very low specimens to improve your correlation.

If the correlation is still below 0.95 after doing this, I would have serious reservations about accepting the instrument that just arrived. I would be discussing the problem with the Service Rep and telling the Service Rep there seems to be a problem with the new instrument. It looks like lack of precision on the part of the new instrument and I am thinking about asking for a replacement for the new instrument.

When carrying out a corrective action on a bad correlation, you are allowed to discard all data and start over if you want. However, you can't arbitrarily remove data points just because you don't like them. If you are going to selectively delete data points, there should be a good justification for doing so (clerical error, miscalculated dilution for that data point, etc.).

CLIA speaks vaguely of "performance specifications comparable to those established by the manufacturer". In my experience, most CMS inspectors interpret this broadly enough that it prohibits arbitrarily keeping data points which result in good correlation and discarding data points which result in poor correlation. Thus, most CMS inspectors would give this an inspection citation. In any event, this is considered bad laboratory practice and should be avoided.

E. Do calibration, verification of calibration and check linearity

CLIA requires the lab to define each test system's calibration and control procedures, criteria for acceptability of calibrators and controls, etc. My advice is to adopt the manufacturer's recommendations. For any given analyzer the manufacturer typically makes available to you everything you will need in regards to controls, calibration and verification of calibration.

A calibrator is a sample containing a known quantity of an analyte. CLIA requires a minimum of 3 calibrators – low, normal and high. Calibrators are typically purchased, usually from the manufacturer of the instrument that will be calibrated using that calibrator. When you purchase calibrators, they will come as a set of at least 3 and possibly as many as 5 of the calibrator material.

The low calibrator should test the low end of the Analytical Measurement Range (AMR). This is near zero for most analytes. There should be a middle calibrator that roughly corresponds to the middle of the reference range. The high calibrator should be just below the upper end of the AMR.

Calibrators typically come from the manufacturer with the mean and acceptable range stated by the manufacturer. The calibration is typically done by a bench level lab tech or the section supervisor of the lab section where the equipment is situated. The calibrators are tested on the analyzer being calibrated. The results obtained from the testing are compared to the known/expected values of the calibrator specimens. If the instrument gives results in the acceptable range the lab tech accepts things as they are. If the instrument gives results that are outside the acceptable range, the lab tech reprograms the instrument so that it gives out the expected results.

Calibration verification refers to testing specimens of known concentration in the same manner as patient specimens to verify the instrument's calibration throughout the AMR. CLIA requires that you perform verification of calibration at least every 6 months, when changing all reagents to new lot numbers, when there is major preventive maintenance or parts replacement, when control materials reflect an unusual trend or shift or are outside of acceptable limits and this can't be fixed otherwise and when the laboratory's established schedule calls for more frequent verification of calibration. The reference is 42 CFR § 493.1255. You will need to perform calibration and verification of calibration prior to setting your new piece of equipment into service.

Calibration verification is easy. All the lab tech has to do is re-run the same calibrator materials after the calibration. Since you've already calibrated the instrument to that calibrator, you're almost guaranteed to pass the calibration verification. If you want to challenge yourself, use a different set of calibrators to perform the verification of calibration. If you pass calibration verification using a different set of calibrators, you can be sure your calibration is very accurate. If you fail calibration verification you should repeat the calibration, then repeat the verification of calibration. If it still fails this typically prompts a troubleshooting call to the manufacturer of the analyzer.

For some analytes, you will receive only 3 calibrators. If you are doing calibration verification and want to test the entire AMR using multiple different known amounts of analyte, you can draw an aliquot from the various calibrators, and mix them to make multiple different samples of known quantity.

For example if the low calibrator has zero of the analyte and the middle calibrator has 100, you can mix the low and middle calibrators 1:1 and assume that the resulting mixture has 50 of the analyte. If the middle calibrator has 100 of the analyte and the high calibrator has 300, you can mix the middle and high calibrators 1:1 and assume that the resulting mixture has 200 of the analyte. If the low calibrator is not zero, you can use saline as a zero calibrator, etc. You can mix saline 1:1 with any of the three calibrators (low, middle and high) to make a mixture of known concentration. You are allowed to use any specimen with a known concentration of the analyte being tested (PT material, etc.). In this manner it is possible to perform calibration verification by testing multiple points throughout the AMR.

Precision is defined as having multiple repeat results closely approximating each other. Precision is tested by making multiple repeat tests of the controls. In my experience the minimum is 3 repeats of each of the controls. Most labs prefer at least 20 data points, in which case you can test the three controls seven times each to get 21 data points.

Allowable imprecision under CLIA is given in a series of tables printed in the Federal Register, the reference is February 28, 1992;57(40):7002-186. In looking over these tables, CLIA allows a huge amount of imprecision. For example for HDL cholesterol you are allowed to be up to 30% off from the target value. In my experience when repeating the HLD cholesterol middle and high controls over and over, they will not usually be off from each other by more than a percent or two. Multiple repeats of the HDL cholesterol low control (i.e. not a zero control) may be off from each other by a few percent.

Aiming to pass the CLIA criteria for precision is like trying to shoot a barn door; it is so wide you can't miss. Hence, I have never seen an analyzer fail testing for precision. The requirements for controls being within 3SD of target are much narrower than the huge variation allowed in precision. Hence, when an analyzer starts having problems it is bound to fail controls before it fails precision.

Linearity refers to the range in which the test result holds a directly proportional, straight line relationship to the analyte. The Analytical Measurement Range (AMR) is defined as the range of analyte concentration that the instrument can measure accurately without pretreatment (i.e. dilution) of the sample. Linearity is very similar to AMR.

Let me explain how linearity and AMR are similar. For example let's say the upper limit of linearity for HCG on your analyzer is 100,000. Below 100,000 HCG if you increase the "true" concentration of HCG by +1, the instrument will report a +1 increase in HCG. However, at the extreme upper range of an analyte most lab analyzers begin to give non-linear results.

In this example, above 100,000 HCG the testing capability of the instrument gets saturated. These tests are typically enzymatic or immunoassays, and above 100,000 HCG most of the enzymes or antibodies used for testing are already saturated with HCG. In this range a +1 increase in the "true" HCG concentration may result in less than a +1 increase in the test result. If this happens, the instrument is now outside its linear range.

The test results for these extremely high, non-linear HCG measurements tend to be inaccurate. The AMR is defined as the range for which test results are accurate. Thus, these extremely high HCG results should be outside the AMR. In other words, any result that exceeds the linearity of the analyzer is typically inaccurate and therefore also exceeds that AMR. Thus, the linear range tends to be identical to the AMR.

CLIA has no requirements for linearity but does have requirements for AMR, so I will spend more time discussing AMR than linearity. In order to set your new piece of equipment into service, you should order one linearity PT event.

When the instrument is being set into commission it is very uncommon to have problems on a linearity PT in my experience. The linearity is identical to the AMR, and the manufacturer has already set the AMR, so you should be good to go. See below. If you fail any part of the linearity PT, do corrective action as outlined in a prior chapter.

While the instrument is in use the linearity proficiency testing will be repeated every six months or year. If the instrument becomes non-linear for any analyte this could be an early warning sign that you are having problems with that particular test. The linearity tends to go out first, before the test goes out of control. See the prior chapter on corrective actions to deal with this situation.

F. Set the Analytical Measurement Range (AMR), Reference Range and Critical Values

The Analytical Measurement Range (AMR) is defined as the range of analyte concentration that the instrument can measure accurately without pretreatment (i.e. dilution) of the sample. The reportable range refers to the range of test results for which the laboratory can verify the accuracy of the test.

I will use again the example of HCG given above. If the test becomes non-linear above 100,000 then the AMR is set by the manufacturer as zero to 100,000. If a specimen has an HCG above 100,000, the instrument will flag the specimen as too high to test, and printout a result of ">100,000".

The lab can either report the specimen as "Greater than 100,000" or dilute the specimen and run it again in a diluted state. Let's say the specimen is diluted 1:1 with saline and rerun. The instrument now reports a result of 76,000. You multiply the result by 2 (the dilution factor in this example) to come out to the "true" HCG result of 152,000. This can be reported with the caveat (usually in a comment) that the test result exceeds the AMR of the instrument and the specimen had to be diluted in order to test it.

In the example of the diluted HCG specimen given above, the AMR of the instrument is 0 to 100,000 but the reportable range of the test is 0 to 200,000. CLIA requires that in order to use this expanded reportable range, the lab needs to run calibration and calibration verification for the expanded reportable range (100,001 to 200,000 HCG in this example).

In regard to setting a new piece of equipment into service, all you need to do is accept the manufacturer's AMR. If you passed all parts of a linearity proficiency test, you have already verified the instrument's AMR, since the linear range and the AMR tend to be identical.

As mentioned above, the calibrators come from the manufacturer designed to test the lower, middle, and upper end of the AMR. When you pass verification of calibration, you simultaneously verify the AMR, since the verification of calibration tests the lower, middle and upper end of the AMR.

I have never seen any lab determine an in-house AMR for each analyte. This would be very difficult to do, very time consuming, and would not add much value. All you have to do is accept the manufacturer's AMR and move on.

The term "reference range" refers to the range of test results that you would expect to see in a normal, healthy individual. For the most part labs simply accept the reference range of the manufacturer.

I have seen a few labs make their own reference range for a few analytes, but this is uncommon. The reference range is frequently defined as the central 95% of test results of normal, healthy individuals. To make your own reference range, you will need to draw 40 normal, healthy people and test their specimens. The 38 median results are the reference range. In other words, starting with 40 normal people's test results discard the highest and lowest outlier from the 40 normal tests. The highest and lowest of the remaining 38 represent the reference range.

Any multiple of 40 normal people can be used to make a reference range. You could stick 80 normal people and discard the two highest and two lowest outliers; you could stick 120 normal people and discard the three highest and three lowest outliers, etc. to make a reference range. The literature prefers 120 normal people, but I will use 40 for this example.

There is very little variation in serum chemistries, hematology, etc. in normal, healthy people. Thus, making an in-house reference range is like re-inventing the wheel - it has been done before. You have to stick 40 normal people to get specimens just the same way that the manufacturer had done when making the manufacturer's reference range.

In my experience any reference range made in-house tends to be almost identical to the manufacturer's reference range. You are measuring the exact same thing - chemistry and hematology tests in normal, healthy people, so it is not unexpected that you get the same results.

You have just stuck 40 people to get specimens, and the whole exercise was a waste of time and effort anyhow. You are right back where you started, with essentially the same reference range. It is much easier to accept the manufacturer's reference range from the start. Regardless of how you obtain the reference range, make sure to document the origin of the reference range in use. You could be asked during an inspection how you obtained your reference range.

CLIA mandates that you verify that the manufacturer's reference intervals (normal values) are appropriate for the laboratory's patient population. This can be done by a simple clinical study in which you pick 20 patients that have lab results available for the analyte in question, but do not have any disease that would be expected to affect the analyte in question. If all 20 of these patient lab results fall within the reference range, you have just verified that your reference range is appropriate for your patient population.

The term "critical values" refers to any lab result that could be life threatening. This was formerly referred to as "panic values". Most labs accept the manufacturer's critical values. I have seen a few labs set critical values for some tests different from the manufacturer's critical values.

The CLIA requirements regarding critical values are given at 42 CFR § 493.1251 and 42 CFR § 493.1291. These require the lab to immediately report any critical values and have a procedure documenting the protocol for reporting critical values. All other requirements given below are from the CAP and TJC. Depending on which agency inspects you, you may or may not have to do a large amount of work setting up a critical value policy.

Your lab should have a policy on critical values. This policy should list all critical values in your lab and require all critical values to be called to the provider with read-back by the provider and documentation of the call. You do not need to have a critical value for every test. For example, most hospitals will not call hemoglobin A1c (HbA1c) or prostate specific antigen (PSA) no matter how low or high the test result.

The time frame for making this call (typically within one hour) must be stipulated in the policy. Only one critical value call is needed per analyte per hospital admission. In other words if the same patient had a critically high glucose previously called on the same hospital admission, you don't need to call any subsequent critically high glucose levels for the remainder of that hospital admission.

If your lab is freestanding, you can set your critical values as you like without needing any approval from any Medical Staff. If your lab is a hospital lab, the critical values must be approved by the hospital's Medical Staff. Before going live with the new analyzer, if any critical values are going to change a hospital lab will need to present the proposed new critical values to the Medical Staff for approval. In my experience, you can present the Medical Staff with the manufacturer's critical values, and the Medical Staff will vote a rubber-stamp approval with little discussion.

Once the Medical Staff approve of the critical values they are all bound by this decision unless and until they collectively agree to change the critical values. In my experience it is not uncommon for one doctor to want his or her own critical values different from the rest of the Medical Staff. For example one OB/GYN doctor wants to be called for all chlamydia results, even the negative ones. The other OB/GYN physicians only want to be called for positive chlamydia results. If the Medical Staff had agreed that only positive chlamydia results get called, all physicians should abide by this decision.

Although there is no regulatory requirement prohibiting multiple critical values for one analyte, it would be too cumbersome and time consuming to have a different set of critical values for each physician. Thus, all physicians must accept the critical values approved by the Medical Staff, or else ask the Medical Staff to change the critical values.

A common problem is providers not answering the phone call. If the provider does not answer calls and pages in a reasonable amount of time, this is typically documented in a comment in the test result. The critical value policy should list the alternates to call in case a physician does not answer a critical call. Typically, if a physician does not respond to a critical call the Departmental Chair or on-call physician is called and given the critical information intended for the physician that did not answer.

You will occasionally have to deal with physicians that missed critical calls, and are upset with the consequences (Departmental Chair informed, on-call physician informed, lab result with a comment indicating that physician was paged but did not answer, etc.). The physician involved may be very upset with lab for doing this. Keep in mind that you have met your regulatory requirements, and that physician has not.

Critical values are distinct from critical tests. According to The Joint Commission, a critical test is any test that requires rapid reporting, even if the results are normal (e.g. a normal CK-MB in an ER patient with chest pain). In contradistinction, a critical value is any result that is so abnormal it requires rapid reporting.

G. Write the procedures for the new equipment

When putting a new piece of equipment into commission the manufacturer will oftentimes supply you with procedures. These are fill in the blank forms in which you paste the name of your hospital in the blanks, print out the procedures, and file them in a procedure manual.

If the manufacturer won't supply you with procedures, you can try the following. Numerous hospitals keep their procedure manuals online, such that it is possible for anyone anywhere to download their procedures. All you have to do is find a hospital that is using the same equipment, download their procedures, change the name to your lab's name, change all the specifics to the way your lab does things, print out the procedures, and you've got a procedure manual.

If the above doesn't work, you will end up writing the procedure manual yourself. See the chapter below on how to write a procedure.

H. Controls, final preparations, going live with the new analyzer and retiring the old analyzer

In most labs the Lab Supervisor is responsible for ordering all the supplies, reagents, PT events, etc. When a new instrument comes on line, the Lab Supervisor will need to set up standing orders (orders for routine delivery) of supplies, reagents, PT events, etc. for the new instrument, and discontinue ordering of supplies, reagents, PT events, etc. for the old instrument.

The standing orders should include orders for controls. A control is a specimen with a known amount of an analyte. This is very similar to a calibrator. The difference is that calibration is typically done at 6 month intervals and designed to set the instrument's results to match the calibrator. Controls are run on each day of testing (or more often) to verify that the instrument is giving good responses. Running controls does not reset the instrument's results while running calibration does. Otherwise calibrators and controls are similar.

Controls can be either assayed or unassayed. Assayed controls are typically made by the manufacturer of the analyzer and are specific to that manufacturer's analyzer. In other words if your chemistry analyzer is made by Siemens, you can't use Abbott assayed controls on it, you can only use Siemens assayed controls on it. An assayed control has a known amount of the analyte. The mean, standard deviation and expected range are provided by the manufacturer. Assayed controls are more expensive, but they are generally worth it since the manufacturer has done extensive testing on that control before sending it to you.

Unassayed controls do not have a known amount of analyte. The mean, standard deviation and expected range are not provided by the manufacturer. This is typically limited to microbiology where a culture is either positive or negative for an organism.

Essentially all hematology and chemistry controls are assayed controls. If you used an unassayed control on hematology or chemistry analyzers, you'd have to determine the mean, standard deviation and expected range of the control on your own analyzers. You would then use that control to check if your own analyzers were in control. You would be comparing your own analyzers to your own analyzers, not the rest of the world. Thus, an unassayed control would be useless in this setting. For the remainder of this book, when referring to a "control" I will be referring to an assayed control.

All labs that I am aware of purchase their controls from a vendor, typically the manufacturer of the analyzer. It is possible to make your own controls in-house but I have never seen a lab do this. Making your own controls would be too time consuming, costly and the controls would be unassayed controls.

CLIA allows the lab to set the QC limits for controls. In theory it would be possible to set your limits so wide you are bound to pass. In other words, for a glucose control with expected mean of 100 your lab could set the acceptable limits of the control as 1 to 1000. If you did this you would never fail QC, but it would make the entire QC process pointless as you would be unable to detect problems with the test. Your inspecting agency is bound to object if you did this. Thus in regard to controls it is best to set everything exactly as specified by the manufacturer. The inspectors cannot question a QC mechanism that is identical to the manufacturer's specifications. The manufacturer's specifications were approved by the FDA when the analyzer was approved by the FDA. As a general rule, one government agency (e.g. the CMS) cannot question something that has already been approved by a different government agency (e.g. the FDA).

CLIA requires the lab to verify the criteria for acceptability for all controls. The reference is 42 CFR § 493.1256(d)(10). The way this is usually handled is to run all newly purchased controls 20 times on arrival. It is best to spread this testing out over time so that different techs run this testing on different shifts. If you test the controls using 20 repeats at the same time this may not be representative of the variation in results seen with multiple lab techs operating the analyzer over multiple shifts.

If the mean, standard deviation and range of these 20 runs are within the specifications given by the manufacturer, the control is accepted as the new control. The new control replaces the old control and the analyzer is programmed with the new control's mean, SD and range. If these test results do not meet the specifications set by the manufacturer this prompts a troubleshooting call to the manufacturer usually with a request for the manufacturer to replace the newly arrived control.

The mean and SD of the control are periodically recalculated while the control is in use. Most modern-day analyzers have software that can calculate the control's mean and SD automatically so that the lab tech does not need to do this by hand. The control's mean and SD should not change significantly over the life of the control. If the control's mean or SD changes significantly this implies a problem, usually deterioration of the control, but sometimes a problem with the analyzer.

The test is said to be "in control" if the results of testing correspond to the expected values from the known amount of analyte in the control specimens. If not the test is said to be "out of control". In general, troubleshooting for out of control tests falls first on the bench level lab tech operating the instrument, next on the section supervisor and then on the Lab Supervisor. If not fixed relatively quickly, calls will be made to the analyzer manufacturer's headquarters and/or the Service Rep for the instrument.

CLIA requires that controls must be run once each day patient specimens are tested or more often if the manufacturer's requirements are more stringent. For each quantitative test (i.e. produces a numeric result), use at least two controls of different concentrations, usually a high and a low control. For each qualitative test (i.e. produces a negative or positive result), include a negative and positive control. For tests giving graded or titered results, include a negative control and a control with graded or titered reactivity. For each test that has an extraction phase, include two controls, including one that is capable of detecting errors in the extraction process. For each molecular amplification procedure, include two controls and if reaction inhibition is a significant source of false negatives, a control material capable of detecting the inhibition. The reference is 42 CFR § 493.1256.

CLIA has two exceptions to the rule regarding daily use of controls. These exceptions are the Equivalent Quality Control (EQC) procedure and the Individualized Quality Control Plan (IQCP). EQC has been phased out and discontinued. IQCP is the replacement for EQC. I will go into more detail about EQC and IQCP in the Advanced topics in Lab Directorship, Chapter 32, Topic #4.

In my experience a new analyzer is almost always in control. I have seen one or two instances where a new instrument arrived out of control, but was easy to bring back into control. I have never seen a new analyzer repeatedly fail controls. If your new analyzer is out of control, and none of the lab techs can get it into control, and the Service Rep can't get it into control, it would mean that you had just received a defective analyzer. Reject this instrument and tell the manufacturer to take it back and replace it with a new one.

If you are testing the same analytes on the new instrument as the old instrument you don't need to rearrange the PT ordering. You do need to inform the PT manufacturer of the change in equipment. The calibrators tend to be specific to one type of analyzer, so you may need to change the ordering of calibrators.

If there are any tests added or deleted from the test directory, the ordering of PT, calibrators, etc. should follow the test directory of the new instrument. If you are adding or deleting tests, you must notify your regulatory agency (CMS, CAP, etc.) before making the change. You may need to receive regulatory approval back before you can put added tests into service.

If you are adding tests and anticipate a significant increase in test volume with the new instrument, you may need to hire additional lab staff. In my experience adding a few tests will not increase test volume enough to justify new hiring.

The staff must be trained on how to operate the new analyzer with documentation of this training. The documentation of training is usually kept indefinitely and stored in each employee's personnel file. Usually this training is done by the Service Rep after he or she has done all other work in preparing to set the new analyzer in service. If the testing is particularly complicated, one or more of your techs may be asked to go to off-site training. This is typically held at the headquarters of the company that made the analyzer. Alternatively the training could be from a third party.

There are limited numbers of seats at the off-site training, typically only 2 or 3 seats. This off-site training is typically seen as a free vacation by the junior techs. The senior techs typically see it as a prestigious perk. The distribution of these seats can be very contentious. For the most part, you are obligated to send the section supervisor of the section where the analyzer will be located. The other one or two seats are up for grabs, but usually go to the next highest ranking techs in the section where the analyzer will be located.

Any tech that wants to go to the off-site training and is not chosen will be very upset. Be prepared to give something of significant value to the techs passed up for the off-site training - raises, bonuses, etc. It is not uncommon for techs to threaten to quit when they find out they have not been chosen for the off-site training. I have seen at least one tech leave for a different company when passed up in this manner.

A peace offering given in appeasement is known as a "sop". In a few places in this book, I will indicate situations where something of value should be offered to employees passed up for promotion, made to work in sections of lab they don't prefer to work in, made to work excessive overtime, etc. In each instance this is an example of a sop.

Immediately before the new equipment is put in service, the hospital's information technology office should be called in to interface the new instrument with the hospital computer system. For every lab test offered, Current Procedural Terminology (CPT) codes are necessary for billing. Is there a CPT code in the computer for billing any new tests offered?

Under CLIA each test report must include the patient identification (either name or a unique identification number), name and address of the laboratory where the test was performed, report date, test performed, specimen source when appropriate, the test result, the units of measurement and/or interpretation and any information regarding the condition and disposition of specimens that do not meet the laboratory's criteria for acceptability. The reference is 42 CFR § 493.1291.

Ask the hospital's information technology office to show you an example of how the test report will appear when using the new analyzer. Check the report to make sure all necessary information will appear in each report issued. Look at how the reports will appear when testing is done on the new instrument. Is the report neat and easy to read? Once you have this worked out, you are ready to go live with the new instrument.

You must inform the Medical Staff whenever any test has a change in specimen requirements, reference range, critical values, etc. If you are getting a new analyzer from the same manufacturer as the old analyzer, the ordering instructions, specimen requirements and the critical values usually stay the same. However, the reference ranges tend to be slightly different from one analyzer to another, even among analyzers from the same manufacturer. In this case, send a memo to all Medical Staff listing the affected tests, the new reference ranges for these tests and effective date of the changes.

If you are getting a new analyzer from a different manufacturer virtually all aspects of the testing could be different. The reference ranges could change considerably for some tests. In this case send a memo to all Medical Staff listing the affected tests, new ordering instructions, specimen requirements, reference ranges, critical values, etc. and the effective date of the changes.

Initially the old instrument and new instrument run alongside each other, until the old instrument uses up all its remaining supplies and reagents. This allows time to make sure the new instrument is running properly.

After a few weeks to a few months the old instrument will use up all its remaining reagents and supplies. If the new instrument is working well without problems, the old instrument is then surveyed out (decommissioned and disposed of). The old instrument's procedure manual is retired to the retired procedure file.

CLIA requires that the lab conduct maintenance and function checks as defined by the manufacturer and with at least the frequency specified by the manufacturer. Function checks must be within the manufacturer's established limits before patient testing is conducted. The reference is 42 CFR § 493.1254.

The new instrument will have a schedule of maintenance set by the manufacturer. It is very important to follow this schedule. Failure to follow this schedule can void the warranty.

The daily to weekly maintenance is usually simple such as cleaning the instrument's surfaces with 10% bleach. This is usually done by the tech prior to the testing, and documented in a logbook. The preventive maintenance (PM) is usually done quarterly to annually and is usually much more complex such that only the Service Rep knows how to do it. Usually the PM scheduling and documentation fall on the section supervisor of the section where the instrument is located. In a few labs the Lab Supervisor is tasked with the PM scheduling and documentation.

The function checks are usually done automatically by the analyzer when it first starts up. Most modern-day analyzers will only do testing if the function checks come in as expected. If the function checks fail, the analyzer will give off error codes and refuse to do any testing. The results of the function checks are documented by the tech doing the testing, before starting that day's testing.

All maintenance records must be stored for at least 2 years. This is usually accomplished by keeping these records in a three ring binder stored in the same place as the procedure manuals for the analyzer. There is no statutory requirement mandating the Lab Director to review the maintenance logs. Although there is no requirement for Lab Director review of these records, I generally review these documents once every 2 years in the run-up to the CMS or CAP inspection.

CLIA requires the retention of all quality control records for at least 2 years. This includes the results of all PT testing and all daily controls. The main part of lab is required to retain a copy of all test reports for at least 2 years. Blood Bank and Anatomic Pathology must retain test reports at least 10 years including donor and recipient records. Pathology and cytology slides must be retained at least 10 years. Employee competency testing, training and continuing education records must be retained for at least 2 years. Test requisitions must be stored for at least 2 years, but can be stored in the patient charts and do not need to be stored in lab. The reference is 42 CFR § 493.1105.

This is usually accomplished by keeping the PT records and control logs as paper documents in three ring binders stored either in the Lab Supervisor's office or in the same place as the procedure manuals for the analyzer. The patient test results are typically stored electronically, not as paper records. The lab must be very careful to have adequate backups of any essential records stored electronically.

The new analyzer will typically come with an operator's guide or owner's manual. Make sure all the lab techs that will be operating the analyzer are familiar with this manual. This manual typically lists everything to avoid, which if done to the analyzer will void the warranty. Examples include putting a different manufacturer's parts into the analyzer, allowing anyone else but the Service Rep to put parts into the analyzer, using tap water in a analyzer that requires distilled water, etc.

It is imperative that you and the lab techs that operate the analyzer know what is not allowed by the manufacturer. You do not want to void the warranty as that would cause a whole series of problems. In my experience, no insurance company would ever insure an analyzer with a voided warranty. No bank would ever lend you money using that analyzer as collateral which means the lease might have to be unwound.

Chapter 8 – How to put a new test onto an existing analyzer

Putting a new test onto an existing analyzer is similar to putting a new piece of equipment into commission but involves fewer steps and fewer analytes.

Let's say that you have a chemistry instrument that is capable of doing serum radon levels, but there really hasn't been much interest in this particular test. You get one test request per year, and you send it out.

Then a few studies come out linking serum radon levels to lung cancer. The health news media runs huge numbers of stories. Suddenly your lab is swamped with specimens for serum radon testing, and sending out dozens per week. The pulmonologist tells you that given the recent journal articles, he will be ordering serum radon levels dozens of times per week forever.

In this scenario, if you can do the test on your existing equipment, you are pretty much obligated to implement the test in house. Here's how to do it.

The first thing to do is to make standing orders for the testing reagents, controls and calibrators as well as enrolling in PT. As mentioned above lab ordering of materials is usually the responsibility of the Lab Supervisor; however, at some labs these duties fall on the section supervisors. When the reagents, controls and calibrators arrive, do the calibration, calibration verification and make sure the test is in control.

Use 20 split specimens to correlate your instrument. If anyone else in the vicinity is doing the test, split 20 specimens, test a split in house, and send a split to the outside lab. Correlate your equipment with their equipment. If no one else in the vicinity is doing the test, split 20 specimens, test a split in house, send the other part of the split specimens to the reference lab, and correlate the results. A correlation coefficient higher than 0.95 is preferable but not required.

Adopt the manufacturer's reference range and AMR. In order to check linearity before going live with this testing, you'd likely have to order an entire new PT event for linearity. I generally don't do this, as it is not required. My approach is to add the analyte to the list of analytes getting routine linearity PT testing so that the next time a routine linearity PT event arrives this analyte is tested.

Once you enroll in PT you will receive the PT once every 4 months. You can start doing the test in-house after you have enrolled in PT, but before the first PT event has arrived. You must notify your regulatory agency before starting the testing. If you are inspected by CMS, use CMS form 116 Application for CLIA Certification. This is the same form as is used to apply for a Certificate of Compliance, but in this case it is being used to modify your existing Certificate of Compliance to add on the new testing. The CMS should acknowledge receiving the new form 116. You can start testing before this acknowledgment comes back. The verification work will usually be checked at the next biennial CMS inspection.

The in-house test is likely to have different specimen requirements, ordering instructions, reference range, critical values, etc. compared to the send-out test that it replaces. If you are in a hospital lab, any changes to the critical values must be approved by vote of the Medical Staff. In my experience, you can present the Medical Staff with the manufacturer's critical values, and the Medical Staff will vote a rubber-stamp approval with little discussion. If you are in a freestanding lab, you can set the critical values as you like without needing any approval from any Medical Staff.

The remainder of setting the new test into service follows the same steps as outlined in Chapter 7 - make a procedure for the new test, train the staff on how to perform the new test, document this training, make sure the new test results will display properly in the hospital's information system, make sure there is a CPT code and billing mechanism for the new test, and go live with testing.

When you go live with the new test, you should send a memo to all the Medical Staff informing them of the new in-house test and any changes in ordering instructions, specimen requirements, reference range, critical values, etc. and include the effective date of the changes for the test.

Chapter 9 – How to deal with analyzer breakdowns

If a test is critical, you are going to have at least 2 analyzers capable of assaying that analyte. Typically, one is used as the primary analyzer, doing most of the work, and the other is a backup, used only when the first analyzer goes down or is taken down for maintenance. In a well funded hospital lab, the existing analyzers are replaced with new analyzers typically every 5 to 7 years, so that the analyzers never get old enough to have frequent breakdowns. In a well funded hospital it is extremely rare for both analyzers to go down at the same time.

In my 29 years experience in Pathology and Lab Medicine I have worked at two very underfunded municipal hospitals. Both put off purchases of new analyzers until the old analyzers were well past their usual lifespan and having frequent breakdowns. I requested new analyzers on several occasions. On each occasion the analyzers were budgeted for, but later the budget was readjusted with the money for the analyzers reallocated for an urgent need elsewhere in the same hospital. As a result, I have seen almost every type of analyzer breakdown imaginable. The list includes:

1. The analyzer gives off error codes and refuses to do anything.
2. The analyzer is out of control and can't be brought back into control.
3. The hospital has not paid its bills to the vendors. The vendors have put the hospital on "credit hold" meaning that they will not send more reagents until the prior shipments are paid for. The hospital lab has run out of reagents for that analyte.
4. Reagents have been paid for and are in transit, but the new reagents do not arrive before the existing reagents run out.
5. The analyzer has been damaged/destroyed by an electric power surge or outage.
6. Every moving part (arm, belt, etc.) is subject to wear and breakdown
7. The software is subject to viruses, corruption, hard drive failure, etc.
8. Other hardware problems (failure of the motherboard, CPU, monitor, etc.) not listed above.

If one analyzer goes down, there is some urgency in getting it fixed, since you dread having both analyzers down at the same time. As a Lab Director you will become very proficient at dealing with analyzer breakdowns if you have to deal with them frequently. The same applies for all other lab disciplines - I spent a year at a Veteran's Hospital and became extremely good at looking at prostate biopsies. I spent 16 years in an underfunded municipal hospital and became extremely good at dealing with analyzer breakdowns.

When an analyzer breaks down, the bench level tech will be the first one to try to fix it. The first thing to do is to diagnose the analyzer's problems. The analyzer may give symptoms such as an error message, funny noise, restricted motion on an arm, etc.

If it is giving off an error code, look up the error code in the analyzer's owner's manual. An analyzer has an owner's manual which is usually stored in a binder in the same area as the procedure manuals. Look up the error code. It will give you a description of the problem, usually with suggested fixes. A common problem is plugged tubes. This usually gives off an error message related to high pressure in the tubing as the analyzer tries to pump fluids through the blocked tube.

If the problem is a funny noise, or restricted motion on the swing arm, this indicates a mechanical problem. This should prompt an immediate call to the hospital's BioMedical Department.

If the only problem is that the analyzer is out of control the lab tech can usually solve this on his or her own. The lab tech will first try rerunning the control. If the first or second rerun is in control, discard the original control results and accept the rerun control results.

If the two reruns are still out of control the lab tech will then try changing disposables (pipettes, cuvettes, etc.), recalibration, ordering new controls, new reagents and/or new calibrators and sending a split of your existing controls and/or calibrators to an outside lab for testing to see if your controls and/or calibrators have deteriorated. If this does not fix the problem the next step is to call the analyzer manufacturer's headquarters.

The manufacturer's corporate headquarters should have techs available 24 hours a day 7 days a week that specialize in handling these sorts of trouble calls. These techs are usually very helpful in guiding you through the corrective process over the phone. If the analyzer still can't be brought back into control with their assistance, it usually means the analyzer has developed a hardware problem. The Service Rep is called and asked to come in person to fix the analyzer.

The tech must be very careful not to release any patient test results generated on an analyzer that is out of control. Those results are assumed to be erroneous and are discarded. If you have two analyzers, use the one that is in control until such time as the other analyzer is brought back into control. If both analyzers are out of control, the specimens must be sent out, or stored until such time that one analyzer or the other is brought back into control

If the analyzer refuses to boot and the power light does not come on check the electric cord, electric outlet, circuit breaker, universal power supply, and/or any special electric supply for the analyzer.

If the power light comes on, but the analyzer does not boot properly, or freezes up and reboots in an endless cycle, this usually indicates a software problem. This should prompt an immediate call to the hospital's Information Services or BioMed department, whichever handles the analyzer software issues.

If the bench level lab tech, and anyone called in by the bench level lab tech, is unable to fix the analyzer they call in the section supervisor who in turn calls in the Lab Supervisor. Each person called in will try to diagnose the problem. BioMed will come and open up the analyzer's cover, such that all the tubes and wires will be visible. They will visually inspect to try to identify the problem.

The next step is a conference call to the Service Rep. This conference call will occur in the same room as the analyzer. The Service Rep typically gives instructions to the BioMed personnel "Try flushing the serum radon line and tell me what happens". BioMed will respond over the phone "we tried flushing the line and the flow is good. It was not blocked". This series of diagnostic maneuvers will continue until the problem is identified.

After diagnosing the problem, you have to fix it. If you are lucky the analyzer will have a problem that can be fixed easily, such as a blocked tube. If the problem is a broken part BioMed will try to fix the part.

If BioMed can't fix the part, you need to have a new part flown in. It is very unlikely that anyone in the same state as you has the part available. Everyone with this analyzer needs that particular part for their analyzer to work. You would need to find a lab that has the exact same equipment as you, and has enough backup analyzers that they could take one analyzer down to give you the part. In my experience, this never happens.

In this situation, you are going to have to order the part from the manufacturer and it will have to be flown in. The manufacturer usually doesn't allow anyone but their Service Rep to put a new part into their analyzer. Thus you will have to wait for the Service Rep to arrive to put the part in. The analyzer will be down until both the part and the Service Rep have arrived. In the remote places where I have been working, that could be 5 days or more.

You will have a very nervous 5 days waiting for the part and Service Rep to arrive. If you are lucky you will get the malfunctioning analyzer up and running before the other analyzer can break down. If the other analyzer breaks down before the first one can be fixed, follow the diagnostic steps above for both analyzers. In this situation it is imperative that you get one analyzer or the other up and running as soon as possible.

If both analyzers break down at the same time you cannot do an essential test. You are in a world of hurt and you have to improvise. Your patient's lives depend on you being able to do the test. You will be scrambling, and you will improvise any way you can.

If patient results are delayed the provider must be notified of the delay. The priority for calls to the providers should be based on the urgency of the tests requested. In other words call the ER providers first to notify them the STAT troponins are delayed and call the outpatient clinic providers last to inform then that the routine labs are delayed. Be prepared that many of the providers on the other end of these phone calls will be very upset about the delays.

After the repairs are completed the analyzer should have QC done to ensure that it is in control before resuming patient testing. If the Service Rep had been called in, ask for a copy of the Service Report for the repair work done. The Service Report should be filed with the other maintenance paperwork for that analyzer. The hospital's accounting department and/or administration may ask for a copy to justify the work done, Service Rep's travel expenses, etc. In theory, you could be asked to produce the Service Report in an inspection to document that the analyzer is in good working order for patient testing.

Before the Service Rep leaves, I usually ask how much life the analyzer has left. The Service Rep should have at least a general idea of the condition of the analyzer and how much lifespan it has left before it becomes completely unrepairable. This will help to guide procurement decisions and can be used to justify the purchase of new analyzers.

If the analyzer turns out to be unrepairable, you will need to purchase a replacement. This is typically considered to be an emergency purchase given the urgency of the need. See chapter 7 on new analyzer acquisition.

Once while I was working at an underfunded, remote municipal hospital both CBC analyzers went down at the same time. One had its motherboard fried by an electric power surge, the other needed a part. The parts could be flown in within about 3 days. However, the Service Rep was in Singapore on a trouble call there and it would be at least 5 days before the Service Rep would arrive. There was a military hospital in that municipality, but it was a 45 minute drive to get there. This is how we handled the CBCs while the analyzers were down:

1. Any patient so critical as to be unable to wait the added 45 minutes drive time would get a spun crit. The tech would make a slide and do a microscopic platelet estimate, WBC estimate and manual differential. These would be called to the patient's Attending Physician as STAT results. The tube of blood was then sent out for the automated CBC.

2. Any patient that could wait the added 45 minute drive time had their tube of blood couriered over to the military hospital for a routine automated CBC.

The same underfunded, remote municipal hospital had ABG analyzer breakdowns. This hospital was doing its ABG's on Cobas analyzers. Both went down at the same time due to a reagent outage. This happened on a Saturday morning with the reagents in transit by air freight due to arrive Sunday night, about 36 hours later. This hospital lab borrowed an Abbot I-stat from the military hospital in the same municipality. This was done as an "emergency" borrow which would need the Admiral's approval when he arrived to work on Monday. The Admiral arrived to work Monday morning and disapproved of the military hospital's lending of the Abbot I-stat. By this time the reagents had arrived for the Cobas analyzers.

I must confess, this episode was the only instance in my career where a laboratory I headed was not able to follow CMS rules. The Cobas ABG analyzers went down in the hospital where I worked. There were 8 patients in ICU on ventilators. These patients needed ABG's at least daily and some as often as every 8 hours. Some or all of them could die if they didn't get ABG's. The only option is to borrow the Abbot I-stat from the military hospital to do the ABG testing. The testing was done without doing any of the necessary work described above for setting a new methodology into place (correlation, calibration, etc.). We could not do this after the fact, since the military hospital demanded the return of the Abbott I-stat analyzer the next working day.

The tech doing the testing manually entered the ABG test results into the hospital computer, and verified them as if they were done on the Cobas, when in fact they were not, they were done on a borrowed Abbot I-stat.

The CMS inspector did not catch this at the next inspection. This could have been caught in two ways. First, test results were generated on a day for which we had not done controls on the Cobas ABG analyzers. Second, results were present in the hospital computer that were not present in the Cobas analyzers. It would take a very astute inspector to notice this, and luckily the CMS inspector missed this at the next inspection. If the inspector had caught this, both the lab and I would have been in deep trouble.

I can tell these stories now that I am more or less retired. My experiences may have been unique. Most other Lab Directors work at better funded hospitals that are able to replace analyzers earlier in their lifespan, before they enter the phase of repeated breakdowns.

As a Lab Director, make sure that all the equipment in your lab is properly maintenanced according to the manufacturer's schedule and in good working order. Make sure all critical equipment is on an Uninterruptible Power Supply (UPS) and all the UPS's are tested as often as the manufacturer recommends. You do not want to find yourself in situations similar to those described above. At the time these events were gut-wrenching; and even now, many years later, they are an unpleasant memory.

Chapter 10 – How to read a linearity proficiency test report

I have discussed linearity a number of times in prior chapters. It is very similar to the Analytical Measurement Range (AMR). CLIA has requirements for AMR but is silent on linearity, so linearity tends to take a backseat to AMR.

Although CLIA has no requirement for linearity proficiency testing, most labs will test linearity twice a year. Linearity PT is particularly associated with chemistry analyzers but is also done in hematology. As a Lab Director you will need to know how to read a linearity proficiency testing event.

In this chapter I will give examples of failed linearity PT and how to remediate failures. Because CLIA is silent on linearity there is no regulatory requirement to correct failed linearity. You can continue testing an analyte in-house even if you repeatedly fail linearity testing. My advice is that failed linearity may indicate an underlying problem with the test, and you should make a good faith effort to determine what went wrong.

An example of a recent linearity PT event on an older analyzer is given on the next page. The data points used to measure linearly are also used to measure calibration verification, so the PT report will come back with both linearity and calibration verification on it.

EVALUATION ORIGINAL	Chemistry/Lipid/Enzyme Calibration Verification/Linearity

Executive Summary

Analyte	Calibration Verification	Linearity Evaluation	Page #
Albumin g/dL	Verified from 1.40 to 8.50	Linear from 1.40 to 8.50	2 - 3
Calcium mg/dL	Verified from 6.80 to 18.65	Linear from 6.80 to 18.65	4 - 5
Chloride mmol/L	Verified from 56.0 to 188.0	Linear from 56.0 to 188.0	6 - 7
CO2 mmol/L	***	Linear from 6.05 to 34.65	8
Creatinine mg/dL	Verified from 0.300 to 31.000	Linear from 0.300 to 31.000	9 - 10
Glucose mg/dL	Verified from 19.0 to 720.0	Linear from 19.0 to 720.0	11 - 12
Iron µg/dL	Verified from 12.5 to 850.0	Linear from 12.5 to 850.0	13 - 14
Magnesium mg/dL	Verified from 0.50 to 9.65	Linear from 0.50 to 9.65	15 - 16
Phosphorus mg/dL	Verified from 0.70 to 13.45	Linear from 0.70 to 13.45	17 - 18
Potassium mmol/L	Verified from 1.60 to 9.30	Linear from 1.60 to 9.30	19 - 20
Total Protein g/dL	Verified from 1.65 to 10.35	Linear from 1.65 to 10.35	21 - 22
Sodium mmol/L	* Verified from 91.5 to 173.0	Linear from 91.5 to 193.5	23 - 24
Urea Nitrogen (BUN) mg/dL	Verified from 2.0 to 183.0	Linear from 2.0 to 183.0	25 - 26
Uric Acid mg/dL	Verified from 0.90 to 24.35	Linear from 0.90 to 24.35	27 - 28
Direct Bilirubin mg/dL	Verified from 2.30 to 10.30	Linear from 2.30 to 10.30	29 - 30
Total Bilirubin mg/dL	Verified from 0.00 to 23.00	Linear from 0.00 to 23.00	31 - 32
Cholesterol mg/dL	Verified from 54.0 to 548.5	* Linear from 54.0 to 466.0	33 - 34
Triglyceride mg/dL	Verified from 20.0 to 622.0	Linear from 20.0 to 622.0	35 - 36
HDL Cholesterol mg/dL	**Different**	Linear from 5.0 to 29.0	37 - 38
ALT (SGPT) U/L	* Verified from 174.0 to 926.5	Linear from 23.5 to 926.5	39 - 40
Alkaline Phosphatase U/L	Verified from 49.0 to 1737.5	Linear from 49.0 to 1737.5	41 - 42
Amylase U/L	Verified from 25.0 to 758.0	Linear from 25.0 to 758.0	43 - 44
AST (SGOT) U/L	Verified from 11.0 to 938.5	Linear from 11.0 to 938.5	45 - 46
CK-2 (CK MB)-Mass ng/mL	Verified from 30.70 to 230.60	Linear from 30.70 to 230.60	47 - 48
Creatine Kinase U/L	Verified from 25.0 to 2119.0	Linear from 25.0 to 2119.0	49 - 50
GGT U/L	Verified from 19.0 to 1048.5	Linear from 19.0 to 1048.5	51 - 52
LD U/L	* Verified from 398.5 to 2083.0	Linear from 49.0 to 2083.0	53 - 54
Lipase U/L	Verified from 92.5 to 1358.5	Linear from 92.5 to 1358.5	55 - 56

Note: For results of Different, see the Calibration Verification Troubleshooting Guide and Investigation Checklist.

* This range does not include all reported specimens. Review your results to determine if excluded specimens reveal possible analytical problems.

*** No Peer Group

Reviewed by_____ Date_____

Notice that HDL cholesterol has failed calibration verification. On an older analyzer that is showing its age, it is not uncommon to fail calibration verification and/or linearity on one or more analyte. As mentioned in a prior chapter, if the instrument becomes non-linear for any analyte this could be an early warning sign that you are having problems with that particular test. The linearity tends to go out first, before the test goes out of control. As with all other problems, follow the corrective action procedure outlined in Chapter 5.

You are probably starting to notice by now that every time something goes wrong, I refer to the corrective action procedure, like a broken record playing the same note over and over. The fact of the matter is that the corrective action procedure is about the only thing you can do to correct a quality control failure on an analyzer. The only alternative would be to follow the analyzer breakdown procedure, but that procedure wouldn't be as applicable for failed linearity or other failed PT.

The carbon dioxide has three asterisks in the calibration verification field. At the bottom, the three asterisks indicates there is no peer group. No peer group means that no other lab is using the same particular combination of equipment and methodology you are using. In my experience, when you have no peer group it means you are the last lab using that equipment. In this circumstance your equipment is outdated and the manufacturer will likely soon stop supporting it forcing you to switch to a newer methodology (i.e. buy a new analyzer).

When there is no peer group, you have to look in the accompanying participant summary to see what the intended answers were. If you were acceptably close to the intended result, make a handwritten note to that effect on the evaluation report. If you were too far away from the intended result, make a corrective action. See page 32 for examples of how to handle ungraded PT.

Here is the sodium calibration verification:

EVALUATION ORIGINAL	Chemistry/Lipid/Enzyme Calibration Verification/Linearity Sodium mmol/L Calibration Verification Evaluation

Evaluation Result: Verified from 91.5 to 173.0

Peer Instrument: ▮▮▮▮▮▮▮▮▮▮
Peer Method: ▮▮▮▮▮▮▮▮▮

Allowable Error: 2.5% or 2 mmol/L, whichever is greater

Specimen	Assay 1	Assay 2	Your Mean	Peer Mean	Peer N	Difference	Allowable Error
LN-28	92	91	91.5	90.8	43	0.8%	± 2.5%
LN-29	111	111	111.0	110.1	43	0.8%	± 2.5%
LN-30	132	132	132.0	129.4	43	2.0%	± 2.5%
LN-31	152	152	152.0	149.1	43	1.9%	± 2.5%
LN-32	173	173	173.0	168.8	42	2.5%	± 2.5%
LN-33	194	193	193.5	186.9	41	3.5%	± 2.5%
LN-34	> 214	> 214		206.9	26		± 2.5%

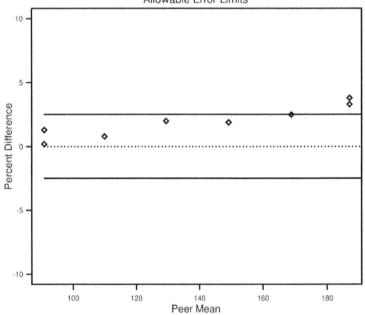

Calibration Verification Plot: Percent Differences with Allowable Error Limits

Peer Results Summary Table Your evaluation may not be included in the peer results. Peer Group Size: 43

	Calibration Verification		Linearity Evaluation		
Range	% Verified	% Different	% Linear	% Nonlinear	% Imprecise
LN-28 - 34	44.2	9.3	53.5	0.0	0.0
LN-28 - 33	32.6	4.7	37.2	0.0	4.7
LN-28 - 32	4.7	0.0	2.3	0.0	0.0
LN-28 - 31	4.7	0.0	2.3	0.0	0.0

The sodium passed the five lover levels, but failed the most extreme high levels, reporting greater than 214 mmol/L on a specimen that should have reported 206.9 mmol/L and reporting 193.5 mmol/L on a specimen that should have reported 186.9 mmol/L. As a result, the verified range for sodium is 91.5 to 173 mmol/L. That is not a big problem. The reference range for serum sodium levels is between 135 and 145 mmol/L. Anything above 155 mmol/L is a critical high.

We will assume that the linearity PT material does not exceed the AMR of the analyzer. It wouldn't make sense for the linearity PT material to be outside the AMR of the analyzer. If it exceeded the AMR it would have to be diluted to be run on the analyzer. This would complicate things unnecessarily such that it isn't generally done for this type of PT.

Making the assumption the linearity PT material does not exceed the AMR of the analyzer, a corrective action might get this test back to being able to read extremely elevated serum sodium levels. Most people won't bother with a corrective action for this since it is not necessary to measure serum sodium at a concentration that is not compatible with life. However, failed calibration verification can be an early warning sign of problems with a test, so I will do corrective action for this type of PT failure.

After you do the corrective action repeat the test for any linearity PT specimen that failed if any of that specimen remains. If the repeat results are now in the expected range, you have just verified calibration for the entire AMR for that analyte. You can keep the same AMR as before, in this situation the AMR does not need to be adjusted.

Let's say we do the corrective action, but still fail on the sodium levels of 186.9 and 206.9 mmol/L. This means the range of calibration verification is 91.5 to 173 mmol/L. CLIA requires that all clinical labs perform calibration verification, but does not set minimum criteria for passing. You as Lab Director can decide if you want to reduce your AMR accordingly. At labs I helm, we try to keep the AMR within the linearity and calibration verification range of the analyte. Given the outcome of the above calibration verification, any sodium level above 173 mmol/L we report as "greater than 173 mmol/L" or dilute and repeat. If a living person really did have a serum sodium above 173 mmol/L, we could dilute the specimen, repeat the test and measure the sodium. Alternatively, we could report it as a "greater than 173 mmol/L" panic value. Either way, this is a critically high sodium level.

In this example, I would recommend that if you plan to dilute and repeat any patient specimen with a sodium above 173 mmol/L you should first dilute and repeat the linearity PT material and obtain results within the acceptable range of the linearity PT material. If you dilute and repeat the linearity PT material and the results are still outside the expected range, you should not dilute and repeat patient specimens. You should instead report patient sodium results as "greater than 173 mmol/L"

Here is the sodium linearity from the same PT event:

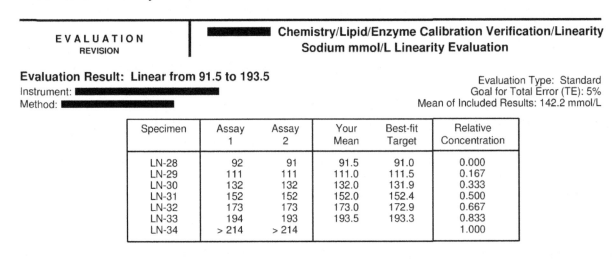

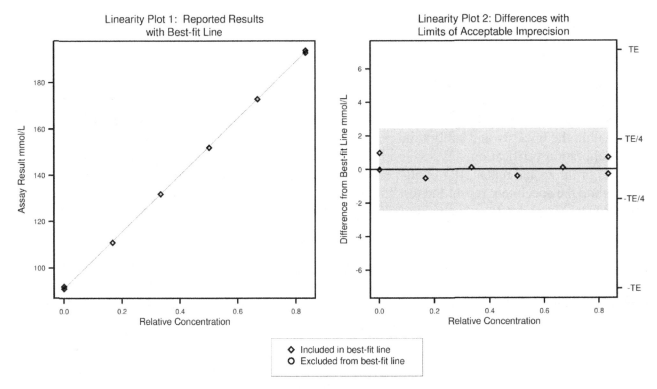

This is an example of what a linearity graph should look like. Every data point is within the allowable error limits, and all data points are very close to a straight line. The sodium did better on the linearity compared to the calibration verification graph given on page 69. In this situation the sodium testing is probably not having problems in its upper ranges. If there was a problem with the testing, both the linearity and the calibration verification should fail.

In the above linearity evaluation, the shaded area in plot 2 is quite narrow, typically within 1 SD. The allowable error when running a control is typically 3SD. Hence, linearity is more sensitive at picking up problems with a test. Linearity also has more "false alarms" of data points falling outside the shaded area by random chance. Hence, an outlier on plot 2 above is not likely to be significant. The sodium linearity above has no outliers, hence I am suspicious that the problems with the sodium calibration verification discussed on pages 69 and 70 are a "false alarm".

Next let's take a look at how we did on the cholesterol calibration verification:

EVALUATION ORIGINAL	Chemistry/Lipid/Enzyme Calibration Verification/Linearity Cholesterol mg/dL Calibration Verification Evaluation

Evaluation Result: Verified from 54.0 to 548.5
Peer Instrument:
Peer Method:

Allowable Error: 4.5% or 3 mg/dL, whichever is greater

Specimen	Assay 1	Assay 2	Your Mean	Peer Mean	Peer N	Difference	Allowable Error
LN-41	< 29	< 29		29.2	76		± 3.0 mg/dL
LN-42	54	54	54.0	54.9	156	-0.9 mg/dL	± 3.0 mg/dL
LN-43	142	142	142.0	143.2	156	-0.8%	± 4.5%
LN-44	258	259	258.5	258.1	156	0.2%	± 4.5%
LN-45	363	363	363.0	362.3	156	0.2%	± 4.5%
LN-46	467	465	466.0	467.3	156	-0.3%	± 4.5%
LN-47	549	548	548.5	549.1	155	-0.1%	± 4.5%

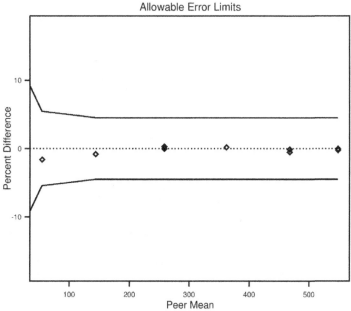

Calibration Verification Plot: Percent Differences with Allowable Error Limits

Peer Results Summary Table — Your evaluation may not be included in the peer results. — Peer Group Size: 156

Range	Calibration Verification		Linearity Evaluation		
	% Verified	% Different	% Linear	% Nonlinear	% Imprecise
LN-41 - 47	21.8	17.9	12.2	0.0	0.0
LN-41 - 46	3.8	0.0	32.7	0.0	0.0
LN-42 - 47	30.1	5.1	14.7	0.0	0.0
LN-41 - 45	1.3	0.0	1.3	0.0	1.3
LN-42 - 46	6.4	0.0	35.3	0.0	0.0
LN-43 - 47	8.3	0.0	0.0	0.0	0.0
LN-41 - 44	1.9	0.0	1.3	0.0	0.0
LN-42 - 45	0.6	0.0	1.3	0.0	0.0
LN-43 - 46	2.6	0.0	0.0	0.0	0.0

This is an example of what a calibration verification graph should look like. Every data point is within the allowable error limits, and most data points are very close to the mean. For LN-47 our mean is 548.5 mg/dL and the peer mean (i.e. everybody else in the world testing the same PT material using the same instrument and methodology) got an average of 549.1 mg/dL. We are off by about 0.1%. As far as I am concerned, we hit the bullseye. The next chart shows the cholesterol linearity.

| EVALUATION | Chemistry/Lipid/Enzyme Calibration Verification/Linearity |
| ORIGINAL | Cholesterol mg/dL Linearity Evaluation |

Evaluation Result: Linear from 54.0 to 466.0
Instrument:
Method:

Evaluation Type: Standard
Goal for Total Error (TE): 9%
Mean of Included Results: 256.7 mg/dL

Specimen	Assay 1	Assay 2	Your Mean	Best-fit Target	Relative Concentration
LN-41	< 29	< 29			0.000
LN-42	54	54	54.0	58.9	0.050
LN-43	142	142	142.0	141.3	0.200
LN-44	258	259	258.5	251.2	0.400
LN-45	363	363	363.0	361.1	0.600
LN-46	467	465	466.0	470.9	0.800
LN-47	549	548	548.5	580.8	1.000

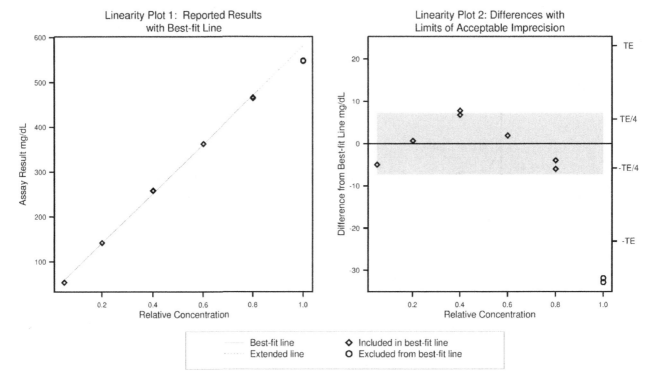

Your plot has one or more points within your linear range that fall outside of the shaded area. Since your evaluation is Linear, no remedial action is necessary.

Points can fall outside of the shaded area for two reasons:
1) an average is used to estimate imprecision, so many small differences can offset a few large differences, and
2) clinically insignificant nonlinearity (curved fit) can contribute to differences between your results and the best-fit straight line. Larger differences may be an early warning sign of nonlinearity, poor repeatability, or poor fit.

The cholesterol linearity graph falls away from a straight line for LN-47, the extreme high cholesterol. Our result is 548.5 mg/dL however the best fit target is 580.8 mg/dL cholesterol. As far as I am concerned, we hit the bullseye with an average almost exactly the same as every other lab using the same equipment and method.

The manufacturer of the PT material thinks they spiked enough cholesterol into LN-47 that it should report 580.8 mg/dL cholesterol. However, every lab in existence using the same analyzer and method we are using reports 549 mg/dL cholesterol. I am suspicious that the problem is with the manufacturer of the PT material, and not with every analyzer in the world.

Let's give the benefit of the doubt to the PT maker. Every lab in the world using the same analyzer and same method we are using got the wrong result. Most chemistry tests are enzymatic or immunoassays, and at extreme high concentrations of the analyte most of the enzymes or antibodies used for testing are already saturated with analyte. In this range a +1 increase in the "true" analyte concentration may result in a less than +1 increase in the test result. Thus our linearity for cholesterol really is from 54.0 to 466.0 mg/dL.

This implies that the PT maker really did send us a PT specimen which exceeded the AMR of our analyzer. Since our results are almost identical to all other labs using the same analyzer, it further implies that the PT material exceeded the AMR of all similar analyzers in the world, with all the attendant problems that creates. Every other lab in the world will have to reduce its AMR or else dilute and repeat the linearity PT specimen to try to obtain acceptable results for this PT event. The PT maker should have known better.

Although our analyzer is not linear at 549 mg/dL, our results are almost exactly the same as every other lab in the world using the same analyzer and method. The results are reproducible, both runs gave very close numbers. I would feel comfortable turning out cholesterol test results up to 549 mg/dL on this analyzer, since it is accurate, precise and reproducible. However, the CMS inspectors would likely object that the linearity of the analyzer has been exceeded, so I do not do this. Instead the AMR for cholesterol is set from 54.0 to 466.0 mg/dL.

Similar to the sodium testing discussed above, the cholesterol testing is in the same situation of reduced AMR upper limit. It is possible to dilute and rerun any specimen with a cholesterol over 466.0 mg/dL. The difference between 466 mg/dL and 549 mg/dL cholesterol is probably not that significant anyhow; they are both critically high values. The AMR of the test is set at the limits of linearity determined by this PT event from 54.0 to 466.0 mg/dL.

In this circumstance, doing a corrective action would likely be a futile maneuver. We have already hit the bullseye, reporting results within about 0.1% of every other lab in the world using the same analyzer and method. You really can't improve on this. Hence, a corrective action should not be able to accomplish anything.

Here is the calibration verification for HDL cholesterol.

EVALUATION ORIGINAL | Chemistry/Lipid/Enzyme Calibration Verification/Linearity
HDL Cholesterol mg/dL Calibration Verification Evaluation

Evaluation Result: Different

Your Instrument:
Your Method:
Peer Instrument:

Allowable Error: 10% or 2 mg/dL, whichever is greater

Specimen	Assay 1	Assay 2	Your Mean	Peer Mean	Peer N	Difference	Allowable Error
LN-41	< 4	< 4		4.2	128		± 2.0 mg/dL
LN-42	5	5	5.0	6.6	154	-1.6 mg/dL	± 2.0 mg/dL
LN-43	11	11	11.0	13.3	160	-2.3 mg/dL	± 2.0 mg/dL
LN-44	17	16	16.5	20.6	160	-19.9%	± 10.0%
LN-45	21	22	21.5	26.3	160	-18.3%	± 10.0%
LN-46	25	24	24.5	31.8	160	-23.0%	± 10.0%
LN-47	29	29	29.0	35.7	160	-18.8%	± 10.0%

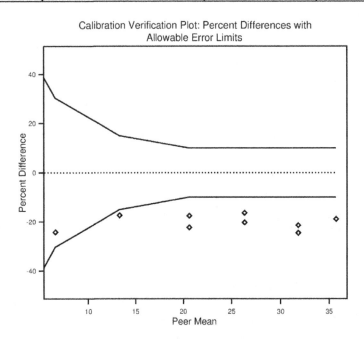

Calibration Verification Plot: Percent Differences with Allowable Error Limits

Peer Results Summary Table   Your evaluation may not be included in the peer results.   Peer Group Size: 160

Range	Calibration Verification		Linearity Evaluation		
	% Verified	% Different	% Linear	% Nonlinear	% Imprecise
LN-41 - 47	41.9	18.1	15.6	0.6	1.3
LN-41 - 46	5.6	0.0	31.9	0.0	0.0
LN-42 - 47	5.6	5.6	13.1	0.6	0.6
LN-41 - 45	6.3	0.0	18.8	0.0	0.0
LN-42 - 46	0.6	0.0	1.3	0.0	0.0
LN-43 - 47	5.0	1.9	3.8	0.0	0.0
LN-41 - 44	8.1	0.0	11.9	0.0	0.0
LN-42 - 45	0.6	0.0	0.6	0.0	0.0
LN-43 - 46	0.6	0.0	0.0	0.0	0.0

The HDL cholesterol calibration verification is quite a disaster. Every result has a huge negative bias. As with linearity, CLIA does not set minimum performance criteria for calibration verification. You as Lab Director could accept such a bad calibration verification if you wanted to. My advice is that you should make a corrective action for any analyte with a calibration verification evaluated as "different" from the expected. As with all corrective actions, be careful to look through the recent controls to make sure this test really is in control. Given how badly it failed calibration verification, it is surprising that the controls were in.

The corrective action was carried out for the HDL cholesterol calibration verification on the prior page. There was no problem with the testing; the problem was that a wrong method code had been filled in on the form returned to the proficiency testing provider. This one small mistake in filling out the form caused our HDL cholesterol results to be measured against the results generated by a different methodology on a different analyzer. In other words, the calibration verification shown above is comparing apples to oranges; our results using our method are not directly comparable to the results generated by a different method or analyzer.

One has to pay attention to the smallest details. The smallest mistake in filling out the proficiency testing form caused us to badly fail HDL cholesterol calibration verification. In this case, we informed the proficiency testing provider of our mistake, asked them to re-grade the HDL cholesterol, and send us a new proficiency testing evaluation, so as to have a passing calibration verification in the file to show the inspector.

Here is a disastrously bad linearity. It is from a different PT event than the above graphs:

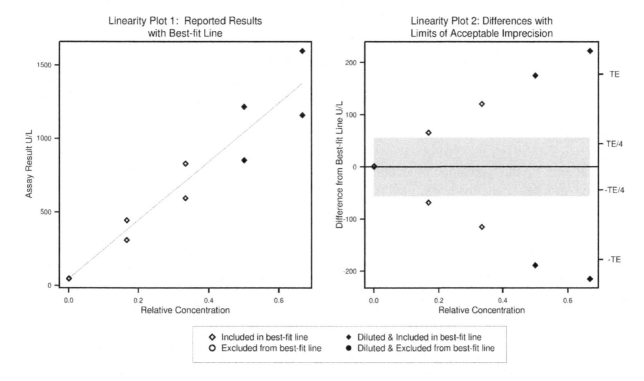

The corrective action was carried out for this alkaline phosphatase linearity. The second set of data points were amylase results incorrectly transcribed in place of the alkaline phosphatase results. In other words, all data in the column "Assay 2" represent data points for the amylase linearity, not alkaline phosphatase. Hence, the huge deviation of the two runs, which progressively widens with higher values.

After replacing the incorrect data points with the correct ones, the test is now showing a high bias that worsens from the low end of the assay range to the high end. The test was in control at the time of this linearity PT event. There were no problems with calibration, proficiency testing, etc. The high bias was not present on repeat testing of the same specimens. The source of the high bias on this linearity was never identified. It was ascribed to "inexplicable, random error".

After the two different types of data entry error shown above, I put in a rule that for all external PT events, a second person must verify that there are no transcription errors, incorrect method codes, etc. in the data entered. This must be done before the results can be reported to the PT provider.

Chapter 11 – How to write a policy and/or procedure

A policy is a statement of intent. It is usually dogmatic, broad and vague, stated in very general terms. For example: "The Lab will uphold quality patient testing". "The Lab will not tolerate unacceptable practices".

A procedure is a written document used to implement policy. It usually lists step by step instructions on how to do things, similar to a cookbook. For example: "add reagents and 2ml patient serum to the test tube. Mix gently then centrifuge at 1000 RPM for 5 minutes". Deviations from the lab's procedures can only occur under extreme circumstances, and usually require permission from the Lab Director or other authority.

A memorandum is a written document containing information usually of a temporary nature. For example: "Lab has run out of reagents for the CRP test. Please store all specimens for CRP testing in the refrigerator until the reagents arrive. The reagents are expected to arrive tomorrow". If a memorandum produces a permanent change, this change must be incorporated into the relevant policies and procedures.

The "procedures" in the typical lab procedure manual are really a mix of both policy and procedure. When I say "procedure" in this book, I am referring to the written documentation in the typical lab manual. Everyone refers to this as "procedure" even though it really is a mix of both policy and procedure.

The original copy of a lab procedure is referred to as the "controlled copy". Access to the controlled copy of the lab's procedures is strictly limited. Usually only the Lab Director, Lab Supervisor, Lab Secretary and possibly the section supervisors are allowed access to the controlled copy. No one else is allowed access to the controlled copy.

The controlled copy is usually stored electronically on the Lab Secretary's computer. The Lab Secretary's computer is usually password protected with the Lab Secretary's office locked at night. The Lab Secretary will have to retype all changed procedures once every 2 years in the run-up to the CMS or CAP inspection, so it makes sense that the original copy of the procedures should be kept on his or her computer.

The Lab Secretary is usually given an unofficial designation as "manual guardian", "procedure protector", etc. It is his or her responsibility to maintain the integrity of the procedure manuals. Be sure to emphasize how important this is and not to allow any unauthorized individuals access to the procedure manuals, secretary's computer, etc.

There is usually a numbering system for the procedures with each procedure given a unique number. The Lab Secretary should maintain a master list of the procedures including the effective date of each procedure.

One often overlooked point is backing up the procedures. I have seen one hard drive crash wipe out hundreds of pages of procedure manual. It is imperative that you make backups at least monthly. I prefer optical media such as CD-R and DVD-R, however others prefer thumb drives, etc. The procedure manuals are thousands of pages; however, text documents are quite compact in terms of computer bytes. The entirety of the lab's procedure manuals should fit on one DVD-R or thumb drive.

The Lab Secretary's computer is not accessible to the lab techs but CLIA requires that the testing personnel have access to the procedures in the testing area. Usually this is accomplished by making a hardcopy printout of the procedures and putting them in multiple 3 ring binders in each section of lab.

This is less commonly done by having copies available on the computers in the work area of lab. If you are going to keep the procedures "paperless" you have to be very careful that all techs are able to access the procedures in the testing area. If the CMS inspectors see that your procedures are "paperless" they are bound to ask several techs to look up several procedures. If even one lab tech can't find one procedure your lab will be cited. This is a favorite citation of the CMS inspectors. Hence, in my experience, you are better off with multiple 3 ring binders.

The reviewing and updating of each lab section's procedures is typically the responsibility of the section supervisor. The Chemistry supervisor has the most knowledge of Chemistry procedures compared to anyone else in lab. The Blood Bank supervisor has the most knowledge of Blood Bank procedures compared to anyone else in lab, etc. It makes sense that they should oversee the work on the procedures for their areas. The general lab procedures are reviewed and updated by the Lab Supervisor.

After being downloaded, written or changed by the section supervisor, the procedure may or may not be signed off by the Lab Supervisor and is always signed by the Lab Director. Both CMS and CAP require that the Lab Director approve of any new or changed procedure in lab. CAP requires the Lab Director to sign all procedures once every 2 years, but CMS does not require this biennial review.

Lab procedures are usually written in simple easy to understand language that tells the tech how to do the testing in a one step at a time, cookbook manner. The procedure has to be understood by the least intelligent tech in lab, so the language tends to be simple and clear. The procedure has to reflect what you are doing in real life and what you are doing in real life has to be documented in the procedure.

If the way your lab does things changes, even a little, you have to change the procedure in the manual. The change is typically written into the hardcopy printout of the procedure present in the work area. It must be signed and dated by the Lab Director in order to be valid.

For example, a citation on one of my recent CMS inspections involved the procedure for urinalysis. The vendor supplying lab had switched dipsticks from one manufacturer to another. The testing was the same, the interpretation was the same, but the name of the manufacturer switched. My lab had the name of the old manufacturer written into the procedure manual. The inspector caught this and cited us.

Once every 2 years in the run-up to the CMS or CAP inspection, the procedure manuals are brought one at a time into the Lab Secretary's Office. Any written changes are typed into the original copy of the procedure on the Lab Secretary's computer. The re-typed procedures are then printed out, signed by the Lab Director and put in the procedure manuals in place of the procedures with handwritten changes. When the work on each procedure manual is completed it is returned where it came from and the next manual is brought to the Lab Secretary's Office. This continues until the work on all procedure manuals has been completed.

Depending on how many procedures have changed, this could be a huge amount of work on the part of the Lab Secretary. Make sure to give the Lab Secretary something of value (overtime, comp time, etc.) in exchange. As mentioned previously, a peace offering given in appeasement is known as a "sop".

As Lab Director, you want all testing to meet regulatory requirements. The techs would prefer the easiest procedure possible. If the lab is adding a new test or modifying an existing test, you will likely be making more work for the lab techs. As Lab Director you may have to do some negotiation with the lab techs who will be doing the testing. It is best to offer them something of value (overtime, comp time, etc.) in exchange. This is yet another example of a sop.

Once the procedure has been signed by the Lab Director it goes in the procedure manual. You have to make sure that all the lab techs are aware of the new or changed procedure. This usually entails calling all the lab techs into one room at the same time and informing them of the new or changed procedure. It is best to buy pizza or otherwise serve food at this meeting. The lab techs may be very unhappy that you are making more work for them.

CLIA mandates that a procedure is needed for every test offered in lab. The lab also needs to have procedures for calibration, verification of calibration, running controls, corrective action to take when controls are out, a description of the course of action to take if a test system becomes inoperable, quality assurance, etc.

The procedure for each test should include requirements for patient preparation; specimen collection and processing, criteria for specimen acceptability and rejection, instructions for step-by-step performance of the procedure, interpretation of results, preparation of all materials used in testing, the reportable range for test results, limitations in the test methodology including interfering substances, reference intervals (normal values), critical results (panic values) and the laboratory's system for entering results in the patient record and reporting patient results. The reference for this is 42 CFR § 493.1251.

CLIA is silent on Safety Data Sheets (SDS) but the Occupational Safety and Health Administration (OSHA) regulations require that for all toxic substances used in the workplace, the SDS has to be readily available in the workplace. SDS are quick reference guides for chemical hazards with information on spill control measures, health hazards, PPE required for safe handling, etc. This requirement is typically met by having each section of lab store a 3 ring binder with all the relevant SDS sheets in the same cabinet as that section's procedure manuals. The older term for these guides, Material Safety Data Sheets (MSDS), is currently considered obsolete.

The SDS are typically separated into their own 3 ring binders, and not mixed in with the procedures. Make sure your lab has one SDS for each toxic substance used in the workplace. If you use bleach for cleaning, you need to have an SDS for sodium hypochlorite present in the SDS binders. At present some analyzer manufacturers are making SDS sheets for their cartridges and test kits. Make sure that for every analyzer you are using all relevant SDS are present in the SDS binder. Neither OSHA nor CLIA require the Lab Director to sign the SDS sheets. I have never signed an SDS binder nor have I ever been asked to.

In the typical hospital lab the procedure manuals can run into thousands of pages. Typing that amount of documentation would take an eternity and would be impractical. Most labs get their procedure manuals from the test manufacturer or download the procedures from the internet. Another source for procedures is nearby hospital labs using the same equipment.

As a Lab Director, you will not be writing procedures, but will be reviewing them for accuracy. Things to check are:

1. Oversights and skipped steps are a common problem. Is the procedure complete? Does one step lead to the next, or is something missing in between?
2. Is it easy to understand? Is the least intelligent tech in lab going to have a hard time reading and understanding it?
3. Could a lab tech new to this workplace read the procedure, and do the test without supervision and without asking for help?
4. Does the written procedure reflect what is being done in real life? If a specific manufacturer is named, are we still using that manufacturer?
5. Does it accurately convey the manufacturer's instructions and lab best practices?
6. Has anything changed since the time the procedure was written?
7. Make sure the procedure includes the CLIA required components as applicable: requirements for patient preparation; specimen collection and processing, criteria for specimen acceptability and rejection, instructions for step-by-step performance of the procedure, interpretation of results, preparation of all materials used in testing, the reportable range for test results, limitations in the test methodology including interfering substances, reference intervals (normal values), critical results (panic values) and the laboratory's system for entering results in the patient record and reporting patient results.

If you are not satisfied with the procedure, you can change it as you see fit. Keep in mind that the techs will have to follow the procedure exactly. Try not to put anything onerous in the procedure.

The Blood Bank Emergency Release of Blood procedure is given on pages 81 to 83 as an example of a procedure.

For each procedure, the date of creation and each date of modification is typed into the procedure. After a procedure is no longer needed, it is retired to the retired procedure folder. The retirement date is logged in the retired procedure logbook. CLIA mandates that retired procedures should be kept at least two years. The reference is 42 CFR § 493.1105.

In my experience the retention of retired procedures is indefinite. They tend to sit forever in a filing cabinet in the office area, never to be disposed of, unless there is a desperate need for space in the filing cabinet.

MY LAB
BLOOD BANK PROCEDURE MANUAL

CATEGORY: **OPERATIONS/MANAGEMENT**	CODE: **3144**
SUBJECT: **Emergency Release of Blood**	EFFECTIVE: **12/20/2013**
RESPONSIBLE DEPARTMENT/DESIGNEE: **BLOOD BANK**	PAGE: 1 of 3

POLICY: Experienced personnel are available in the Blood Bank on a 24-hour basis to assist with the provision of blood and blood components during emergencies. Only Blood Bank employees are allowed access to the blood inventory, or are permitted to issue blood for transfusion.

Procedure to request blood during an emergency:

1. Call Blood Bank at XXXX.

2. Describe the urgency of the situation. "The ER/OR/ICU has a patient with an emergency need for transfusion".

3. Provide the patient's name and medical record number. For multiple patients with unknown names, see the Mass Casualty Disaster procedure.

4. Indicate the blood component and amount required. Indicate how quickly it is needed - immediate, 10 minutes, 45 minutes, etc.

5. Provide the number and name of the ordering physician.

6. Indicate the location of the patient.

7. Blood Bank will read back orders and patient identifiers to assure accuracy.

The Blood Bank will check if it already has crossmatched blood for the patient. If crossmatched blood is not currently available, the Blood Bank can then determine the extent to which compatibility testing can be performed. As the amount of compatibility testing decreases, the possible risk of transfusing incompatible blood increases. Depending on the availability of a specimen and current status of testing blood may be released as:

1. **Uncrossmatched red blood cells:**
   - Available immediately
   - Should only be requested in situations where the transfusion cannot wait 10 minutes for patient typing.
   - Type O-negative blood is the universal donor blood. It is rare and hard to obtain. It should only be used in life-or-death emergencies.

2. **Type specific blood:**
   - Available after typing the patient (10 minutes required for typing).
   - Should be used in situations where transfusion can wait 10 minutes but cannot wait about 45 minutes

3. **Full crossmatch blood:**
   - The full crossmatch requires about 45 minutes to complete.
   - A fully crossmatched unit has the least risk of causing a transfusion reaction.

4. **Least Incompatible blood:**
   - In a patient with an unexpected antibody, it may not be possible to obtain a crossmatch negative unit.
   - This type of transfusion comes with significant risks of a transfusion reaction. It should only be given if the benefits outweigh the risks.
   - The patient should be informed of the risks of this type of transfusion, and should sign an informed consent form.

Release of Blood:

1. The nurse or other authorized person will come to Blood Bank.

2. The release of blood will follow the same procedure as described in the Issue and Release of Blood and Blood Components procedure.

3. For uncrossmatched blood, the crossmatch will be completed after the transfusion. The patient's Attending Physician will be notified promptly if the crossmatch is found to be positive.

4. For least incompatible units, the antibody identification and donor unit typing will be completed after the transfusion. The patient's Attending Physician will be notified promptly of the results.

REVIEWED AND APPROVED BY:

_____   _____
Blood Bank Supervisor   Date

_____   _____
Lab Supervisor   Date

_____   _____
Lab Director   Date

Reviewed Last
(Date and Initial)

_____
_____
_____

CLIA is silent on retention when a procedure is changed, for example a change of reference range, but not completely discontinued. In this situation, my advice is to keep a copy of the unmodified procedure for at least 2 years from the date of modification. This copy should be clearly marked as an old, superseded procedure to avoid confusion with the current procedure. At a subsequent inspection, the inspector may review old records and notice you were doing things differently than the current procedure. In this circumstance you must be able to produce the old, superseded procedure and document the date of modification in order to prove that you really were following the correct procedure in place at the time.

Chapter 12 – Quality Assurance, complaints, incident reports and root cause analysis

Quality Control (QC) is typically done daily to ensure the quality of lab testing and is typically limited to the testing process (i.e. testing of controls). Quality Assurance (QA) looks at broader time frames and looks at processes that occur before, during and after testing. CLIA requires that all labs have both a QC and a QA program. The daily QC requirements have already been discussed in prior chapters.

In most larger labs there is a QA coordinator who takes care of all the QA work. I have spent most of my career working in small labs in remote areas which do not have a QA coordinator. In the absence of a QA coordinator, the work falls on the Lab Supervisor and the Lab Director.

The usual list of QA indicators to measure include:

1. Greater than 90% of STAT tests turned around within 1 hour
2. 100% of tests marked "Routine" turned around (or canceled) within one day (24 hours) of ordering.
3. 100% of tested specimens properly labeled as to patient name, identification, etc. All unidentified specimens rejected by lab and not tested. All specimens with illegible and/or incomplete test requisitions rejected by lab and not tested.
4. Corrected (modified) test results
5. 100% of specimens are acceptable (all lipemic and/or hemolyzed specimens rejected if lipemia and/or hemolysis would affect test results).
6. 100% of critical values (panic values) called to the provider in the time allowed (typically one hour).
7. Complaints and/or incident reports involving Lab.
8. Inpatient AM lab draw turnaround time (goal is more than 95% reported by 9AM).
9. Phlebotomist hand hygiene (handwashing or use of alcohol based hand rub) between patient contacts (goal is 100% compliance). This should only be on lab's list of monthly quality assurance indicators to review if it is not already part of the hospital-wide infection control quality assurance program.
10. Culture contamination rate (i.e. percent of blood, urine or other cultures contaminated with extraneous organisms)
11. Crossmatch:transfusion ratio
12. Specimen rejection rate less than 5% (i.e. more than 95% of specimens are acceptable)
13. Expiration rate of red blood cell units (goal is less than 1% expiration rate).
14. Customer satisfaction surveys.
15. Lab analyzer downtime, tests unavailable and/or outages of reagents, supplies, etc.
16. Appropriateness of test orders (e.g. daily CBC's ordered on a patient with normal hematologic parameters and no known hematologic disease).

CLIA is silent on what exactly your QA program has to measure. In theory, you could pick only one QA indicator from the above list, measure it, and you would have a QA program. In reality, most labs pick about 5 of the above 16 QA indicators. If you pick the entire list, you are going to be working very hard. You are not limited to this list. You can measure anything you want to in lab and call it QA.

Although CLIA is silent on what a lab's QA program must measure, CMS places requirements on the hospital as a whole. These state that the hospital must develop, implement, and maintain an effective, ongoing, hospital-wide, data-driven quality assessment and performance improvement program. There must be an ongoing program that shows measurable improvement in indicators for which there is evidence that it will improve health outcomes and identify and reduce medical errors. The hospital must set priorities for its performance improvement activities that focus on high-risk, high-volume, or problem-prone areas. The reference is 42 CFR § 482.21.

Thus, if you are in a hospital lab the hospital-wide QA program may mandate the QA indicators for you to measure. If you are in an outpatient lab there is no specific requirement on what your QA program should measure. You should pick QA indicators that relate to problems your lab has, or had in the past, or could potentially develop. If you are in an outpatient lab without a Blood Bank it is pointless to try to measure crossmatch:transfusion ratio as one of your QA indicators. If you tried doing this you would end up dividing zero crossmatches by zero transfusions every month.

You need to set criteria, usually expressed in terms of percent or ratio, that is considered passing for each of these QA indicators. You should document the significance of the indicator and why the indicator was chosen to be studied. In other words, what is the impact on patient care of passing or failing this QA indicator. If you know at the start that you are not passing for that QA indicator, you should set a goal or target with an explanation of what you are trying to achieve and why.

For patient safety indicators, only 0% is acceptable (i.e. no patient falls in lab). For other QA indicators the CMS has no set criteria. The suggestion is that your QA numbers should be comparable to similar hospitals elsewhere. In other words, you can ask similar sized hospital labs in the region what their QA indicators are and what they consider to be passing. The goals should be realistic and attainable. My advice is to only set 100% as the goal if the indicator is life-or-death for the patient.

The method of data collection (observation, retrospective review of lab records, etc.) and the frequency (typically monthly) must be specified. If any QA indicator is found to be in the unacceptable range you must devise and implement a plan to intervene. You then measure the success of the intervention. If the intervention is successful the QA indicator goes from active management to assessing if success is sustained. If the intervention is unsuccessful, new interventions must be devised and implemented. This cycle of devising plans, intervening and measuring the outcome must continue until the problem is resolved and the QA indicator returns to the acceptable range. Then the active intervention stops but the QA indicator should continue to be measured indefinitely. I will give examples of this process below.

Laboratory testing can be divided into three analytical phases. The preanalytic phase is everything that occurs before the testing – identifying the patient by wristband, putting the correct patient's bar-code label on the tubes, etc. The analytic phase is the testing. The postanalytic phase occurs after the test – reporting the correct patient's test results in a timely manner to the correct provider, etc. The sum of all three phases is known as the Total Testing Process (TTP). The QA plan should be set up to measure preanalytic, analytic, and postanalytic quality.

I like to measure test turnaround time, calling of critical values, crossmatch:transfusion ratio, blood culture contamination rate, and complaints received. Generally the collection and evaluation of the data is done monthly.

CLIA requires that all complaints and problems reported to the lab are documented and investigated with corrective actions implemented as needed. The reference is 42 CFR § 493.1233. This does not specifically require that complaints and incident reports should be handled as part of the monthly QA. However, at most hospital labs, complaints and incident reports are on the list of monthly QA indicators to review in addition to the immediate work done at the time the complaint or incident report is received. I will go into greater detail about complaints and incident reports later in this chapter.

For some QA indicators it is not likely that any lab will ever achieve perfection. For example no lab will ever maintain 0% blood culture contamination rates for long. In this circumstance, you are looking for improvement over time, or at least maintaining the rate in an acceptable range (preferably less than 3% and definitely less than 5% blood culture contamination rate).

If any QA indicator is in the acceptable range, but is slowly deteriorating within the acceptable range, it is best to be proactive. Take action before the numbers deteriorate into the unacceptable range.

Most hospitals have a monthly, quarterly, and annual QA form to fill out. One form is used for each QA indicator for each time period under evaluation (monthly, quarterly or annual). Lab typically uses the hospital-wide forms and does not have its own separate forms for QA. An example of a monthly QA form is given on page 87.

Let's say that you calculate the blood culture contamination rate for the last month and find that it is 6%. This is in the unacceptable range. The data is presented at the relevant committee meetings (Infection Control Committee, Quality Management Committee, etc.).

The corrective actions to take include educating the phlebotomists who draw the blood cultures on aseptic technique for drawing. Have the most senior phlebotomist or the Lab Supervisor watch the more junior phlebotomists to make sure they really are swabbing the alcohol or iodine for 30 seconds and allowing it to air dry. The 30 seconds and air dry rules tend to be shortcut, as the phlebotomists are usually in a hurry. The information (high blood culture contamination rate, 30 seconds and air dry rules, etc.) is typically presented to all lab staff at a lab-wide meeting. The signed attendance sheet from the lab-wide meeting is kept as evidence of corrective action.

The Lab cannot carry out corrective actions on the nurses without the approval of the nursing administration. If the nurses draw blood cultures, the Lab should inform the Director of Nursing that there is a problem, and ask him or her to address the issue. Usually, the information (high blood culture contamination rate, how to draw a blood culture, etc.) is passed down from the Director of Nursing, to the departmental nursing heads to the individual nurses. Alternatively, the nurses can have one big educational meeting where this information is presented to everybody at once, usually with the infection control nurse present at this meeting as well. Keep a copy of the meeting minutes as evidence of corrective action.

Monthly Quality Assessment and Performance Indicator Monitoring Report
Please use one form per indicator being studied

Month of: _____ **Department:** _____ Laboratory

Study Start Date: _____ Study End Date: _____
(Note dates that data monitoring/collection started and ended for given month)

Quality Indicator being studied: _____

Significance of Quality Indicator: _____

Goal/AIM of Quality Indicator: _____

Does this indicator focus on one or more of the following areas: please check all that apply

☐ High Risk ☐ High Volume ☐ Problem Prone Areas

☐ Other: Please Describe: _____

<u>Data Statistics</u>: Attach data collection method for month with report.

Target Goal: _____ %

Total met (numerator): _____

Total sample size (denominator): _____

% of target actually met in a given period: _____ % $\left\{ \dfrac{Total\ met}{Total\ sample\ size} \times 100\% \right\}$

Monthly Data Comparison (Please note previous month[s] % of target actually met):

1st Month % of target met	2nd Month % of target met	3rd Month % of target met	Quarter Average of target met {1st month + 2nd month + 3rd month % of threshold met} ÷ 3 months x 100%	Comments/Action Taken:

Quality and Performance Management Services Comments/Recommendations:

Monthly Quality and Performance Indicator Monitoring report is to be submitted to the Quality and Performance Management Services Department by the 7th of the month.

Handwritten reports are acceptable but must be in ink & legible. Illegible copies will be returned to the department for correction.

Submitted by: _____ Date: _____
Department Supervisor/Manager

Continue doing this and check how the next month's blood culture contamination rate comes out. If it is improved, and in the acceptable range, you can stop active intervention. If it is still not in the acceptable range, you have to keep working on improving it. You will need to continue with the education of the drawing staff. You can add on a policy of collecting a waste red top tube prior to collecting the blood culture bottles.

Continue doing this and see how subsequent months' blood culture contamination rates come out. If it is improved, and in the acceptable range, you can stop active intervention. If it is still not in the acceptable range, you have to keep working on it. You can track the contaminated blood cultures back to who drew them. If there is one or a few people that drew most of the contaminated blood cultures, they are singled out for more intensive education and scrutiny on their technique for drawing.

If the employees having problems drawing blood cultures improve their technique, and the contamination rate drops into the acceptable range, you can stop active intervention. If these employees do not improve their technique, and still have an unacceptably high contamination rate, they should be sidelined from further drawing of blood cultures.

Eventually, the problem will be fixed, and the blood culture contamination rate will come back into the acceptable range. You may upset many people while trying to fix the problem, and that may be unavoidable. The alternative is sticking your head in the sand and ignoring the problem, which is even worse. Once the problem is fixed, the blood culture contamination rate goes from active intervention to watching the numbers every month. This monthly review of the numbers should continue indefinitely. If the problem recurs, repeat the corrective action steps given above.

The information on your efforts to fix the problem, your results and the relevant QA forms are presented on a monthly basis to the relevant committees with quarterly and annual summaries. There is usually a due date for the monthly, quarterly and annual reports. Be careful of these dates and submit all reports on time. At most hospitals, the hospital QA office circulates a list of the departments with delinquent QA reports, and you don't want lab constantly on the delinquent list.

In these reports, document the improvements made, opportunities for further improvement, constraints to improvement and how you have or will overcome the constraints to improvement. The paperwork is filed in the relevant file folders. The same is done for each and every QA indicator that you have picked from the above list.

Let's say that we picked crossmatch:transfusion ratio as a QA indicator, and set a target of no more than 1.5 ratio of crossmatches to transfusions. Here is an example of what the crossmatch:transfusion data will look like after it is compiled:

Blood Utilization and Transfusion Review Committee

DATA COLLECTION for October 2013

Ward	ER	Peds	NICU	Hemo	ICU	Med	OB	L&D	OR
PRBC units crossmatched	50	33	11	0	2	13	7	3	5
PRBC units transfused	45	28	9	0	1	11	5	2	4
Ratio	1.11	1.18	1.22	N/A	2.0	1.18	1.40	1.50	1.25

	Hospital wide total
PRBC units crossmatched	124
PRBC units transfused	105
Ratio	1.18

After compiling the data you then review it. In the above example, the hospital wide crossmatch transfusion ratio is quite good. You want it to be less than 1.5 and it came in much better than this. The ICU falls out with a ratio of 2.0. However with only one unit transfused the ratio for ICU is not really meaningful.

The data is presented at the relevant committee meetings (Blood Utilization and Transfusion Review (BUTR) Committee, Quality Management Committee, etc.). If there are no significant fall-outs the data is then filed in the relevant file folder.

If you have a significant fall-out, for example the hospital wide crossmatch:transfusion ratio comes out higher than the 1.5 target you must try to correct the situation. For crossmatch:transfusion ratio this would entail informing the providers that they should only order crossmatches if they are relatively certain that the patient will need transfusion within the next 72 hours.

Next month check to see if this QA indicator has improved. If it is improved, and in the acceptable range, you can stop active intervention. If it is still not in the acceptable range, you have to keep working on improving it. Continue educating the providers. If this doesn't improve things, you can have the BUTR Committee send letters to offending providers, refer egregious cases to the various departments of the hospital for peer review, etc. A copy of any documents generated should be kept in the lab's QA file as evidence of corrective action.

If you persist eventually you will fix the problem. You may upset many people while trying to fix the problem, and that may be unavoidable. The alternative is sticking your head in the sand and ignoring the problem, which is even worse.

The information on your efforts to fix the problem, your results and the relevant QA forms are presented on a monthly basis to the relevant committees with quarterly and annual summaries. There is usually a due date for the monthly, quarterly and annual reports. Be careful of these dates and submit all reports on time. At most hospitals, the hospital QA office circulates a list of the departments with delinquent QA reports, and you don't want lab constantly on the delinquent list.

In these reports, document the improvements made, opportunities for further improvement, constraints to improvement and how you have or will overcome the constraints to improvement. The paperwork is filed in the relevant file folders.

Once the problem is fixed the crossmatch:transfusion ratio goes from active intervention to watching the numbers every month. You should keep measuring the same QA indicator (in this example crossmatch:transfusion ratio) indefinitely to make sure the problem never recurs. If the problem recurs, repeat the corrective action steps given above.

The same is done for each and every QA indicator that you have picked from the above list. Choose your QA indicators carefully, or you will be working very hard.

You are allowed to change your QA indicators over time. If some of the QA indicators you are watching come out good month after month for an extended period, it may not be worthwhile to continue measuring these QA indicators. The assumption is that your hospital doesn't have a problem in these areas and won't ever have a problem in these areas. If you drop one QA indicator, it is best to add a different QA indicator, or the inspector may think you are slacking off.

The lab Quality Assurance program typically includes complaints and incident reports involving lab. As Lab Director, you will spend a significant portion of your time answering complaints. A complaint is typically defined as an allegation that lab has not followed its own policies and procedures. I define a complaint even more broadly as any customer dissatisfaction with lab.

For example a doctor comes to me complaining that a routine lab test ordered at 3PM was not ready by 4:30PM. I inform that doctor that lab policies allow 24 hours for a routine test to be completed. If you need faster turnaround time, order the test as a STAT so as to have results within one hour. To me this counts as a complaint, even though the lab followed its own policies and procedures.

Most complaints are petty, such as the example above. As a Lab Director you will spend a good amount of your time answering to clinicians upset about everything imaginable. In my experience this includes the computer screen is too small to read, the lab did not FAX the results I wanted, I want the lab to print out the test results and courier the printout to my clinic, etc. As you can see there is quite a bit of overlap between complaints and unreasonable clinician demands on lab. I will discuss unreasonable clinician demands on lab at greater length in a later chapter.

More significant complaints are less common and typically involve a clinician's suspicion that there is something wrong with one or more test. An ER doctor has 10 consecutive patients with low platelets and calls you to ask if there is a problem with the platelet testing. A call of this nature should send you into the hematology section immediately. Look at the controls for that day and the prior days of the same month. Did the controls come in on the first try? When was the last calibration? Was the lot changed recently? Does the lot number on the control bottles match the lot number the analyzer is programmed with? Are all the reagents in date with no expired reagents?

Other possibilities include problems with the specimens such as clotting, hemolysis, lipemia, inadequate centrifugation, inadequate rocking, etc. Pull out the specimens in question, examine them for integrity and retest them.

Once you are satisfied that there are no problems with the testing, you can call back the doctor in question and reassure that doctor there was no problem with the testing. In this example you'd be calling back the ER doctor and telling him or her that there was no problem with the platelet testing, and yes there really were 10 consecutive patients with low platelets.

The next type of significant clinician complaint involves a problem with one patient's testing. In this scenario the clinician calls and tells you "Patient X has secondary polycythemia, but today's CBC shows severe anemia. Please double-check the results". In this case, when there is only one patient result in question, you have to rule out a switched specimen, or some other type of misdrawing in which the wrong patient's results are being assigned to the patient in question.

In my experience clinician calls asking "is there a problem with this one patient's test?" are a false alarm more than 90% of the time. However, you are obligated to follow up on these calls as urgently as possible. If your lab ever does release erroneous results this is the first and most likely way it will get caught. Thus every complaint of this nature is taken seriously and followed up with urgency.

Incident reports are a little different than a complaint. An incident report is an internal hospital document that records information relating to an accident or other unwanted event at the facility. An incident report is filled out by hospital staff whereas a complaint is typically made by a lab customer. Incident reports tend to be of a more serious nature than a complaint. There is some overlap, as it is possible for a complaint to be written up as an incident report.

The most serious incidents I have seen involve switching one patent's specimen and/or lab results with another patient's specimen and/or lab results. This typically occurs at the time of drawing with the wrong barcode label put on the wrong tube. This is typically caught when a "delta check" shows wide swings in the patient's results for certain analytes since the prior testing. Delta check is the mandatory comparison of current lab results with any prior lab results to make sure that the current results are consistent with the prior results. I have also seen switched specimens caught when the patient is blood typed and found to have a different ABO blood type than the Blood Bank records indicate.

In my experience if a switch occurs, it is usually caught before the results go out from lab. If switched patient test results get released, you will likely get a call from one or both clinicians involved that today's lab test results for a patient do not fit the clinical picture.

Pull out the tube of blood used for the testing and check the label against the patient identifying information in the computer. Some hospitals require the patient's name to be handwritten on the tube before applying the barcode. In this case, peel back the barcode label to ensure the handwritten name matches the name on the barcode. The phlebotomists are required to initial all labels on the tubes they draw. Talk to the phlebotomist who drew this specimen and ask if it is possible there was a switch. Check the other test results on that run, to see if some other patient has an unexpected test result that would fit better for the patient in question. If so, this would be evidence of a switch.

If you are trying to rule out a misdraw or switch, you can type the tubes of blood for ABO and Rh, minor blood group antigens, etc. A change in ABO, Rh or minor blood group antigens confirms a specimen misdraw or switch. Unchanged ABO, Rh and minor blood group antigens indicates a switch or misdraw is less likely, but does not completely exclude this. Have the patient in question redrawn and compare the redraw results to the results in question.

The phlebotomist who drew the switched specimens should have immediate corrective action. For such a severe incident, this counseling is done in a closed-door meeting usually by the Lab Supervisor with the section supervisor and Lab Director present in the room. Be as nice as possible. The Lab Supervisor will inform the phlebotomist involved that a switched specimen has been identified and that phlebotomist drew the switched specimen. The phlebotomist involved will usually be very apologetic. The phlebotomist will be informed of the requirement for two patient identifiers before drawing and that switched specimens have the potential to be life-threatening to the patients involved. Further occurrences are considered unacceptable.

Another less common error is testing the right patient, but using the specimen from the wrong time of collection. Let's say I'm in the ICU getting heparinized. My 3AM INR is 1.2 and I am drawn again at 3PM. The 3PM specimen has an INR of 2.5 due to heparinization. The 3PM specimen is drawn and put on a refrigerator rack next to my 3AM specimen. My 3AM specimen is pulled out of the refrigerator inadvertently and run in place of my 3PM specimen. The incorrect result of 1.2 INR is given, and I get a whole lot more heparin than I really need. Later the mistake is caught and the 3PM results are corrected to a 2.5 INR. This sort of mistake indicates carelessness and/or inattention and should prompt immediate corrective action as described for the phlebotomist above.

Any public disturbance in the hospital will generate an incident report. At one hospital I worked at, there were several incident reports involving the Morgue. On several occasions, the family of a deceased patient had a reaction interpreted by the hospital staff as a public disturbance. These were duly written up.

Incident reports are used to document a wide variety of problems, from computer outages to power outages to analyzer breakdowns. If an unexpected event stops the lab or part of the lab from doing testing, it probably needs an incident report. I have seen incident reports generated by earthquakes and hurricanes.

The lab must report to OSHA all accidents, spills, chemical exposures, injuries and biologic exposures. An incident report should be generated for any untoward event in these categories, so as to be able to keep track of any occurrences.

As Lab Director all incident reports involving lab should come across your desk. The incident report form typically has fields to be filled out for investigation, Root Cause Analysis (RCA) and plan of correction to prevent recurrence. You can do the investigation, RCA and plan of correction yourself or more likely delegate this off to the Lab Supervisor.

As the name implies, an RCA tries to identify the root cause of the incident. In one of the examples above the root cause of the problem was that the phlebotomist switched specimens. In order to do an RCA properly you must examine the entire system involved. Why did the phlebotomist put the wrong barcode labels on two different tubes of blood? Is there a policy in place mandating the phlebotomist to use two patient identifiers? Is there a policy in place requiring all patients to have a hospital wristband in order to be drawn? Is there a policy in place requiring the phlebotomist to label each tube of blood before leaving the patient's room? Can the delta check process be improved so as to be more likely to catch a switched specimen before the results are released from lab? Are the phlebotomists overworked and making fatigue errors?

In order to do an RCA correctly, you must examine the entire process of drawing: The patient comes in to the hospital and has the wristband put on. The patient should be instructed to never alter or remove this wristband. The doctor orders the test in the hospital computer system. The request prints in the phlebotomy printer. The phlebotomist arrives at work and collects up the list of patients to draw. The phlebotomist goes to that patient's room, draws the patient, and somehow gets the wrong barcode label on that tube of blood. The process repeats at the next patient's room. Alternatively, the phlebotomist may have drawn two patients, and applied the barcode labels after the fact. The lab does the testing not realizing that the wrong patient's blood is being used for the testing.

When doing an RCA it is not sufficient to take the easy way out and say "it's all the phlebotomist's fault". This would not be considered an adequate RCA. If your CMS inspector caught you doing this, you'd be cited in the inspection, in effect being told by the inspector to do it the right way.

Another technique for doing an RCA involves repeatedly asking "Why?" until one comes to the root cause of the problem. This technique is mentioned in the COLA literature. In my experience, there is no way to know when you have reached the root cause and it is time to stop asking "Why?". Instead, one could ask "Why?" forever. I prefer the systematic approach given above. It has a defined start, systematic way of looking at the problem, and a defined end point.

After making the RCA you then make a plan of correction to prevent recurrence. For the above example of switched specimens, the plan of correction is to counsel the phlebotomist that made the switch, monitor that phlebotomist's performance closely, and remind all phlebotomists to check two identifiers on all patient's wristbands and label all tubes before leaving the patient's room.

Write the RCA and plan of correction into the appropriate fields of the incident report form. Sign off on the incident report form, and forward it to the next person in line to receive it, typically the hospital Risk Manager or hospital-wide Quality Assurance Coordinator.

In most hospitals it is forbidden to make copies of an incident report form. The completed forms for lab incident reports are usually not stored in lab but instead are stored in the hospital Risk Manager's Office.

Chapter 13 – How to deal with personnel problems

The reason I went into Pathology and Lab Medicine is because it tends to be relatively sheltered from interaction with others. As a Lab Director you will almost never see a patient directly and never have to tell anyone horribly bad news such as "You have cancer", "You have 3 months left to live", etc.

The Lab Supervisor is tasked with enforcing the rules and regulations on the lab staff including all disciplinary matters. As such the Lab Supervisor will have much more contact with a problem employee than you will. However, as Lab Director one still has to interact with the various personalities found in the typical hospital lab.

In most of the labs I am familiar with the lab staff works together like family. The most frequent problem is the late to work or lazy employee not getting the job done in the time allotted. Significant arguments between 2 employees are rare. Employees with significant behavioral and/or performance issues are very rare. I have seen less than 10 for-cause terminations in my entire career. In the vast majority of these, I was in the Pathologist position, not the Lab Director position and did not directly supervise the termination. I have only directly supervised two for-cause terminations in my entire career, both for performance issues.

Potentially homicidal or suicidal employees are so rare that I have only seen one each in my 29 years in Pathology and Lab Medicine. It is imperative to spot a potentially homicidal or suicidal employee. The consequences of missing warning signs could be devastating. I will cover these two topics first.

A. How to spot a potentially homicidal employee

Workplace violence typically involves an adult acting alone. There are typically a series of warning signs given off prior to the event:

1. Male gender. This is really the strongest risk factor. Workplace violence perpetrated by a female is virtually unheard of.
2. The offender is typically a socially withdrawn loner with no friends and no interest in making friends.
3. Gun ownership. Fascination with guns and war. Tends to stockpile ammunition.
4. Prior history of violence. Prior history of incarceration.
5. Psychiatric history, especially the types of personality disorder that cause the sufferer to dehumanize others.
6. History of drug and/or alcohol abuse.
7. Indirect threats are more likely than direct threats in the run-up to workplace violence.
8. Triggering event, such as loss of the job, divorce, etc.

My assessment: I would recommend against knowingly hiring any employee with a prior history of violence. If any employee has 3 or more of the above risk factors, I will refer them to counseling. In a separate phone call to the counselor I will ask the counselor to evaluate the employee for potential workplace violence.

In my 29 years in Pathology and Lab Medicine only once have I had contact with a potentially homicidal employee. His name is Fred. I will not mention his last name. He moved from Las Vegas in the late 1990s and took jobs in two different labs in my community. His day job was a full time position in the lab where I worked, which I will refer to as "my lab" for the purpose of this story, even though I don't own this lab. His other job was a part time night job at an outside lab I will refer to as the "other lab" for the purpose of this story.

Fred's performance at my lab was perfectly acceptable. A few people in my lab though he was a little strange, but most people liked him. He didn't seem to be having any major problems. He got good evaluations from the Lab Supervisor at my lab, and got a few routine salary increments over the course of the next few years.

However, Fred was having major problems at the outside lab. The Lab Supervisor at the outside lab had a reputation for being excessively tough, and excessively writing up the subordinate lab staff. Fred got into an escalating series of arguments with this Lab Supervisor sometime around the year 2000. The more Fred argued with this Lab Supervisor, the more this Lab Supervisor wrote Fred up.

This escalating series of arguments and write-ups ended with Fred shouting at the Lab Supervisor "I am going to go home and get my gun. I'll be back" and then storming out of the outside lab. The Lab Supervisor called the police. The police came to the outside lab, took down the complaint, went to Fred's house and arrested Fred.

No one at my lab was aware of what was going on at the outside lab. The way we found out is that Fred didn't show up for work at my lab as scheduled. The lab staff of my lab called Fred's house to see why he no-showed work. The staff were shocked when they found out Fred was in jail because of his confrontation with the Lab Supervisor at the outside lab.

When we found out about this, my lab quietly dropped Fred from the employee rolls. The Personnel Office presumably send a letter to his address telling him he was no longer an employee. He was in jail at the time so likely didn't get the letter. We never heard from Fred again, and this was probably for the best.

I got some follow up from an acquaintance that works at the outside lab. Fred spent about a month in jail waiting for his case to come in front of the Judge. When he came in front of the Judge, the Judge ordered a 30 day psychiatric evaluation. After the 30 day psychiatric evaluation was done the Judge heard the case again. The Psychiatrist said that Fred was not a threat to the outside lab or its Lab Supervisor. The Judge released Fred based on time served, and made a restraining order that Fred is not allowed to come within 500 feet of the outside lab or the outside Lab Supervisor.

Fred moved back to Las Vegas shortly after being released from jail. I had no further contact with him nor did anyone else from my lab.

B. How to spot a potentially suicidal employee

The following are warning signs of a potentially suicidal employee:

1. Adverse or traumatic life event, especially divorce or death of a spouse.
2. Mental illness, especially major depression. The clinical manifestations of depression include deep sadness, loss of interest in things one used to care about, making comments about being hopeless, helpless, or worthless, trouble sleeping and eating, sudden weight gain or loss.
3. History of alcohol and/or substance abuse.
4. Talking or writing about death or suicide.
5. One or more prior suicide attempts.
6. Family history of mental disorder or substance abuse.
7. Gun ownership, with gun kept in the home.
8. Chronic physical illness, including chronic pain.
9. Gender is not a risk factor. Suicides occur at about equal rates in both genders.

My assessment: If any employee has 2 or more of the above risk factors, I will refer them to counseling. In a separate phone call to the counselor I will ask the counselor to evaluate the employee for potential suicide.

In my 29 years in Pathology and Lab Medicine only once have I had contact with an employee I thought was potentially suicidal. In September, 2013 I was acting as an off-site Lab Director for a small hospital lab. I was remote from the Lab and communicating by E-mail. In mid-September the Lab Supervisor E-mailed me that an employee showed up late for a scheduled 3 to 11 PM shift arriving approximately 4:30PM. According to the Lab Supervisor, she is going through a divorce and has to pick up her children from school and can't make it in to work until after 4PM.

On September 12, 2013 from me to the Lab Supervisor: I think the best way to handle this is to sit down with her, and try to work out a schedule that will accommodate her without unduly inconveniencing lab. If she has to pick the children up from school at 4PM, and there is no one else that can pick her children up from school, then we should try to arrange things so that she starts work at 5PM. Ask the day shift if there is anyone willing to work an extra two hours every day at the end of their shift, to cover the 3PM to 5PM block.

On September 18 from the Lab Supervisor to me: She came to me in tears the other day. In labs where no one wanted to work odd shifts, holidays, etc a monthly rotational schedule was implemented.

On September 19 from me to the Lab Supervisor: I do not know her personally. Where I work, there is counseling on site for employees having personal problems. If an employee was having the same problems as her (getting divorced, repeatedly late for work, crying at work, etc.) that employee would get mandatory referral to the internal counselor. She is sending out a lot of red flags that she is having personal problems and may need help. If you have an internal counseling service, please refer her.

As an epilog written many years later, this lab staff survived her depressive episode. About five years after this episode, her daughter committed suicide while a junior in high school after the daughter had a failed romantic relationship. This was unforeseeable and no one in lab could have prevented this.

C. How to deal with two lab employees that do not get along

Minor disagreements between two employees can usually be resolved by the next person up the chain of command. Usually it is a negotiating process in which the supervisor offers one of the two disagreeing employees something of value (e.g. overtime pay) in exchange for doing something that person otherwise wouldn't want to do (e.g. work in a different section of Lab).

The situation where two people in lab truly hate each other is uncommon in my experience. However, when it happens you will never forget it.

I graduated from training in 1996 and went to work in a hospital where two Blood Bank techs had been having a long-running argument. I was hired into the Pathologist position at that hospital. The Lab Director at that hospital was older, nearing retirement, and tired of constantly having to referee the arguments between these two Blood Bank techs.

The Lab Director had long since given up on getting these two quarreling techs to agree on anything. When I started work there, he immediately delegated me Blood Bank. This meant that he could distance himself from the two quarreling techs and I would have to deal directly with them.

When I started work at that hospital the Blood Bank was divided into donor side and transfusion side. One of the Blood Bank techs was on the transfusion side and the other was on the donor side. Each of them kept accusing the other of making more work for the other.

It was my assignment to try to get these two Blood Bank techs to bury the hatchet. First, I spoke to them individually. The tech working the donor side of Blood Bank said that the tech working in transfusion side is making more work for the donor side of Blood Bank. The tech working the transfusion side of Blood bank said that the tech working in donor side is making more work for the transfusion side of Blood Bank.

While meeting individually with the techs I explained to each of them that yes, transfusion side makes more work for donor side, and yes, donor side makes more work for transfusion side, but if both sides stop working, the Blood Bank as a whole would stop working.

This did not help. The next approach that I tried is called "one big meeting". In this approach, the two quarreling techs are called into a meeting along with their respective supervisors, the Lab Supervisor, and the Lab Director. I called everyone in for one big meeting. In this meeting the supervisory people tried to negotiate away all the problems, and tried to cajole and coerce the two quarreling techs to stop arguing so much.

This approach of having one big meeting is popular in the management literature. In my experience it does not work. The techs may pretend to get along for the course of the meeting. However, as soon as the meeting is over they will go back to arguing. That is exactly what happened. In this case the two techs were back to arguing within one week of this one big meeting.

I proposed merging the donor side and transfusion side of Blood Bank, so that it would not appear that one side was making more work for the other. This was not possible due to the different credentials of the people working on the different sides of Blood Bank.

I proposed hiring more techs for Blood Bank or reshuffling techs from the main part of the lab into Blood Bank so as to spread the workload around. The Lab Supervisor felt there wasn't enough work to justify more techs in Blood Bank and the two quarreling techs in Blood Bank did not have excessive workload. In other words, the Lab Supervisor felt that the quarreling Blood Bank techs were not justified in their complaints about their workload, each making more work for the other, etc.

The next thing to try is to separate the two arguing techs in time and space as much as is possible. If one tech can "float" send that tech to a different section in lab such that there is minimal contact with the other tech. Reassign one or both of the techs to the swing shift and/or graveyard shift such that the only time they see each other is at change of shift.

In reality what happened is that these two techs continued their arguing throughout the remainder of the 1990s. It did not end until the donor side tech moved to a job in a different part of the same hospital around the year 2000.

In my career of 29 years in Pathology and Lab Medicine I have not seen lab techs argue so much before or after this episode. Thankfully this was an isolated episode.

D. How to deal with a disagreement between employees inside and outside lab

In this permutation, the disagreement is between one or more lab staff and one or more employee that works in a different part of the same hospital. This is relatively common and I could give multiple examples. In order to keep this chapter brief I will only give one example.

One of the hospitals I have worked at was a small community hospital with only one doctor staffing the ER at night. This one doctor was older, but very energetic. The ER had a heavy volume. Most nights there were fairly large number of patients coming in, but a lot of the work was routine. In this small community the clinics all closed at 6PM. All the minor cough, cold and flu cases came to the ER after 6PM and the ER was loaded with routine work.

This doctor insisted on having a phlebotomist by her side the entire night so that as this doctor went from patient to patient the doctor could order lab tests and have them drawn on the spot. The lab policy allows the phlebotomists to take a 30 minute meal break at the midpoint of the 8 hour shift as long as there is no STAT work to be done. This ER doctor would object to the 30 minute meal break. This ER doctor wanted a phlebotomist by her side the entire 8 hours she was working.

There is only one phlebotomist scheduled on the night shift, and the night duty would rotate among a pool of 5 phlebotomists. Most of the phlebotomists did as told, skipping their 30 minute meal break and working 8 hours straight to keep this ER doctor happy. One phlebotomist objected. This resulted in a mutual write-up in which the ER doctor wrote up the phlebotomist for "attitude" and the phlebotomist wrote up the ER doctor for "attitude".

As a Lab Director, all write-ups and incident reports related to lab should come across your desk. If it is important you will usually be informed at the start of the next working day. The mutual write-up between the ER doctor and the phlebotomist was seen as relatively unimportant; the paperwork came across my desk with other routine paperwork well after the fact.

I dutifully carried out my part. I talked with the phlebotomist and asked her side of the story. She is diabetic and needs to eat at regular intervals. The ER doctor gave the phlebotomist "attitude" when the phlebotomist said that she had to take off for a 30 minute meal and that the routine testing can wait.

The ER doctor works the night shift, and I did not speak directly to the ER doctor. I left a message for the ER doctor to call me during the daytime hours regarding the phlebotomy coverage of ER. The message was left for me that the ER doctor considers it essential to have a phlebotomist present the entire time, with no breaks.

Let's think this through. The lab policy says that the phlebotomist gets a 30 minute meal if there are no STATs to be drawn. The routine work can wait 30 minutes. I have never heard of any other ER doctor needing to have a phlebotomist right by their side the entire shift. At this point, I make the judgment call that the ER doctor is being unreasonable.

As Lab Director your authority begins and ends with lab. You can rearrange the phlebotomist schedule such that the diabetic phlebotomist only works the day shift, and the other phlebotomists work the night shift with the ER doctor in question.

As Lab Director, you do not have authority over an ER doctor. The chain of command is such that the ER doctor answers to the ER department head who in turn answers to the hospital Medical Director.

The best thing to do at this point is to call the ER department head and inform the ER department head that there has been a mutual write up between the ER doctor and a phlebotomist. The lab thinks that the ER doctor is being unreasonable. Even so, the lab will schedule a different phlebotomist at night so hopefully this will not recur. The Lab considers the case to be closed, unless and until there are further write-ups between this ER doctor and the phlebotomists.

In general for a situation such as this it is important to resolve the disagreement as quickly as possible. If you leave the same phlebotomist working with the same ER doctor, the result is likely to be intractable arguments and a firestorm of write-ups. From an administrative perspective, a firestorm of write-ups between two employees is very difficult to deal with, a real headache. It is best to separate the two before the situation comes to this.

The switching of the phlebotomists solved the lab's problem with this ER doctor. The other phlebotomists did not mind working 8 hours straight.

Let's suppose the same ER doctor and the other phlebotomists start doing mutual write-ups. In this situation the best approach is to call a meeting with the ER department head and the ER doctor in question. Talk to the ER department head in advance of this meeting and make sure the ER department head will back you in this meeting. In the meeting explain to the ER doctor in question that the phlebotomist really is allowed to take a 30 minute meal break if there are no STATs to be drawn. Ask the ER to accommodate this by assigning a nurse or other ER staff to do the phlebotomy for the 30 minutes the phlebotomist is on break.

E. How to deal with the chronically late to work employee

Work ethic is not distributed evenly among mankind. I am relatively hardworking, putting in an average of 10 hour days five days a week. That is slightly more than the typical Pathologist/Lab Director, but not as hardworking as a surgeon.

At the other end of the spectrum are people who consider 6 or 7 hours of work a day and/or three day weekends to be the normal and natural state of affairs. I have no problem with this as long as it is acknowledged that the person is working part-time by the definition the lab uses. Full time is defined as 40 or more hours per week, part time is anything less.

If a person shows up late to work in Lab it creates a problem for the other people working in Lab. The Lab staff schedule typically has to be rearranged at the last minute with someone on the prior shift asked to keep working until the late employee shows up. I will refer to this late arriving employee as CLTW for Chronically Late To Work. In my experience the CLTW employee is the most common problem employee in Lab.

When an employee in lab is CLTW it can be very demoralizing to the other lab staff. A lab tech or phlebotomist has to stay late every time the CLTW employee arrives late. The other lab techs and phlebotomists have family, children to pick up from school, etc. If the situation is not corrected the other lab staff will eventually come to believe that they should not have to work hard if the CLTW employee does not have to work hard. Once an employee becomes CLTW they will not usually start showing up on time until they receive one or more corrective actions. In this circumstance, the corrective action reassures the other lab staff that something is being done to fix the problem.

The Lab Supervisor is generally the person tasked with the scheduling of the lab staff. The CLTW employee can be a big headache for the Lab Supervisor, but is usually not a big problem for the Lab Director.

As a Lab Director you will only see the CLTW employee if the Lab Supervisor and/or section supervisor have been doing multiple write-ups on the CLTW employee. In my experience this is uncommon and the CLTW employee will show up on time to work after the first write-up or two.

Motivating the CLTW employee to work hard is another story. This falls first on the section supervisor. If the section supervisor fails it then falls on the Lab Supervisor. You will only see the CLTW employee if the section supervisor and/or Lab Supervisor have been doing multiple write-ups on that employee.

In my 29 years in Pathology and Lab Medicine there have been only one or two instances where this came across my desk in the form of multiple write-ups that I had to sign off on. In these cases, I asked the CLTW employee to get a medical evaluation to make sure there was no correctable condition (hypothyroidism, anemia, diabetes, etc.) that was curtailing their ability to work hard. I did not document this request in writing.

If the employee refused medical evaluation or if the medical evaluation came back with nothing wrong, I would sign off on the write-ups and forward them to the Personnel Office. The Lab Supervisor and the Personnel Office would do the dirty work of removing the CLTW employee, or renegotiating the CLTW employee's position as a part-time position.

Another variation of this occurs when a lab employee chronically abuses leave time. In one of the labs I worked at, there was a lab tech named John who liked to take annual leave the entire week between Christmas and New Year. Any year that he did not get scheduled for this leave, he would call in sick the entire week.

The problem is that everyone else also wants time off at Christmas. The scheduling of leave is on a first-come, first-served basis. At this particular lab, the annual leave scheduling calendar opens in January. I encouraged John to put in his Christmas leave request 11 months in advance, when the annual leave calendar opens, so that he could get his wish of leave time at Christmas.

One year John lost this race to other techs, who put in their request for Christmas leave first. When Christmas time came, John called in sick the 4 working days between Christmas and New Year's Day. The hospital's policy on leave time requires a doctor's sick excuse when sick leave time is used for 3 or more consecutive working days. John was asked to produce his doctor's excuse but he could not produce one. The hospital's administrative manual will tell you what to do in this circumstance. In this particular lab, if the lab tech cannot produce a doctor's excuse the lab tech is assigned leave without pay for the days missed.

A lab tech who does this once a year is not a major problem. Any lab tech doing this frequently will quickly become a problem. In most labs the Lab Supervisor is tasked with all lab tech scheduling issues to include employees who abuse leave time. As Lab Director, all you have to do is sign off on the write-ups done by the Lab Supervisor and/or section supervisor.

F. How to deal with an employee with performance and/or behavioral issues

The textbook definition of behavioral problems is behavior representing symptomatic expressions of maladjustment. I define behavioral problems more broadly as any behavior that bothers or annoys co-workers.

Performance issues are defined as inability to complete one's assigned tasks with accuracy, speed and/or completeness. This is virtually synonymous with incompetence. The only difference as far as I can tell is that performance issues are seen as temporary whereas incompetence is seen as a permanent state that can't be corrected.

Behavioral issues are generally much less serious than performance issues. Minor behavioral issues do not affect patient care and only represent an annoyance to co-workers. Behavioral issues have a great deal of overlap with the types of disagreements discussed in the section on lab employees that do not get along. As far as I can tell the only difference is that the dispute is not over anything that relates directly to work. Usually these sorts of disagreements can be mediated.

For example, in virtually every lab I have ever worked at, all lab employees share the same breakroom. Most employees bring their own lunch to work and microwave it when lunchtime comes. In one lab I worked at, one employee used excessive garlic in her lunches. When microwaved this would make the whole lab smell like garlic. The other lab employees would complain and tell her to stop adding so much garlic to her lunches. Every time the employee involved was told this, she would add even more garlic to her lunch the next day. This resulted in a recurring cycle of more complaints and more garlic. The employee involved was acting passive aggressive, by adding more garlic to her own lunches when told by co-workers not to do this.

The dispute could not be settled among the lab techs involved and was elevated to lab management. In this situation there are a limited number of things you can do. Many options are a bad idea. Do not call in this employee and tell her to stop adding garlic to her lunches. As I see it, she has a right to add whatever she wants to her own lunches. I called Facilities Maintenance and asked them to make the lab breakroom negative pressure and/or vent the exhaust air away from main lab. Maintenance wasn't able to get negative pressure in the lab breakroom, but they were able to turn up the ventilation enough that the garlic odors in the lab breakroom did not permeate the whole lab. This solved the dispute among the lab techs involved.

Most minor behavioral issues can be negotiated away in a similar manner. Anyone showing more significant behavioral problems should probably be referred to the employee health office for a psychiatry consult.

Performance issues are much more serious, since they can impact patient care. Each hospital should have an employee corrective action (i.e. disciplinary action) procedure in the hospital-wide administrative manual. I will go into detail on lab tech performance issues and disciplinary action in Chapter 16. The typical hospital's disciplinary action pathway as described in Chapter 16 could be used for all lab employees (lab techs, phlebotomists, secretaries, etc.) except Pathologists. Because Pathologists are privileged physicians, they have a different pathway for disciplinary action. Pathologist performance issues are discussed in chapter 21.

Everyone makes mistakes. No one is perfect. It is almost always a judgment call as to whether one employee is making too many mistakes too often and the mistakes are serious enough to justify disciplinary action. Be prepared that anyone receiving disciplinary action will claim he or she is being singled out, treated unfairly and his or her mistakes are being taken more seriously than other people's mistakes. Thus, when investigating any mistakes, you must take a fair and even-handed approach.

When investigating mistakes start with the basics. Did the incident deviate from lab best practices? Is there a written policy that was violated? Is there conclusive evidence that this employee (as opposed to someone else) was responsible? Is the proposed discipline proportional to the severity of the offense? The investigation must be fair and equal. It must be done fairly without regard to whether you do or do not like the employee in question, whether you do or do not like any group the employee belongs to, etc.

I will give an example of this process. One hospital I worked at did not have a FAX policy when I started work there. An outside clinic headed by Dr. S called and asked lab to FAX the most recent lab results for one patient. A phlebotomist FAXed lab results to the outside clinic. The clinic called back and complained that the results have Dr. K's name as the ordering physician not Dr. S's name. It turns out the FAXed results were for the right patient, but for the wrong day (an ER visit and not the clinic visit in question). Apparently, the patient had made an ER visit and didn't tell the clinic about the ER visit. The lab FAXed the most recent results as requested by the clinic, but it was not what the clinic wanted. The immediate corrective action is to ask the outpatient clinic to shred the FAX since it does not contain the results they want (right patient, wrong day) and FAX the correct results to the clinic.

The phlebotomist involved was written up for HIPAA violation. At this hospital HIPAA violation calls for termination on the first offense. The paperwork went to the Hospital Administrator. The Hospital Administrator determined this was not a HIPAA violation since it involves lab tests for the same patient (but on a different day than requested). The decision was made not to fire the phlebotomist over this incident. I asked the Hospital Administrator to make a FAX policy for the entire hospital, since there was no FAX policy in place.

In my opinion, for the FAX incident described above the best corrective action is to make a lab-wide or hospital-wide FAX policy (before FAXing you must check the patient name, check the ordering provider's name, check the date of testing, etc. Do not FAX unless all details match. Any discrepancies must be resolved before FAXing). Provide a copy of this policy to everyone in lab and make sure everyone is familiar with it.

In this situation, corrective action toward the one employee involved would not likely prevent recurrence of the problem. The clinic is likely to keep calling for patient results, and one by one the lab staff will receive these calls and FAX results. If you took this approach, you would end up doing the corrective action on the lab staff one at a time as they receive calls asking for FAXes.

Chapter 14 – Physician and administrator demands on lab and physician ordering practices

This is really the most onerous part about being a Lab Director. Most hospital administrators see lab as a cost center and are constantly looking to cut costs. Most physicians expect to have unlimited access to lab testing. As Lab Director, you are caught between a rock and a hard place.

As Lab Director, you don't have enough time to police every test ordered by every physician. Thus the most expensive and most esoteric tests are the ones that come under the most scrutiny. Even so most doctors are upset when I call to ask the indications for doing this testing, or question the need for any given test. If the doctor says that it is a medical necessity, I generally allow the testing.

I have seen many instances where doctors made unreasonable demands on lab. In one such instance, a hematologist/oncologist wanted to do bone marrow exams during the nighttime hours. In this episode, the hematologist/oncologist was at her clinic during the 8AM to 5PM time frame, went home, ate dinner then came in to the hospital between 7PM to 9PM to do rounds. If any patient needed a bone marrow, she wanted to do it at that time.

The problem with this is that the lab's day shift is long gone by 7PM and the swing shift is a skeleton crew. There were only 3 or 4 people on swing shift, and none of them could be spared to assist with the bone marrow exam. Part of the bone marrow testing was sent out, and the reference lab would not send a courier after 5PM. The specimen would wait for pickup until the next working day.

This hematologist/oncologist was insistent that lab had to accommodate her schedule, and not the other way around. We came to an agreement that the hematologist/oncologist would have to schedule all nighttime bone marrows well in advance so that lab could arrange for an additional person on swing shift. The reference lab agreed to send the courier up to 9PM if we scheduled this in advance.

Hospital Administrator demands on lab almost always come in the form of a generic "cut costs". The labs that I have worked at have no fat left to cut. Cutting costs means cutting services.

When I get called into an administrator's office and told to cut costs, my response is that the only way to cut costs is to cut services. I mention a few things that can be done to save money - close the lab at night, curtail blood bank services, etc. I ask the administrator to pick which one of these to cut. Since cutting any of these would be onerous, and would result in a backlash from the medical staff, the administrator usually backs off at this point.

In the rare instance in which the administrator wants to cut services, I make sure that the medical staff knows where the decision came from. This way the backlash will be against the administrator and not me.

Chapter 15 – Professional relations. Making sure you are not a problem employee

As an employee, the number of possible rule violations is virtually limitless. The Code of Federal Regulations is tens of thousands of pages. Most municipalities have thousands of pages of municipal codes. Most hospital's administrative manual is in the hundreds of pages. I couldn't repeat it all here, to tell you what not to do, or I would end up writing the longest book in history.

However, some basic rules are universal. Obey the laws of the community in which you live. Do not make unwanted advances to another employee in your workplace. Do not discriminate. Do not use vulgar language or dirty words in your workplace. Avoid conflicts of interest. Avoid even the appearance of a conflict of interest. Do not divulge confidential information. In other words, respect the basic rights of everyone around you.

As a Lab Director you will be supervisory to a part of a hospital where maybe 20 to 50 people work. You should try to set a good example for those below you. Lead by example.

    A. What to wear to work

Most hospitals have a dress code that is very vague. The following is a quote of one hospital's entire dress code: "Dress in a neat, clean, professionally appropriate manner". This is so vague as to be useless.

In most hospitals the personnel who will come into contact with patients are held to a higher dress standard than the personnel that will not have patient contact. As a Lab Director, you will not have patient contact on most working days. However, you will be enforcing dress code on the lab staff that does have patient contact. In my opinion, you should be dressed at least as well as the people you are enforcing dress code on; or else your enforcement of the dress code will be seen as hypocrisy.

In my 29 years in Pathology and Lab Medicine I have worked in widely disparate geographic locations. The dress code varies by locale. The description given below should be appropriate for most of the continental US.

For men: Wear dress pants, typically a dark color, without patterns. Wear a lighter colored dress shirt, long sleeve is preferred but short sleeve is acceptable. The shirt should be ironed or pressed. Wear a tie and a jacket or sport coat. The jacket or sport coat should be the exact same color as the pants. Wear dress shoes, typically dark color. This combination of clothes is known as a "business suit".

For women: Skirt or trousers, with matching jacket and a blouse. More variation is allowed than for men.

While in the continental US my usual daily routine is to dress up in the business suit in the morning. When I come to work the first thing I do is to take off the sport coat and set it on a hanger in my office area. The business suit minus the sport coat is called "business casual" or something similar. When going out for lunch and at the end of the day, I put the sport coat back on as the last thing I do before heading out of the office.

In some areas, the dress code is more casual. In the time I worked on Guam, some of the attending physicians came into the hospital in jeans and sneakers, and did their rounds wearing jeans and sneakers. There was even a story about a surgeon who was at the beach on the weekend, and was paged to come in for an appendectomy. He came into the hospital wearing nothing but swimming trunks, and had to change into scrubs to see the patient.

As far as I can tell, the dress code for Hawaii and the US Pacific territories is:

For men: Wear khaki colored cotton trousers and a shirt with floral patterns. Wear sneakers or similar casual shoes.

For women: Wear a skirt with floral patterns.

     B. Always know your relationship to your employer

I graduated from training in 1996 and took my first job as an attending Physician. I was hired into a municipal hospital on a GG1 form, a one page form that did not stipulate any conditions other than my salary and that I was full-time. This is what they offered me and I accepted. I was fresh out of training at the time, and did not have experience in negotiating salary, terms, etc.

The same hospital hired a variety of doctors on a variety of different terms. Some were hired as locum tenens, some were hired on contracts, some were hired on GG1 forms. Depending on the nature of the employment, some did or did not get callback pay, some did or did not have to clock in and clock out in the hospital's computer timecard system.

At the start of my employment, I was told that I had to clock in and clock out in the hospital's computer timecard system. I was not told anything about callback time. Over the course of the next 2 years and 9 months, I was called back a few times in the evenings and on weekends. I clocked in and clocked out as a callback. Some callback pay accrued during this time.

In March, 1999 the Medical Director called me in to his office and told me I was not eligible for callback pay. I had accrued about $3800 in callback pay over the course of the prior 2 years and 9 months. My base pay at the time was $156,000 per year so this was less than one percent of my base pay over the course of that time. I apologized to the Medical Director and said that he could make me a bill and I would pay back the $3800 in disputed callback pay.

The Medical Director was disproportionately upset about the callback pay. I found out later that the hospital was starting to have financial problems about this time. The Hospital Administrator had been repeatedly criticizing the Medical Director in private over excessive physician pay. The Medical Director took it out on me, chewing me out over a trivial amount of callback pay.

I made a point of being as nice as possible to the Medical Director. A few weeks later he made a bill for the $3800. I paid the bill to the Hospital Cashier the same day. When the canceled check came back I gave the Medical Director a copy of the canceled check.

Months later, sometime towards the end of 1999, I was offered a contract at the same hospital. I took the contract to my private attorney for review. I spent a long time in the attorney's office talking about the proposed contract, the GG1 form signed in 1996 and the callback pay. The attorney said that the Medical Director was wrong. I really was entitled to the $3800 callback pay. The attorney offered to sue for the disputed $3800. I said that it was best to take no action. The amount in question is trivial, and any action to reclaim the callback pay would only antagonize the hospital administration.

I have told this story to many people. Most people think I should have come out fighting, and given the Medical Director an argument over the $3800. The decision to turn the other cheek or not to turn the other cheek is a personal decision. I can't tell other people what to do in the same circumstance. Neither can anyone else tell me not to turn the other cheek. There are however a few take home points here:

1. Always know your relationship to your employer. In the above story, I did not know in advance if I was or was not entitled to callback pay.
2. Never antagonize your employer unless it is absolutely necessary.
3. In every situation where you will be negotiating, try to imagine the playing field from the point of view of your counterparty. Imagine that you are the Medical Director and you have just been called on the carpet for excessive physician salary. If you can imagine yourself in the Medical Director's predicament, you will understand why the Medical Director is doing what he does, and you will have some common ground to negotiate.

I worked at this hospital from 1996 to 2012. The story of my departure is relevant so I will include it here. As mentioned in the above story, the hospital had a deteriorating financial condition over time. This was never resolved in the time I worked there and seemed to slowly worsen over the years. By 2011 the hospital was in very poor financial condition and new management took over. At this time I was in the Pathologist position with someone else in the Lab Director position. The new management put in a rule that no physician employee could make more salary than the money he or she brought in to the hospital.

By the time this rule went into effect, there were only two physician administrators left at this hospital, the Nursing Home Director and the Lab Director. Both were laid off immediately after the new management took over. The new management felt that physician administrators had no measurable income for the hospital and the hospital could no longer afford their services. I was in the Pathologist position at the time, and the Lab Director duties were transferred to me after the Lab Director was laid off. The Nursing Home Director duties were transferred to an Internal Medicine physician.

A few weeks later, I was called in to the Hospital Administrator's office in regard to my salary. At the time, I was the only pathologist in this hospital. The Lab Director was already gone by the time of this meeting. I was told that the gross billing from histology and cytology combined was about $455,000/yr. and the collection rate was around 33%. They offered to drop my salary from $188,000/yr. down to $150,000/yr. to match the income I was bringing in to the hospital. I said that the added duties of the Lab Director position have some income. Medicare part B pays an amount for lab administration and part of this is intended for the Lab Director's salary. The Hospital Administrator asked me to document how much of the money was intended for the Lab Director's salary. I said that Medicare does not give a breakdown for this amount; therefore, I could not document how much is for the Lab Director's salary and how much of it is intended for other lab administration.

I also mentioned that the 33% collection rate is quite low compared to other hospitals and the hospital should try harder to collect its bills. A higher collection rate would justify more salary. The hospital was in effect penalizing its employee physicians for the hospital's low collection rate even though the physicians have no control over this. The hospital was not able to raise its collection rates in the remaining time I worked there. The patient base was largely indigent and unable to pay their bills.

The rates for pathology professional fees were low and I recommended that the hospital should raise its rates. The hospital was a municipal hospital and all rate increases had to be approved by the municipal utilities board. This process took years, and by the time the rate increases were implemented I had already left this municipality.

The Hospital Administrator said that I could only document income to the hospital of $150,000/yr. and asked me to voluntarily take a pay cut to this level. I said "no". The Hospital Administrator initiated paperwork intended to drop the salary of most of the physician employees at that hospital. However, this paperwork would take some time to route as this was a municipal government hospital and the paperwork needed approval from the local government Civil Service office. In the meantime, I began to look for other jobs elsewhere. I moved on to another job about a year after being asked to take a salary cut. At the time of my departure, the paperwork for the salary drop had not gone through yet. During this time, I was not in good graces with the Hospital Administrator. He was upset with any physician that did not accept pay cuts.

The moral of this story is that life is tough when you work for a financially troubled employer. Another important point to take home from this story is that a financially troubled hospital will see all physician administrators, including Lab Directors, as a liability. The administration tends to change over quickly in financially troubled hospitals. Be very careful taking a position at such a hospital. The Hospital Administrator that hired you could be gone quickly, and the next Hospital Administrator may see you as a liability.

I had a series of part-time side jobs in addition to my main job while working in that municipality. Before leaving that municipality, I thought about ramping up the side jobs, possibly setting up my own lab, and then quitting the day job. None of these options looked promising. This was a small municipality with only one hospital and no other pathologist job positions. There were already several clinical labs competing against each other in this municipality and the clinical lab market looked saturated. I applied for jobs elsewhere and was accepted at a job in a distant municipality. I made this cross-country move because the new job and new municipality offered much better opportunity.

    C. Avoid conflicts of interest

The term "conflict of interest" refers to when an individual or organization is involved in multiple related interests or transactions, one of which could possibly influence the motivation for an act in the other.

The term "arm's length transaction" refers to when the parties in a transaction are independent, equal and unrelated to each other. Any given transaction is either conflicted or arms length (not conflicted).

In 1996 I graduated from training and took my first attending level job at a hospital in a small community. I was hired into the Pathologist position. The Lab Director of that hospital had an outside job working as the lab director of an outpatient lab. The outpatient lab was a subsidiary of a large reference lab that the hospital had been sending its send-out specimens to.

This relationship was conflicted in two ways. First, the hospital Lab Director could divert specimens to the outside lab. As in any lab, some tests must obviously be sent out and some tests must be obviously done in-house. However, there are also many classes of specimens that are a "judgment call" as to whether to send out or examine in-house.

The conflict of interest arises from the temptation to send as many specimens as possible to the outside lab, so as to have less workload (i.e. less work for the same pay) at the hospital lab and enhanced revenue at the outside lab.

Secondly, the hospital Laboratory Director must determine if the reference Lab is doing a good job examining specimens from the hospital. The conflict of interest arises from the temptation to look the other way and/or cover up mistakes made by the reference lab.

From what I have been told, this small community had very limited numbers of qualified people in most fields, so the same people tend to occupy multiple different positions of authority at the same time.

There are not enough qualified people in this small community for all transactions to be arm's length (not conflicted). In order to have all the Lab Director positions at arm's length, one person would need to be Lab Director at the hospital, a different person Lab Director at each of multiple outside clinics, a different person Lab Director at Public Health, etc. Since there are not enough qualified people to fill all these positions, the Conflicts of Interest are tolerated as the least bad option.

Eventually, that hospital Lab Director position was reshuffled. The hospital Lab Director retired, but retained his lab directorship at the outside lab. I took over the hospital Lab Director position when it was vacated by retirement. Thus the conflict of interest was resolved amicably by reshuffling the position.

Later, I would take a position in a different small community. In August 2013 I was hired to "turnaround" a troubled lab in a remote area. The Lab Director had just quit, and the Lab Supervisor had been fired two years prior. When I started work at that lab, my first priory was to get the lab past an upcoming CMS inspection. After passing that CMS inspection, I went through the records to see how the Lab got into its troubled situation in the first place.

There was only one person in that small community who was qualified to be a Lab Supervisor and willing to take the Lab Supervisor position at the hospital. The hospital had a two other ASCP certified lab techs but they were adamant that they would not take the Lab Supervisor position. They did not want the Lab Supervisor position and the hospital regulations would not allow for involuntary promotion.

The only person who was qualified for the Lab Supervisor position and willing to fill the position also had part ownership in an outside lab in the same community.

Again the problem crops up that a small community has very limited numbers of qualified people in most fields. There are not enough qualified people for all transactions to be arm's length (not conflicted).

In this case, the Lab Supervisor cooked up a scheme in which the paying patients would be diverted from the hospital lab to the private lab he had part ownership of. The non-paying patients coming to his private lab would be diverted to the hospital lab.

This scheme was caught. I do not know exactly how it came to light, but that does not matter for the purpose of this story. This person was immediately forced to resign from the hospital Lab Supervisor position as soon as the scheme was caught. This was a serious blow to the hospital's lab, as there was no replacement for the Lab Supervisor. The hospital administration would not have taken this decision lightly. The lab fell into disarray and later the Lab Director quit. When I took over the leadership role in this lab, I had to carry out both the Lab Director and Lab Supervisor work, as there was no one else available to do it.

The point of this story is to avoid conflicts of interest. Avoid even the appearance of a conflict of interest. There may be situations in which you have to take on two conflicted positions since both positions are necessary and no one else is available to fill them. If you find yourself in this position, never ever act on the conflict of interest. If you act on a conflict of interest you are almost certain to get caught, your punishment will be severe and deservedly so.

Chapter 16 – Lab tech hiring, orientation, competency testing, promotion, retention and discipline

Lab techs are the "testing personnel" as defined under CLIA. Their responsibilities are spelled out in 42 CFR § 493.1475 and 42 CFR § 493.1495. To briefly summarize their job is to do the testing, document and maintain records of their work as necessary, follow the laboratory's procedure manual and quality control policies, identify and correct problems that may adversely affect testing and follow instructions from their supervisors.

Lab techs can be divided into technicians and technologists. Technicians typically have two years of post-secondary education (i.e. an associate's degree) while technologists have four years of post-secondary education (i.e. a bachelor's degree).

The CLIA qualifications for high complexity testing personnel are given in 42 CFR § 493.1489. The requirements for moderate complexity testing personnel are lower and given in 42 CFR § 493.1423. In the typical hospital lab there is a mix of waived, moderate and high complexity testing. A lab tech must be able to go back and forth from one analyzer to another, hence the CLIA high complexity testing personnel requirements serve as the minimum hiring criteria for lab techs at every hospital lab I have ever worked at.

To briefly summarize the CLIA high complexity testing personnel qualifications a lab tech must have an associate degree or higher level degree (doctorate, master's, or bachelor's) in a laboratory science, or MD, DO, or DPM or meet criteria from a list considered equivalent education and training. The equivalent education and training is a high school diploma plus at least 60 semester hours and either completion of a clinical laboratory training program or at least 3 months on-the-job training in each section of lab where the lab tech does high complexity testing. The lab tech must be licensed if licensure is required by the State the lab is located in. Anyone grandfathered under older rules can continue to work as a lab tech.

In my 29 years in Pathology and Lab Medicine, I have only once seen CMS inspectors question a lab tech's credentials. This occurred at a small municipal hospital that had hired me to "turnaround" its troubled lab. The lab was under heavy regulatory scrutiny mainly due to reagent outages. A team of CMS inspectors had been dispatched for a re-inspection.

The CMS inspectors completed this re-inspection relatively quickly, and had some spare time on their hands. They went through the personnel files, which I have never seen done at any other CMS inspection. They found that an older lab tech did not have documentation in his file of his military training as a Medical Laboratory Specialist. This was a 50 week course offered by the US Military prior to April 25, 1995. Without this training certificate in the lab tech's personnel file, it looked like the lab tech was a high school graduate doing high complexity testing.

The lab tech in question was called in during the inspection to speak with the CMS inspectors. The lab tech had a copy of this training certificate at home. The lab tech was sent home to get a copy of his training certificate so as to produce it to the inspectors. The certificate was decades old, and this lab tech had been working at the same hospital for decades. The personnel file indicated that the lab tech had produced a copy of this certificate at the time of hiring. The certificate should have been in the personnel file, but it was not there. Somehow a copy of this training certificate had been lost in the sands of time from this lab tech's personnel file.

The lab tech was able to produce a copy of the training certificate at the time of the inspection. This satisfied the CMS inspectors, they did not issue a citation. Later this lab tech asked the military to produce a copy of the training certificate directly to the lab. The military had a hard time finding the records for this decades old training, but did eventually produce it, mailing it to the lab.

CLIA makes the Lab Director responsible for adequate staffing of the lab. In my experience, recruitment of lab techs is very difficult, especially in the remote areas I have been working. From talking with others in the field, I think that the US as a whole has a shortage of lab techs. CLIA mandates that you have to hire adequate staffing, but frankly, there aren't enough qualified applicants to fill all of America's lab tech positions.

The best source for hiring lab techs is word of mouth. If you tell enough people in the lab field that your lab is hiring techs, you will eventually receive a call from a lab tech interested in working at your facility. While you are telling everyone else in the lab business that you are hiring for your lab, they will likely tell you that they have vacant positions in their labs that they would like to hire for.

If word of mouth doesn't work, try putting advertisements in the magazines most often read by lab techs - Advance for Medical Laboratory Professionals, American Journal of Clinical Pathology (AJCP), etc. Other possibilities include internet-based advertising of the vacant position(s) and paid recruiters.

I prefer word of mouth for hiring lab techs. When using word of mouth you will mostly get applications from techs that have worked at nearby labs. You will probably know that lab tech personally or by reputation. When you call to verify the references, you will personally know the Lab Supervisor on the other end of the phone call. I prefer getting the reference from a known quantity; someone I can trust.

An applicant responding to a journal advertisement will likely be from the other end of the country, an unknown quantity. The references will include an unknown Lab Supervisor from across the country. When you call this unknown Lab Supervisor, he or she will most likely only say positive things about the applicant. This Lab Supervisor doesn't know who you are; and likely would not feel comfortable saying anything negative about the applicant. You will have no idea if you can trust the reference.

Recruiting lab techs right out of school is common. One of the municipalities I worked at had a lab tech program at the local University which graduated about 30 students a year. Most years the entire graduating class of 30 lab techs had hiring arrangements in place months before they graduated. The local hospitals would recruit these students during the middle of their fourth year at school. At the time I was working at a municipal hospital which had a slow recruitment process. As a result of slow recruitment, this municipal hospital lost out on the best and brightest students, and had to take whatever students barely passed.

Later the University involved started having financial problems and closed this lab tech program. The University saw it as a small and unimportant program. All the local hospital labs protested the closing of the lab tech program, but the University stood firm saying that they could no longer afford the program. This only served to worsen the lab tech shortage in that municipality.

Recruitment of lab techs is oftentimes a "hard sell" with the hospital administration. The typical hospital administration is very cost-conscious and always looking to cut costs. Salary is one of the biggest expenses in the typical lab. The hospital administration typically wants to keep this to a minimum.

In this situation, the best thing to do is to keep track of the overtime hours and overtime salary paid to the existing lab techs. The overtime is typically paid at time and a half or more. If the overtime amounts to much more than the salary of a lab tech, you can tell the hospital administration that hiring a new lab tech would be a cost saving measure which would eliminate much of the overtime.

Most hospital labs I am aware of are short of staff and many are very short. I only know of a few hospital labs that have no vacancies in their lab tech positions. The typical hospital lab gets by with the existing staffing by making heavy use of overtime. If staffing drops further, the next step is to send out as much non-essential testing as possible.

Sending a test to a reference lab is typically much more expensive than doing the same test in-house. When the bill comes back from the reference lab, present the bill to the hospital administration. This usually gets the hospital administration's attention, and they will develop a sense of urgency in the lab tech hiring.

If staffing was to drop further, eventually essential services would need to be curtailed. I have only seen a few instances in which a hospital lab become so short of staff as to curtail essential services. In all instances, the backlash from the medical staff was so severe that the hospital administration quickly became motivated to hire lab staff.

There are a variety of certifying agencies for lab techs. The two I am most familiar with are American Society for Clinical Pathology (ASCP) and American Medical Technologists (AMT). CLIA does not recognize any of these certifying agencies. As far as I am concerned any lab tech with US training and an ASCP or AMT certification as a lab technician or lab technologist is good to go. I will not question their underlying education.

If they have work experience I am much more concerned about their recent evaluations than training that may be decades remote. If they are just graduating from training, they will get started out in entry level positions with little responsibility until they can prove themselves.

Occasionally you will be faced with evaluating foreign lab tech credentials. I have seen an occasional international applicant with the ASCPi (international ASCP) certification. My understanding is that the holder of ASCPi certification has training in all areas except US regulatory issues.

It would probably be difficult for someone with ASCPi certification to fill the Lab Supervisor position in the US. The Lab Supervisor position deals with regulatory issues, and the ASCPi certification specifically excludes US regulatory issues. There should be no problem with someone holding an ASCPi certification and filling a bench level lab tech or section supervisor position.

CLIA requires an equivalency evaluation for foreign lab tech credentials. The equivalency evaluation has to be performed by a nationally recognized organization or their affiliates. Such organizations include the National Association of Credential Evaluation Services (NACES), the Association of International Credential Evaluators (AICE) and others.

These organizations charge for the evaluation for foreign credentials. In general this cost burden falls on the applicant. In most labs, in order to consider a foreign-trained applicant for a lab tech position the equivalency evaluation must be submitted along with the job application. Without the equivalency evaluation, it is very hard to compare US and foreign credentials. Thus, the application is not considered complete until the equivalency evaluation is submitted.

In states where lab tech licensure is required, that license is the single most important credential for hiring. In states that do not require lab tech licensure, the most important point to look for is certification by one of the lab tech certifying agencies (ASCP, AMT, etc.). An exception to this certification requirement has to be made for students and recent graduates. They will not be able to sit for the certifying exam until about a year after graduation.

Next most important are the references, recent job evaluations, and grades in school. Be wary of any recent graduate that just barely passed, and had to repeat multiple classes in order to graduate. In my experience any hardworking person of average intelligence should be able to get through lab tech school with no problems. The barely passing student is either lacking in intelligence or lacking in effort or both.

The interview has the least importance in my lab. In my experience, a good talker is unlikely to be a hard worker, and vice versa. In the interview style will win out over substance. In my lab, the interview is done mainly to weed out unacceptable candidates. There are a few red flags in the interview that will disqualify a candidate or reduce their ranking.

In the interview you are looking for a lab tech that can think in a linear, logical manner. Ask the applicant how to do typical lab procedures such as phlebotomy or operating an analyzer. Multiple "I don't know" answers disqualifies the applicant. If the applicant is able to answer, but the steps of the procedure are given completely out of order, the applicant's ranking is reduced. If the response is a completely jumbled "word salad" the applicant is disqualified. If the applicant knows the steps of every procedure by heart and recites them all in the correct order, the applicant is moved up in ranking.

In my experience most people can hold themselves together long enough to get through an interview. I am aware of one lab tech passing the interview, and turning out to have a major alcohol problem. This lab tech was only able to stay sober on the day of the interview. At the other end of the spectrum, I have known very bright students who were so shy that they interviewed poorly. They became so intimidated at the interview they began talking in "word salad". Thus in my experience the interview is of little value.

CLIA makes the Lab Director responsible for ensuring that the lab staff are appropriately trained and demonstrate competency prior to testing patient specimens. In virtually every lab I have ever been to, this is delegated to the Lab Supervisor and/or section supervisors.

In my lab, when a lab tech is newly hired, that tech must go through orientation prior to doing any testing. Orientation usually consists of having the tech read the procedure manual for the section of lab they will be assigned to (this should take no more than 2 working days) and then having the section supervisor show the new lab tech the procedures for testing in that area of lab. Then the section supervisor will watch as the new lab tech does some testing. This should take no more than 2 weeks from the time the lab tech starts. The section supervisor will then sign off on the orientation paperwork, attesting that the newly hired lab tech is competent in that section of lab.

This stage of competency testing is very basic. I have only seen a few lab techs that needed to repeat orientation. I have never seen a lab tech fail orientation on the second try. If anyone repeatedly fails the orientation, inform the Personnel Office and ask for them to remove the employee.

Under CLIA the following are the minimum requirements for competency testing for all laboratory testing personnel. The competency testing must be done for each person, each test, at least semiannually during the first year and annually thereafter. Competency testing must be repeated if the test instrumentation and/or methodology changes, prior to reporting test results by the new instrument and/or method. It should evaluate competency to perform test procedures and report test results promptly, accurately and proficiently. The procedures for evaluation of the competency of the staff must include, but are not limited to:

1. Direct observations of routine patient test performance, including patient preparation, if applicable, specimen handling, processing and testing
2. Monitoring the recording and reporting of test results
3. Review of intermediate test results or worksheets, quality control records, proficiency testing results, and preventive maintenance records
4. Direct observations of performance of instrument maintenance and function checks
5. Assessment of test performance through testing previously analyzed specimens, internal blind testing samples or external proficiency testing samples
6. Assessment of problem solving skills.

The references are 42 CFR § 493.1413 (8) and 42 CFR § 493.1451 (8).

The competency assessment should evaluate the lab tech for all phases of testing, preanalytic, analytic and postanalytic. There should be direct observation of skills, not just a written test.

CLIA requires competency testing for each test done; however, in all labs I am familiar with the competency testing is done by section. In effect all tests done in one section of lab (e.g. chemistry, hematology, Blood Bank) are lumped onto one competency testing form. I will give an example of a Blood Bank competency testing form on pages 114 and 115. All other sections of lab (e.g. chemistry, microbiology, etc.) should have a similar form for competency testing in that section.

If a lab tech "floats" through multiple sections of lab, a competency testing form must be completed for each section that tech "floats" through, no matter how little that tech "floats". For example, if a blood banker "floats" through chemistry and performs only one test in chemistry during the year, that tech needs both blood bank and chemistry section competency testing forms completed.

The situation is not as clear if a lab tech is able to float, but has not actually done so in the last year. Let's say the blood banker in the above example is qualified in chemistry, but has not actually "floated" into chemistry and has not performed any chemistry tests in the last year. CLIA would not require competency testing in chemistry, only in Blood Bank for this tech.

In this situation, my recommendation is that this lab tech should be competency tested in both chemistry and Blood Bank if there is any chance at all this tech could be called upon to "float" to chemistry. I would further recommend that if the lab tech in this example is not competency tested in chemistry, the tech should be limited to Blood Bank and sidelined from chemistry, and this should be documented in writing.

My assessment: The check boxes are all "yes" or "no". Any lab tech that gets a "no" box checked off where it should be "yes" is immediately referred for additional education and/or training, and then re-tested. In my experience there are few lab techs that fail the initial competency testing, and almost none fail the annual competency testing.

I have not seen repeat competency testing failure after reeducation and/or retraining. If this were ever to happen, you would have to call the Personnel Office and/or Human Resources (HR) Department at your hospital to ask what to do. They would likely have policies requiring suspension or removal of any employee that repeatedly fails competency testing.

CLIA requires a lab tech to cease testing in any area of competency testing failure. If a lab tech passes competency testing in some sections of lab but not others, the lab tech must be restricted from testing in any section where that tech failed competency testing but could continue testing in any section where he or she passed competency testing.

The "yes" or "no" checkbox nature of the assessment assumes that competence is binary - all or none. In my experience competency is really a spectrum or continuum, ranging from perfect competence to perfect incompetence with infinite possibilities in between.

In my experience, competence tends to decline very slowly with age. You do not have to worry much about a lab tech that recently graduated from training. In order to get through training, his or her performance was evaluated by numerous professors. Be wary of any lab tech that is working past the usual social security retirement age, currently 66 years old.

MY LAB		COMPETENCY TESTING FORM	MY PROCEDURE MANUAL
Title	**Section**	**Type of Evaluation**	**Employee Name:**
Training and Competency Checklist	Blood Bank	☐ Initial Training ☐ Annual Competency ☐ Other: _____	Position Title: _____ Date of Hire: _____ Date of Assignment: _____

See Page 2 For Instructions to Complete Form

	Policy, Procedure, Function	Y	N	N/A
	TRANSFUSION SERVICE			
1	Fundamental knowledge of Blood Bank: antigen/antibody interaction, technical aspects of blood group system			
2	Familiarity with current recommendation of method, time restriction, sample quantity and type			
3	Familiarity of current guideline for handling, accepting / rejecting specimens			
4	Familiarity with crossmatch procedure			
5	Performance of ABO and Rh typing			
6	Performance of Antibody Screening: determine positive and negative results, identification of positive screen by antibody panel, evaluation of positive antibody and subsequent procedure ie. crossmatch			
7	Direct Antiglobulin Test (Coombs): principle and procedure			
8	Indirect Antiglobulin Test (Coombs): principle and procedure			
9	Transfusion reaction workup			
10	FFP, PC, Platelet, and Neonate set-up: correct paperwork, correct labels on bags, proper expiration dates and incubator temperatures, use of scale to determine weight			
11	Knowledgeable in: maintenance of blood sterility, adherence to expiration dates, storage temperatures- maintaining logs, proper refrigerator operation and temp.			
12	Knowledge of criteria for neonatal transfusion and exchange transfusion selection of blood: age (birth to 4 mos old), selection of blood, set-up procedure label and issue			
13	Knowledge of Emergency Transfusion: selection of blood, set-up procedure, label and issue			
14	Knowledge of compatibility testing: major / minor crossmatch, identification / label of specimens, cell washer procedure (including QC/PM), sample, controls, results, incubation time/temperature, serofuge time/RPM, agglutination determination, visual aid use (light/microscope), sample retention time/place			
15	Daily reagent quality control			
16	Daily QC/PM regarding: cleaning, gloving, safety, infection control, documentation/labeling			
17	Ensures that all procedures are followed exactly for all manual procedures performed.			
18	Knowledge of procedures for resolving technical problems, blood group discrepancies, antigen testing, prewarm technique, mono-specific AHG			
19	Determination of weight of bag, minimum amount, short draw, proc., tubing clamp, sealing tubing, proper component prep. and storage			
20	Knowledge of proper procedure for Therapeutic Phlebotomy: consent, scheduling, procedure, paperwork			
21	Knowledge and complete compliance of all QC and PM, safety and infection control requirements (gloves, cleaning, labeling reagents)			
22	Knowledge of FFP, PC, and Platelet preparation, temperature requirements, operation of centrifuge, use of plasma expressor, QC and log books, time and weight requirements			
	OTHER NOT LISTED ABOVE:			

Comments:
_____
_____

Employee Signature: _____ Date: _____

Supervisor Signature: _____ Date: _____

Lab Director Signature: _____ Date: _____

INITIAL TRAINING AND COMPETENCY CHECKLIST BLOOD BANK
Instructions for Supervisor/Evaluator
- Use correct form. A sample specific for your section should be in your manual.
- Refer to competency testing policy for general information.
- Use the following symbols to indicate competence:

Y: Yes, competent
N: No, needs training
N/A: Item not applicable

- If any failure to demonstrate competence is observed, the evaluator must initiate and complete a "Competency: Remediation Form". See the competency remediation procedure.
- Have employee sign and date the evaluation form indicating that he/she agrees with the evaluation.

Instructions for Employee

If you feel that the training and competency evaluation is inadequate or inappropriate, ask for a conference to include the section supervisor and Lab Supervisor.

Notice that in the lab where I work the form does not have checkboxes for an overall grade, not even "pass" or "fail" checkboxes. CLIA does not require an overall grade. All that is required is that any possible deficiencies are identified and corrected. If any deficiencies cannot be corrected, the lab tech cannot continue with the patient testing.

Although CLIA does not require an overall grade for the lab techs, most hospitals require an annual graded evaluation for every employee. In the hospital lab where I work the Personnel Office makes us use the hospital-wide Annual Employee Evaluation Form to give the lab techs an overall grade. Most labs assign an overall grade to the lab tech as part of the competency testing. If an overall grade is assigned, it may be "pass" or "fail". Alternatively, a variety of gradations may be used such as:

1. Outstanding. The lab tech does more work than is expected, works independently, is able to supervise other lab techs, and/or has skills or knowledge beyond that expected for a lab tech allowing the tech to do something extraordinary such as taking on work in areas a tech would not be expected to work in. The lab tech arrives early, leaves late and has not missed one working day in the time frame being evaluated. The lab tech has made no mistakes at all during the time frame being evaluated.

2. Acceptable. The lab tech does the amount of work expected of a lab tech in the time allotted, functions independently and may or may not be able to supervise other lab techs. The lab tech shows up to work on time and doesn't abuse sick leave. The lab tech will make a very rare mistake that doesn't affect patient care and will correct his or her own mistakes.

3. Barely acceptable. The lab tech may not get all the assigned work done on all days. The lab tech needs frequent supervision to ensure that the job is done correctly and/or all work is done. The lab tech may come in to work late and/or abuse sick leave on occasion, but not consistently. The lab tech makes occasional mistakes that have to be corrected by other lab techs but these do not have the potential to cause patient harm.

4. Unacceptable. The lab tech is not able to get much work done and/or not able to function independently The lab tech requires constant supervision. If not constantly supervised, will not do any work and/or will make frequent mistakes that have the potential to cause patient harm. The lab tech consistently comes in late and abuses sick leave. Other lab techs have to spend a good deal of their time correcting this tech's mistakes.

The evaluation form is filled out behind closed doors. The lab tech is called in to a closed door meeting with his or her supervisor and presented with the findings. The tech is asked to sign the form. There is a field on the form for the lab tech to write in any responses if he or she wants. The form is typically filed with that lab tech's other competency testing documents in a folder kept in a locked file cabinet. The key to that locked file cabinet is kept secure usually by hiding the key someplace where only the Lab Supervisor and Lab Director know to find it. The typical hospital requires a copy of all completed competency testing forms to be forwarded to the hospital's HR department.

The CLIA regulations delegate the competency testing to the technical supervisor position of a high complexity testing lab or the technical consultant position in a moderate complexity testing laboratory. This position is called "Lab Supervisor" in most of the laboratories I have worked in. This creates a problem when the technical consultant and/or technical supervisor is the only person performing the testing. This situation came up in a small, remote laboratory where I was lab director. This lab had a large menu of waived tests but only one moderate complexity test - TB testing by

GeneXpert. The problem is that there was only one lab staff qualified to operate the GeneXpert and this same person was the technical consultant. There were two other lab staff on site, but they were not trained to operate the GeneXpert analyzer. In this situation, I recommended three possible routes of action:

1. Train more of the lab staff on site to operate the GeneXpert analyzer. The technical consultant and the lab staff could then perform competency assessment on each other.
2. Send the technical consultant off site once per year for competency testing.
3. Someone qualified to operate a GeneXpert analyzer flies in every year to evaluate the technical consultant's competency.

Option #1 was chosen as it was the most cost effective. Furthermore, other people at that lab would need to know how to operate the GeneXpert in case the technical consultant was away from work for an extended time.

Another related topic is promotion and retention of lab staff. Most of the labs I have worked at have a core membership of long term techs who have been working at that lab for many years. They tend to occupy the Lab Supervisor and section supervisor positions. This group is older, typically at least age 50, and will stay at the same lab until retirement.

As each one retires, another member of this long term group moves up to the position vacated by retirement. Hence, for this cadre, promotion occurs by the retirement of the person above them. This is not a problem when one of the section supervisors retires. The number two person in that section automatically moves up to the section supervisor position. The number three person in that section automatically moves up to the number two position, etc.

This creates a problem when the Lab Supervisor retires. The Lab Supervisor position is up for grabs and most of the section supervisors will be interested. Only one section supervisor can be promoted to the Lab Supervisor position. You must be prepared to give something of value to the section supervisors who applied for the Lab Supervisor position but were passed up.

There is a group of younger techs working in the bench level positions. They are younger and more mobile. In most labs, the retention efforts are mainly directed to the younger, more mobile lab techs.

At most of the labs I have worked at retention has been difficult. These hospitals were cash strapped and couldn't afford raises or bonuses. Other smaller perks could be offered, such as the off-site analyzer training which tends to be seen as a free vacation.

In my experience, lab tech compensation is determined by the hospital. As Lab Director you do not have much input in determining the hourly salary rates for the various positions in lab. If a valuable lab tech receives a higher paying offer from another lab, you cannot raise the hourly rate for that lab tech's position. The only way you can counteroffer is by offering to promote that lab tech to a higher paying position. In order to carry out this reshuffling, there needs to be a higher paying position vacant in lab.

If the hospital offers annual increments, it is imperative that the lab completes the paperwork in a timely manner. If this paperwork is delayed the techs will likely not receive their increments for that year. These increments will be seen as automatic by the lab techs. If you fail to give out the annual increments, this will be seen by the affected lab techs as a huge affront.

Without much to offer in the way of financial incentives for retention, the best you can do as Lab Director is to ensure a nice, happy working environment where everyone is as friendly as possible. There are numerous points to mention is this regard. In my experience it is best to allow every position in lab as much autonomy as possible. The techs can function independently, so allow them complete autonomy. If you micromanage, and take away their autonomy, it will cause resentment. If a lab tech makes a suggestion for improvement to the lab, take that suggestion seriously. In the majority of situations, treat the lab techs as equals, not subordinates.

Lab staff discipline and termination are among the most contentious issues in lab. No one is perfect and everyone will make an occasional mistake. The Lab Supervisor is tasked with the discipline of the lab staff and as such, it is the Lab Supervisor's judgment call if any person in lab is making significant mistakes too often.

As Lab Director I generally respect this judgment call by the Lab Supervisor. I am not a lab tech whereas the Lab Supervisor is. The Lab Supervisor knows the ins and outs of a lab tech's job and if the Lab Supervisor makes a judgment call that one of them is making too many mistakes, I will back the Lab Supervisor's decision. The only exception is if there seems to be some personal grudge involved. In that circumstance I will ask the Lab Supervisor privately if he or she is sure that the action being taken is the right thing to do.

In theory there is a long list of causes to remove an employee. Aside from mistakes this would include behavior problems, low productivity, alcohol problem, even poor morale. In reality mistakes are almost the only cause I have seen for a lab tech's removal.

Most hospital labs are short of staff and many are very short. They can't be choosey in who they employ. I have known of a lab tech who had an alcohol problem so severe that he was in and out of rehab for more than 2 years. That tech was allowed to work the entire time that he was not locked up in rehab.

I have almost never seen a lab tech removed for behavior problems. I am aware of lab techs with major mental illnesses including schizophrenia and manic depression. If the lab tech is on medication, and the mental illness is under control, they can continue to work. They cannot work if actively hallucinating or having a manic phase. Generally the tech will know the difference and call in sick if they are not able to work. The supervisor will be familiar with the tech's problems, and is usually quickly able to tell if the tech can work on days that tech comes in.

The lab tech mentioned above in the section on spotting a potentially suicidal employee was getting divorced, repeatedly late to work and repeatedly crying at work. The Lab Supervisor decided that this lab tech did not need mandatory referral to a Psychiatrist. This lab tech would eventually sort things out on her own, completing the divorce and moving on with her life.

In some circumstances low productivity is not a cause for removal either. I know of one older lab tech who had a stroke resulting in weakness in his right hand. He was able to return to work, but his productivity was very low, about half of what it had been before the stroke. He applied for disability retirement, but the retirement board said that he could still work and he was not disabled. He continued to work for a few more years until he reached his age based retirement. During that time, the other lab staff pitched in to help with the work, so as to make up for his low productivity.

Let's review the situation discussed in chapter 12 of the phlebotomist who switched specimens, putting the wrong patient barcode labels on two tubes of blood. There is no question this is a huge mistake, and could easily cause patient fatalities. The hospital administrative manual states that grounds for disciplinary action include inexcusable failure to discharge duties in an efficient manner. The progressive discipline scheme is as follows:

1. Verbal warning from supervisor
2. Written warning from supervisor
3. Suspension for 2 weeks
4. Termination for cause.

The hospital administrative manual also states that if the offense is particularly serious, you can skip the first two steps and start with the third step. Although the switching of specimens is a huge mistake, let's say the phlebotomist has been a long term employee with a good track record up to this point. The Lab Supervisor decides for convenience that this can be a four step progressive discipline pathway instead of a two step progressive discipline pathway.

The progressive discipline scheme given above starts with a verbal warning. For less serious offenses, this can be a simple reminder from the Lab Supervisor of the lab's policies, for example "the lab's policies require all employees to arrive at work on time".

For a serious mistake such as switched specimens, the counseling is done in a closed-door meeting usually by the Lab Supervisor with the section supervisor and Lab Director present in the room. Be as nice as possible. At the minimum, you have to inform that person of the offense that person committed, the possible or actual adverse effects to patient care, the lab and/or hospital policy that has been violated, discuss how to prevent recurrences, and the consequences of further violations of that policy.

Usually, that one meeting shakes up the phlebotomist enough that he or she will never switch another specimen. The Lab Supervisor may want to follow up at regular intervals to see how that phlebotomist is doing. This could be done in additional closed-door meetings, and/or the Lab Supervisor can simply ask the phlebotomist in passing "Have you been remembering to check the patient wristbands while drawing?"

If that phlebotomist never again switches specimens, the problem is solved. If that phlebotomist continues to switch specimens, follow the progressive discipline procedure outlined above. Each step of the pathway involves a closed-door meeting with the person being disciplined. The meetings are typically conducted by the Lab Supervisor with the section supervisor and Lab Director present in the room.

Each of these meetings follows the same general outline: recite the list of offenses that person has committed, the possible or actual adverse effects to patient care, the lab and/or hospital policy that has been violated, discuss how to prevent recurrences, and the consequences of further violations of that policy.

Each step of the pathway likely has a form associated with it, e.g. written counseling form, suspension for cause form, termination for cause form. The Lab Supervisor will fill out the appropriate form, sign it and present it to the employee during or after the meeting described above. The employee may sign it or refuse to sign. Either way it is a valid document after you sign it as Lab Director. The final disposition of the form is dictated by the progressive discipline procedure. Typically the completed form ends up in the employee's competency testing folder with a copy going to the employee and another copy going to the hospital's Personnel Office.

In most hospitals the employee is allowed an appeals procedure. It is important to follow the progressive discipline procedure to the letter. If you deviate even one iota from the progressive discipline procedure, the appeals process could overturn your decisions.

No one likes to wave the axe on coworkers. It will make you extremely unpopular with the entire lab staff. If you have worked with this lab tech for many years your participation in the progressive discipline meetings will make you feel like you are Judas, the betrayer. At progressive discipline meetings I will let the Lab Supervisor do most of the talking. I will back up the Lab Supervisor as necessary, but he or she is really in charge of these meetings. As Lab Director you should make someone else wear the black hat to the extent possible.

Chapter 17 – Administration, management, planning and deciding which tests to do in-house

Administration is defined as the process of running an organization. Management is defined as controlling or supervising an organization. I tend to see administration as determining the overall direction and purpose of the organization with management implementing the plans made by administration.

In most hospitals and hospital laboratories, there is no distinction between management and administration. I tend to use these terms interchangeably, as do most other authors writing about clinical laboratory administration and management. The majority of topics discussed in this book would count as lab administration or management.

The clinical lab administration and management literature covers business plans, managed care, marketing plans, health care economics, ownership structure, finances such as calculating return on investment, revenue projections, pricing of lab tests, etc. In my experience hospital labs have little to no input in the hospital's business plans, pricing of lab tests, etc. These are handled by the hospital's administrator, Chief Financial Officer (CFO), etc. Knowledge of these topics would only be required in a freestanding lab not affiliated with a hospital. I will not discuss business plans or health care finance further as this knowledge is not needed in the typical hospital lab. Lengthy discussion of these topics can be found elsewhere in the clinical lab literature. Other topics covered frequently in the same literature include time management, how to prepare your own resume and apply for job positions, delegation, prioritization, etc. I will not go into detail in regard to these topics as there is already abundant literature written on these topics.

In regard to ownership structure, this is typically mandated on the lab by the hospital's administration. At the time most hospitals were built, clinical labs were typically a department of the hospital. Later, in the 1980s and 1990s, the healthcare industry had a large number of mergers, acquisitions, and spinoffs. Other types of lab ownership structures, such as partnerships, joint ventures, not-for-profit corporations, merger with a commercial reference laboratory, etc. were mandated on a few hospital laboratories. The majority of hospital laboratories remain a department of their hospital. As such the hospital's management can change the ownership structure of lab at will, and lab has little to no input in this decision making. The typical laboratorian has no ownership interest in the lab he or she works for. If the hospital's administration decides to change the lab's ownership structure, the typical laboratorian must either play along, or seek employment elsewhere.

I will touch on customer satisfaction briefly, as this is important to all clinical labs. Most of your patients will have no medical knowledge .As such, they will judge your lab based on cleanliness, accessibility, telephone waiting time, telephone etiquette and the interaction with the lab staff they meet. The patients will likely only meet the phlebotomists and never meet the testing personnel. As such, it is important for the phlebotomists to have a professional appearance, compassion and sympathy. Unfortunately, your patients may judge your lab based on the size of the bills they receive, and this billing is largely out of lab's control. The hospital's providers will judge your lab by their perceived quality of the lab test results.

CAP's criteria for the Clinical Laboratory Director lists strategic planning. This is defining the lab's direction and making decisions on allocating its resources to pursue this direction.

In my experience, most labs plan to stay the same forever. The next year's budget is the same as last year's budget with a small increment to make up for inflation. I have not seen an existing lab make a major change in direction. When labs change, it is usually in small steps. Most Lab Directors and lab management are very conservative in this regard.

Testing has changed over the years, and hospital labs have kept up with technology for the most part. When I stated in the field, neither troponin nor BNP testing was readily available to the small community hospital. They were added as they became available on the chemistry equipment in use at the typical hospital lab. Later troponin became available as a point of care test, and the hospitals I have worked at all switched troponin to point of care testing.

During the same time frame, some older tests and methodologies have been discontinued. When a test is discontinued by the manufacturer, it forces the hospital labs using that test to switch to newer methodology. In my first job out of training, I had looked at occasional blood parasite smears to rule out malaria. Now that test is obsolete and replaced by a DNA technique which is much more sensitive than the human eye. Blood parasite smears have been discontinued by most small hospital labs.

My assessment of the field is that everything is moving to waived testing. More and more tests are available as waived tests, and this seems to be the direction that everything is heading.

The decision as to which tests to send out and which tests to run in-house depends on both economic and medical considerations. If there is an overriding medical necessity for putting the test in-house you will have to do so no matter what the cost. This situation is relatively rare, and in my experience for most analytes this decision making is based on economics.

If any given analyte is sent out for testing and you are looking to bring the test in-house do the following. First, determine the medical necessity. Ask the providers that most frequently order the test what their feelings are in regard to the current arrangement. Is the turnaround time fast enough? How heavily do they rely on the results of the test when evaluating patients?

If the providers want a fast turnaround time and depend heavily on the test, you are obligated to put the test in-house, otherwise you are making the decision based on economics.

Here's how to get a rough feel for the economics of testing in-house. Add up the total number of tests for that analyte sent out over the last year. Multiply this by the cost per test to figure the annual amount spent on that testing. Figure out how much the supplies and reagents would have been to do this many tests in-house. Remember to add in the costs of PT testing, controls, calibrators, tech time, capital expenditures for new equipment, depreciation of equipment, etc.

I like to see the in-house testing on paper look at least 10% to 20% less expensive than send out testing before proceeding. Oftentimes there are hidden costs with in-house testing that you don't initially figure on. If the numbers come out favorable for in-house testing, then that is the way to go.

The more often a test is ordered the better the in-house testing does financially. If you put a new test in-house make sure to advertise it – send a memo to the medical staff telling them that the test is available in house with a short turnaround time. Present a grand rounds on the disease associated with that particular test, etc. The more you raise awareness of the test, and/or the disease associated with that test, the more the test will be ordered, and the better that particular test will perform financially.

Chapter 18 – Other duties delegated to the Lab Director

The Lab Director is responsible for everything in lab in much the same way a captain is responsible for everything on his or her ship. I have seen literature indicating that the Lab Director has responsibility for such things as test development, the workflow in Lab, the decor on the walls, billing, keeping the internet connection up, etc. In my opinion, this is perpetuating a myth. A myth is defined as a belief that is persistent, pervasive yet unrealistic.

It is unrealistic to expect the Lab Director to do everything in Lab, such as test development, the workflow in lab, choosing the internal decor, billing, keeping the internet connection up, etc. Few hospitals do their own test development, instead the testing equipment is bought from vendors. The rest of this list is all delegated to the Lab Supervisor, hospital-wide interior decorator, billing department, Information Services Department, etc. The captain of a ship is held up to the same unrealistic expectations, and likewise delegates these duties off to multiple subordinates.

I will give lab workflow as an example. The workflow can be summarized as follows. A doctor comes in for rounds, sees a patient and orders tests. The nurse types the order in the computer. The doctor reviews the order and verifies it in the computer using his or her electronic signature. The nurse may or may not need to prepare the patient (overnight fast, instruct patient on urine collection, etc.). The order is transmitted in the hospital computer to the lab. This will print out a page in the phlebotomy pick up printer. This page will include the patient name, room number, and type of tube to draw (green top). Lab will check the order for completeness.

The phlebotomist will come to the patient's bedside, identify the patient by wristband using at least two identifiers on the wristband, draw the patient, properly label the tube and return to the lab with the specimen. The specimen may or may not need centrifugation. The tube of blood is handed off to the lab tech doing the testing. The lab tech will check the specimen for adequacy. The test is run and the results go from the analyzer to the hospital's computer system. The results are now viewable in the patient's hospital computer chart. Any critical and/or STAT test results are called to the doctor.

Essentially none of this process is under the direct supervision of the Lab Director. Some of the action involves the nurse and doctor on the ward, such that the Lab Director does not have any authority over the action. The workflow pathway is largely determined by the hospital's computer system. In other words, the hospital's computer typically has only one way to handle test requests, specimen routing, and test results such that all tests must follow this pathway. Yet the Lab Director is responsible for the entire process, from start to finish, much the same way the captain of a ship is responsible for everything on the ship.

In this circumstance, do the same thing that a ship's captain would do, optimize everything you can. Make sure that everything under your control is running smoothly and hope that the ship never sinks. If it does, you may be going down with that ship.

Several tasks are made the responsibility of the Lab Director under CLIA. This includes making sure the physical and environmental conditions of the laboratory are adequate and appropriate for the testing performed, the environment for employees is safe from physical, chemical, and biological hazards and safety and biohazard requirements are followed.

In my experience this is almost always delegated to the hospital's safety office, employee health, or other similar office outside Lab. The Lab Supervisor enforces the lab's internal policies such as universal precautions. I have never seen a Lab Director taking an active role in physical or environmental issues within lab. For example, if there is ever a significant chemical spill in lab (not uncommon given the amount of formalin used in histology section) the lab techs call the hospital's Safety Office first and inform the Lab Director after the fact.

Essentially all clinical labs in the US are covered by the Occupational Safety and Health Administration (OSHA) regulations. These regulations require that for all toxic substances used in the workplace, the Safety Data Sheet (SDS) has to be readily available in the workplace. This requirement is typically met by having each section of lab store a 3 ring binder with all the relevant SDS sheets in the same cabinet as that section's procedure manuals. There is no regulatory requirement for Lab Director signatures on the SDS sheets. I have never signed an SDS binder nor have I ever been asked to.

Other OSHA regulations covering lab require that Personal Protective Equipment (PPE) be available for use and in good working order. The lab must train the staff on how to put on, use and take off the PPE. The lab must have procedures for infectious agent containment, ventilation failure, first aid, fires, emergencies and controlling the risk of exposure to chemical and biological hazards. The lab must ensure clean and sanitary conditions. Fire extinguishers, emergency eyewashes and showers must be tested on a routine basis to ensure good working order. The lab must keep a record of all workplace accidents, spills and exposures and prepare an annual summary. The lab must ensure waste disposal meets OSHA regulations. OSHA will inspect each lab annually.

OSHA does not specifically require fire drills, but recommends that they should be conducted at least annually. Most hospitals I have worked at have annual fire drills and disaster drills. These can be a fun diversion from the routine work at hand. The simplest disaster drill consists of herding all the lab staff out into a corridor deemed to be safe from tornadoes. I have been to much more elaborate drills, including mass casualty disaster drills conducted as a joint exercise between the hospital and airport. In these drills actors were painted with red paint at the airport to simulate blood then driven by ambulance to the hospital. One fire drill I went to had a "live fire" exercise in which the trainers took the trainees into the parking lot, set fire to a barrel full of newspapers and the trainees one-by-one had to put out the fire using a fire extinguisher.

TJC and CAP require all labs to have a disaster plan. Most of the lab disaster plans I have seen center on recalling staff, stockpiling enough reagents and supplies to meet an anticipated surge in lab testing after the disaster, stockpiling blood units in Blood Bank, limiting testing to STAT testing (no routine testing until the disaster is over), stockpiling food and water for the hospital staff and patients, stockpiling fuel for the generator, leadership and chain of command delegation (Incident Commander takes over from Hospital Administrator until the disaster is over), increased security presence, communication using satellite telephones, making back-up copies of lab records, plans for shutdown of the lab with evacuation of the building, plans to relocate testing to a different site, etc. The disaster plan is usually kept in the laboratory's general procedure manual. Everyone in lab is required to read and sign the disaster plan as well as the rest of the lab's general procedure manual.

After a major disaster, the most important tasks relate to continuity of the lab's operations. The lab's goal after a community-wide disaster is to continue with the testing and preserve lab records to the extent possible.

In my 29 years in Pathology and Lab Medicine I have been present for four disasters that I consider to be major disasters – the August 6, 1997 crash of Korean Airlines flight 801 on Guam, Typhoon Pongsona on December 8, 2002 on Guam, Typhoon Soudelor on August 2, 2015 on Saipan and Typhoon Yutu on October 24, 2018 on Saipan. In each of these disasters, some the above list of preparations helped somewhat. Most of the above list of preparations would prove unnecessary; while other, unexpected problems cropped up. In other words, in this setting you need to be flexible and find workarounds for problems as they appear.

The only real mass casualty disaster I have attended to was the August 6, 1997 crash of Korean Airlines flight 801. It went down on Guam with 254 people aboard a little after 1AM. At the time of the crash, I was one of three Pathologists working at Guam Memorial Hospital (GMH) and there was a military pathologist at the Guam Naval Hospital. The Guam Medical Examiner was on vacation and unavailable at the time of the crash. At about 3AM I was paged to come in to work at GMH and stationed at the Blood Bank. The other GMH Pathologists were assigned to the site of the crash and tasked with body identification and body recovery. The Navy pathologist was assigned to work at the Naval Hospital Blood Bank to help mobilize their frozen blood supply.

In the first 24 hours after the crash, GMH Blood Bank drew close to 100 blood donors. I did the donor screening and most of the donor interviews. There were 6 lab techs that drew the donors. We all worked non-stop at a frantic pace the first 24 hours after the crash. If anyone told me that it would be possible to do that much work in 24 hours I would not have believed them.

In this particular disaster there were few survivors. Only about 28 of the 254 people on board the aircraft survived. There was little surge in test volume after the crash, since there were few survivors. The main problem for lab related to morgue capacity. The number of deceased remains recovered from the crash far exceeded the morgue capacity of all local hospitals, the Medical Examiner's and all local funeral homes combined. The body recovery and identification occurred over several weeks on the Navy Base. The first intact 75 bodies were brought to a Navy refrigerated storage location and later the bodies and body parts were placed in refrigerator trucks. Many of the remains were fragmented which made identification difficult. In many cases identification was by DNA matching to surviving relatives. In the late 1990s this type of testing took months to complete. Most of the remains were stored in refrigerated trailers until they could be identified and buried.

Here is a picture of the service pin I received from the Government of Guam for my work done after the crash of KAL flight 801.

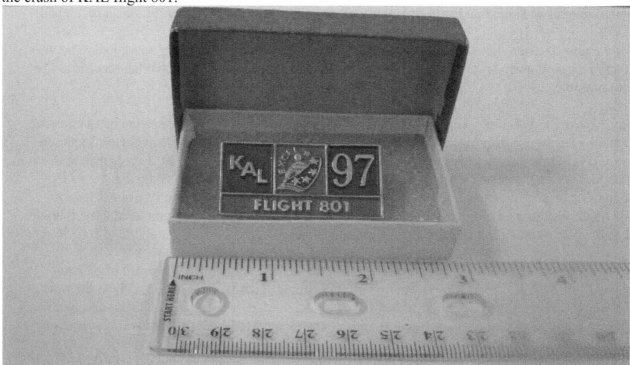

I was on Guam at the time of Typhoon Pongsona which hit December 8, 2002. This storm would have been considered a category 4 hurricane if it was on the Atlantic; however, different terminology is used in the Pacific. It was not a mass casualty disaster on Guam, there were no direct fatalities. However, it did extensive damage to the infrastructure. As is typical of a major disaster, there was no running water for weeks, no electric power for months, and no gasoline at the gas stations for about 2 weeks. The roads were impassable for several days until the debris was removed from the roadways. The telecommunication system also failed with almost all telephone poles and lines downed by the storm. Cellphones were restored in a few days but landlines and internet service took months to restore. Once cellphones came back up we were placing supply/reagent orders using cellphones until the landlines and internet service were restored.

At the time of the storm, the electric grid failed and the hospital went on generator power. The hospital's generator failed in the storm and the hospital was without electric power for about 12 hours. Testing had to be suspended while there was no electric power, but resumed after the hospital's generator was restored. Some parts of lab had flooded from rainwater permeating a damaged roof. This was relatively easy to clean up with no structural damage to the interior of the lab from the storm.

It took weeks to restore the connection to the local electric utility, and during this time the lab was running on the hospital's generator power. Generator power is subject to frequent spikes and outages, which disrupted lab's operations. As mentioned previously, it is imperative to have all critical equipment on UPS's. Any equipment that was not on a UPS would be damaged or destroyed by the power outages and power spikes in this situation.

Under these conditions, the hospital-wide computer system is very problematic. It tends to crash with each power out and power spike. If the hospital-wide computer system is going to be down for an extended length of time, the lab will have to revert to printing paper lab results and hand delivering the paper lab results to the wards, ER, clinics, etc. In this situation, make sure to inventory your stock of printer paper and toner cartridges, as you will be using these up much faster than usual. You may also need to ask for additional secretarial help to hand deliver all the paper lab reports.

The hospital's generator was not powerful enough to fully run the air conditioning system. Several lab instruments began to give overheat alarms. These instruments had their covers removed, and were cooled by fan while still continuing with the testing.

After a major disaster, the airport and seaport will be closed for a few days to a few weeks due to damage at their facilities. All supplies will dwindle during this time and there will be no way to restock. Day five after a major disaster looks worse than day one after the disaster as all supplies dwindle down.

In the immediate aftermath of Typhoon Pongsona, the main problems related to resupply. The airport was closed for about 2 weeks after the storm, and by the time it reopened the lab was running low or running out of most essential items. Some local vendors had their businesses completely destroyed, or had major loss of inventory in the storm. Most local vendors were unable to open their businesses most days because of lack of electric power to run the vendor's computers and inventory system and lack of employees reporting to work. The reason most employees were not reporting to work was because of impassable roads, lack of gasoline at the gas stations making commuting impossible, the large number of damaged/destroyed houses were a more immediate priority than work, and the employees needed to secure food and drinkable water for themselves and their families.

At the start of each working day, the first thing I would do is to check what is working and what is not working in lab, check which testing is available and which testing is suspended due to reagent outage. Next I would inventory all critical supplies in lab, then call all the vendors to see which vendors would be able to open for business that day and which would not. Each time a vendor was able to open, I would ask the hospital's Materials Management Office to buy as much lab-related inventory as possible, since there was no way of knowing if that vendor would be able to open their business again in the short term.

FEMA staff did not arrive at the hospital until about 2 days after the storm passed. They were not present in large numbers until at least 5 days after the storm. Their first priority was ensuring adequate supplies, continuous electric power and potable water for the hospital. Immediately after arriving, the FEMA staff will typically call a meeting with all hospital department heads and separate meetings with hospital administration. Be prepared to give the FEMA staff a copy of your inventory lists and list of reagent shortages/outages the first time you meet with them.

Many of the businesses that were destroyed in the storm never reopened. Instead the owners collected the insurance checks and moved to the US Mainland, relocating their businesses. The reduced number of vendors available after the storm affected procurement.

It is particularly important to keep the microbiology testing functional. The conditions after a disaster are conducive to epidemics - large numbers of people crowded into shelters, lack of running water for basic hygiene, lack of basic sanitation, lack of drinkable water, etc.

Staffing was an issue after Pongsona. In the immediate aftermath of the storm most lab staff were not able to report to work due to impassable roads, no gas at the gas stations, their homes were damaged or destroyed, they needed to secure food and drinkable water for themselves and their families, etc. Lack of gasoline was a greater problem for lab staff that lived further from the hospital as they would need more gas to commute to work. A rule was put in place that each staff member must work until relieved (i.e. until their replacement arrived to work). This resulted in many lab staff having to work two consecutive 8-hour shifts. We tried to arrange things so that no one had three consecutive 8-hour shifts, but this was unavoidable in a few cases.

On a personal level, Guam after Pongsona resembled a death trap. There was little access to food or drinkable water. The hospital reserved its food and water for the patients and did not give any food or water to the employees. There was no way out - the airport was closed. At the time the storm hit, I had about two week's supply of food and water in my apartment. For the first two weeks after Pongsona, I was using up the food and water in my apartment. The next several weeks, it was catch as catch can in a time when stores would reopen, quickly sell out of all food and water, then close again until they could restock. During most of this time frame I had less than a 2 day supply of food and drinkable water available. FEMA eventually provided Meal Ready to Eat (MRE) rations to the hospital staff. This was too little, too late, and the MRE were not very appetizing anyhow. The situation would improve later on as more stores restocked and reopened.

The airport cleared its runway of debris and reopened for flights about 2 weeks after the storm. After the airport reopened there was a mass exodus. I can't count how many going-away parties I went to in the next 3 months. I am guessing about 10% to 20% of the population left and never returned. A few lab staff quit and moved away, but the test volume was down due to mass exodus, so this pretty much evened out. Things did not reach a more normal state until about 3 to 6 months after the storm.

I was on Saipan at the time of Typhoon Yutu which hit October 24, 2018. It was the equivalent of a strong Category 5 hurricane on the Atlantic. This storm hit with sustained winds of 180 MPH making it the second strongest landfalling tropical cyclone in the history of the US and the sixth strongest landfalling tropical cyclone in the history of the world. It did considerably more damage than any prior typhoon I have seen. The usual post-disaster problems of protracted airport closure and staff unable to report to work occurred. The hospital did not lose power or water. However, as is typical of a major disaster there were protracted power outages in the community. The recovery of the water system and gas at the gas stations was faster than for previous typhoons.

After this disaster, the main problem from lab's perspective related to the airport closure. The airport was not able to open for inbound traffic for about a week after the storm. Several shipments were delayed including our hematology controls. The hematology controls arrived warm with the ice packs melted. We contacted the vendor's technical service department and they said to test the controls. We ran 20 repeat runs of the received warm controls and the results were acceptable. The technical service department said to use the received warm controls. Even so, I insisted on a replacement and the vendor replaced the received warm controls with a new shipment of controls which were received cold.

Another problem after Typhoon Yutu involved shipping of specimens off from Saipan for reference testing. For example, the lab receives numerous specimens for tuberculosis testing, but only has a BSL-2 capability. All specimens for tuberculosis culture must be sent out and the nearest reference lab offering tuberculosis culture is in Hawaii. The airport remained closed for outbound shipments for about two weeks after the storm. After about 2 weeks, I received notice from the hospital's preparedness office that the airport had reopened for outbound shipments.

Over the course of the next week, all local couriers were refusing to accept outbound shipments as they had not received the "all clear" from the airport to send outbound shipments. It took several phone calls, meetings and E-mail to inform all the couriers that the airport was open for outbound shipments. In that time we had many specimens waiting for shipping for send-out reference testing. For specimens with short stability (tuberculosis culture, newborn screening, etc.) we informed the patients that we could not collect the specimens due to shipping issues and we would call them back for specimen collection when we are able to ship the specimens out for testing.

In this disaster, my car's rear window was broken by flying debris. However, there was no damage to my apartment. My car insurance was with a local company whose office was almost completely destroyed by the storm. One's car insurance is only as good as the company providing it. There is no way to file a claim with a defunct insurance company. Next, I tried filing with FEMA for the broken car window.

From what I have been told, FEMA only reimburses if there is damage to the house or the car is undrivable. See below. I was told that my damage did not meet FEMA's criteria because my house was undamaged and the car was still drivable with the rear window broken. FEMA did not reimburse my $650 out of pocket expense for the car window repair. Instead, FEMA referred me to the Small Business Administration (SBA) for a loan. See below explanation:

DisasterAssistance.gov   Feedback   Contact Us   Sign Off

| Access Registrations | Status | Correspondence | Upload Center | Upload History | Resources | Referrals | Inspection | Applicant Information |

Your Application Status   Registration ID:
Help for this page   Disaster Number: 4404

When you registered with FEMA, the damages reported did not meet the required conditions to refer you to the Individuals and Households Program. If you have any questions about the programs and your specific registration, please contact the FEMA Helpline at 1-800-

FEMA has sent you correspondence that you should have received or will be receiving soon. These were sent to the mailing address shown on the applicant information screen. Please refer to the correspondence screen for details.

Based on the information you have provided to FEMA, no inspection of your property is required.

Assistance from FEMA
You have not provided FEMA any information regarding specific types of disaster related damages

Assistance from Other Government Agencies

Agency	Form of Assistance	Reference ID	Application Status	Date
U.S. Small Business Administration	Home and Property Disaster Loans		Apply	11/01/2018

Version: 8.01.00.00.1226 | Server: DAC-PROD12C-DC2-PUBLIC

The SBA opened a Disaster Recovery Center on Saipan shortly after the typhoon. It was open seven days a week for about three months. I went on a Saturday as I was off from work that day. I waited in line two hours to meet with an SBA representative. The SBA offered to loan up to the $650 loss at a low interest rate. They said that the loan could not be for more than the $650 damage incurred by the storm. This would have involved filling out paperwork, scheduling an SBA inspector to look at the broken car window, etc. The SBA representative said that for small dollar amount loans, the loan typically has to be paid back within a year or two. I asked what happens if you don't pay the loan back. She said the government would take the money out of my tax refund at the end of the year.

By the time I met with the SBA representative I had already paid the $650 out of pocket to replace the broken rear car window. I told the SBA representative I was still in good financial condition without the $650 and did not want to file for the SBA loan. She said that if I change my mind, I could come back, fill out the form (takes 30 to 45 minutes) and apply. They would need to send an inspector to look at my broken car window.

I spent hours waiting in line at the FEMA and SBA offices while filing the claim for the broken car window and had the opportunity to speak with several of their staff. The FEMA and SBA staff were impressed with the extent of the damage from Typhoon Yutu, This was the worst storm I have ever seen, and some of the FEMA and SBA staff had never seen a category 5 tropical cyclone either. You know things are bad when the FEMA and SBA staff are impressed with the destruction.

At least this time around I got more Meals Ready to Eat (MRE) from FEMA and did not lose as much weight (215 pounds at the time of Typhoon Yutu down to 203 pounds one month later) compared to prior typhoons. I also got some free Disaster Response Training:

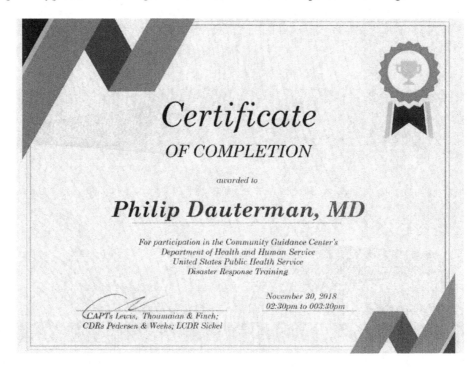

After the disaster was over, the hospital I work for asked me to list the additional work done above and beyond my usual duties. The response was:

1. Ensure the lab has adequate supplies by providing inventory lists to Incident Command (IC) and arranging with IC for alternate routes for supply shipments.
2. Ensure 24/7 coverage of laboratory as several lab staff were not able to report to work due to damaged/destroyed homes. The work schedules were increased for the staff that were able to report to work.
3. Ensure continuity of lab's operations, including outbound shipping of specimens for off-site reference lab testing. Several specimens were delayed in shipping out due to problems at the airport. This was resolved with coordination from IC.

About 3 months after the storm, the landlord of the apartment building where I live sent notice that all units in the building would have a rent increase of $50/month. This letter stated that essentially all businesses on Saipan had incurred significant expenses from repairs after the storm. All businesses on Saipan were passing the costs onto the customer in the form of higher rates. The landlord would have higher costs for all goods and services for the foreseeable future and had no choice but to raise the rent to offset the higher maintenance expenses. In this setting, I paid the higher rent without questioning. The apartment building where I live is made of concrete and survived the storm intact. I am guessing about 15% of the houses on Saipan were completely destroyed (roof gone, walls gone, nothing left but debris) and another 30% were severely damaged (roof gone, walls still standing). With large numbers of displaced people looking for shelter one needs to stay on good terms with one's landlord.

Even the lab staff were not spared from the dislocation. Four of seventeen lab staff lost their homes in the storm and were living in temporary housing arrangements for months after the storm. Several additional lab staff lost their roof in the storm but remained in houses that were considered unlivable because they had nowhere else to go. Still others moved in with relatives whose houses survived the typhoon.

In the immediate aftermath of the typhoon, most of the houses that survived the typhoon ended up with two or more families living in the same house. Two days after the typhoon I called several apartment buildings asking for available units for my co-workers in lab. I was told that every vacant real estate property on Saipan was rented the day after the typhoon. It took months to repair the damaged houses so that the displaced people could move back into their own homes.

In closing, I would like to thank the lab and hospital staff that reported to work during and after the disasters listed above. Many of the lab staff were working despite significant personal hardships including damaged or destroyed homes yet they continued to report to work on schedule. This shows the dedication and determination of everyone in lab. It is an honor to be a part of this.

CLIA makes it the Lab Director's responsibility that test reports include pertinent information for test interpretation. The way I interpret this is that it means each test result must have the reference range displayed. Lab results typically go from the testing equipment to the hospital's computer via some type of interface. The provider views the test result as it appears in the computer, not the analyzer. The appearance of the lab result is thus determined by the hospital's computer and computer support personnel.

Generally, the only time the display changes is when the hospital is getting a new computer system, or lab is getting new equipment. When this happens always remind the hospital's computer support personnel that the reference range must appear next to (or at least on the same page as) the test result.

CLIA states that the Lab Director must be available for consultation concerning test results and the interpretation of those results as they relate to specific patient conditions. In my experience this requirement for availability can be met by being on call (cellphone number available to the hospital operator) and does not require one to be on-site full time.

CLIA makes it the Lab Director's responsibility to ensure each employee's responsibilities and duties are specified in writing. In my experience hospitals delegate the writing of all job descriptions, including lab's job descriptions, to the hospital's Personnel Office, Human Resources (HR) office or other similar office.

Whenever you are called upon by the hospital's HR office to help write a job description, your input is typically limited to a description of the duties and minimum qualifications (degree or certification, years of training, years of experience, etc.) for the job position. All other particulars such as the salary, how to apply for the job, etc. will be determined by the HR office. When writing the list of duties try to specify the duties as broadly as possible for the envisioned job position. Do not specify methodology or instruments as this could change over time such that the lab's job descriptions would need to be updated each time the lab's methodology, instrumentation, etc. changed. Do not specify shift (day shift, night shift, etc.) as this would make it difficult for the person occupying the position to work any other shift. At the end of every list of job duties always add "other duties as assigned" to give added flexibility to the position.

Once written, a new job description is routed for signatures. The completed, signed job descriptions are kept in the HR office possibly with a copy in lab. These job descriptions change very little over time, and are almost never updated. For each individual employee, their job description is kept in a file folder in the HR Office, possibly with a copy in their competency testing file folder in Lab.

CAP's list of criteria for a clinical Lab Director lists research and development. In my 29 years in Pathology and Lab Medicine, I have only had very limited research duties. The hospital Lab Director typically sits on the hospital Institutional Review Board (IRB). Under the Code of Federal Regulations, any human subject research requires approval of the IRB of the institution where the research is to be done.

While sitting on the IRB committee, my involvement consisted of voting "yes" on all the human subjects research that the local university wanted to do at the hospital. Their projects involved counseling patients on weight loss, smoking cessation, etc. Since these projects were non-invasive, a "yes" vote as an IRB committee member was not difficult.

My only direct involvement in research was with a brain research project. My involvement ran from the late 1990s to around 2004. My participation consisted of doing autopsies on request. I had no other participation in the project. Over the course of about 8 years, I did only about 6 autopsies for this research project. The project had a hard time getting families to consent to autopsies with use of their loved one's brain for research. As a result, the numbers of autopsies were very low.

In my experience, most Lab Directors at community hospitals have no research duties whatsoever. Only Lab Directors at university hospitals will be expected to do research.

CAP lists educational duties in its list of criteria for a clinical Lab Director. There have not been any pathology fellows, pathology residents or medical students at any hospital I have worked at. My entire career has been at small community hospitals, not directly affiliated with an educational program. Educational duties of this nature are only expected of the Lab Director at an academic hospital. On occasion I provide some education to the Lab staff, such as reviewing pictures of urine sediment crystals, synovial crystals, blood cells, etc. at the time of PT testing or PT corrective action.

CAP mandates that the Lab Director must select the reference laboratory. In every hospital I have worked at, the hospital lab had been affiliated with its reference lab for many years before I arrived. The only time that a hospital lab will change its reference lab is when the reference lab drops the hospital lab.

In the time I have been working on Saipan one of the reference labs, Ascent Lab of California, pulled out from the local market. This sent several labs on Saipan scrambling to find a new reference lab. Thus, in my experience the reference lab chooses to affiliate with the hospital lab, and not the other way around.

CLIA does not specifically require a contract to be in place between a lab and its reference lab. However, the CMS places this requirement on the hospital as a whole. The reference is 42 CFR § 482.27(a). Based on the way the regulations are set up, a hospital lab must have a contract with its reference lab, but outpatient clinic labs do not have this requirement. Before every inspection make sure you can find the contract between your hospital and the reference lab. The original contract likely stipulates that it renews automatically every two years if not altered by either party. If this is the case a decades old contract is still good. However, finding a copy after that length of time is problematic. Such things tend to get lost in the sands of time.

Find a copy of this contract and set it in your office in a place where you can easily produce it if an inspector shows up unannounced. If no one at your hospital can find the contract, ask the reference lab for a copy. If the reference lab can't find the contract either, it is time to make a new contract. The same applies for the contract with your blood supplier. The CMS requires all hospitals to have a contract in place with their blood supplier governing the procurement, transfer, and availability of blood and blood products. The reference is 42 CFR § 493.1103 (a).

The CAP makes the Lab Director responsible for selecting the equipment, reagents and supplies used in Lab. Most hospitals I have worked at have been government hospitals where these were purchased in a bidding process. The only input I had was writing the specifications for all new analyzers and sitting on the steering committees for the purchase.

The supplies and reagents are typically determined by the type of analyzer you have. For example, you cannot use Siemens reagents in an Abbott analyzer or vice versa. Once you have purchased an analyzer you are committed to using that company's reagents and supplies for the life of that analyzer. This can be a major drawback if you or the company you work for has a falling out with the vendor.

CAP mandates that the Lab Director must monitor the performance of the reference laboratory. I have seen a reference lab make a significant mistake only once in my 29 years in Pathology and Lab Medicine. This episode occurred in 2000 or 2001. At the time the technology used for Acid Fast Bacilli (AFB) culture involved incubating culture bottles. Once every day, the bottles would be tested for growth by an instrument that sticks a needle into the bottle, sucks some air out, and checks for carbon dioxide as evidence of growth.

The needle has to be cleaned very carefully, so that if one bottle has AFB in it the AFB doesn't get into the subsequent bottles that are tested with the same needle. Apparently, someone at the reference lab didn't clean this needle properly and there was a specimen positive for tuberculosis at the front end of this line of bottles to test. As a result, all subsequent bottles were contaminated with tuberculosis. One by one these bottles grew tuberculosis even though the patients whose specimens were in those bottles did not have tuberculosis (i.e. false positive tests).

A handful of false positive tuberculosis results were turned out, and several patients were told that they had tuberculosis when in fact, they really did not have tuberculosis. This problem was later identified and several corrected reports were issued, correcting AFB results from positive to negative.

When this happened I called the reference lab to express my displeasure. I also sent them a few letters and memos in regard to this episode. The reference lab was apologetic. They acknowledged that they had made a significant mistake, and promised that it would not happen again.

In my formal communication with the reference lab, they said that confidentiality issues prevented them from discussing what internal actions were being taken to prevent recurrence, or what they would do to the lab tech who had made the mistake.

Later, I met with officials from this lab privately. They said that they had fired the lab tech involved. They switched to DNA testing for AFB which does not have the same problems as the older culture technology.

In this same meeting, they asked me privately if any damage was done, and if their lab was going to get sued. I said that a handful of people got put on isoniazid and other antituberculous medications for about a month, and were then taken off of the medications when it was discovered they didn't really have tuberculosis. None of them had any complications from the treatment, and none of them was interested in suing that I knew of. Most of them were glad that they didn't really have tuberculosis.

The problem of false positive AFB results never recurred. Frankly, if it had recurred I would have very quickly been looking to switch reference labs.

CLIA has no specific requirements to monitor the performance of a contractor. However, the CMS places such requirements on the hospital as a whole. The reference is 42 CFR § 482.12 (e). Each hospital typically will ask all departments to provide input on all their contractors' performance on an annual basis. Typically all departments are asked to fill out a hospital-wide annual Contractor Quality Assessment Form. The routing of this form is typically to the hospital-wide Quality Assurance committee.

For most vendors being reviewed, there is nothing major wrong and the Quality Assurance committee will sign and file the documentation without further action. If there is something major wrong, such as the reference lab disaster described above, the hospital-wide Quality Assurance committee will forward the paperwork to the hospital's Board for action (termination of the contract, legal action against the vendor, etc.).

As a reminder, an incident of the magnitude described above should be immediately reported as an Incident Report to the hospital's Risk Manager as well as added to the annual Contractor Quality Assessment Form turned in at the end of the year.

Chapter 19 – How to be a Lab Supervisor

Under CLIA the Lab Director is allowed to take on the responsibilities of several lower ranking position in lab including the clinical consultant, technical consultant, technical supervisor and general supervisor as long as you meet the personnel qualification requirements.

As mentioned before, in most labs the Lab Director and clinical consultant are the same person. Only once in my career have I also had to fill in as the Lab Supervisor. In August 2013 I was hired to "turnaround" a troubled lab in a remote area. The Lab Supervisor position had been vacant for most of the prior 2 years. When I took over the leadership role in this lab, I had to carry out both the Lab Director and Lab Supervisor work, as there was no one else available to do it.

This was a very unusual situation. In my 29 years experience in Pathology and Lab Medicine I never had to take on the Lab Supervisor position before. I am only aware of one other instance where a lab had no Lab Supervisor for an extended period of time and the Lab Director had to fill in.

As mentioned above this is allowed under CLIA. It has happened in real life and is more than just a theoretical possibility. You as Lab Director should be prepared and able to take over the Lab Supervisor position should that be necessary.

The Lab Supervisor position is essentially equivalent of the "technical supervisor" position of a high complexity testing lab which in turn is essentially equivalent to the "technical consultant" in a moderate complexity testing laboratory as defined under CLIA. The qualifications are given at 42 CFR § 493.1449 and 42 CFR § 493.1411. The qualifications can be summarized as must possess a current license issued by the State in which the laboratory is located, if such licensing is required. There are several permutations of educational and training requirements that would be acceptable:

1. Board Certified pathologist licensed to practice in the State in which the laboratory is located or else
2. doctor of medicine, doctor of osteopathy, or doctor of podiatric medicine licensed to practice in the State in which the laboratory is located with at least one year of laboratory training or experience or else
3. earned doctoral degree in a chemical, physical, biological or clinical laboratory science with at least 1 year of laboratory training or experience or else
4. a master's degree in a chemical, physical, biological or clinical laboratory science or medical technology with at least 2 years of laboratory training or experience or else
5. a bachelor's degree in a chemical, physical, or biological science or medical technology with at least 4 years of laboratory training or experience.

In most small hospital labs the Lab Supervisor position is filled by someone with a bachelor's or master's degree. In such a lab the Lab Director is typically the only person with a doctorate level degree. In larger university hospital labs you must typically have a PhD to be considered for the Lab Supervisor position.

Under CLIA, the Lab Supervisor's responsibilities are given at 42 CFR § 493.1413 and 42 CFR § 493.1451. These stipulate duties such as selection of the test methodology, verification of the test procedures, establishment of the laboratory's test performance characteristics, etc. This list largely overlaps with the duties CLIA requires of the Lab Director. In my experience, at most hospital labs the "command decisions" are made by the Lab Director not the Lab Supervisor. At most hospital labs, the Lab Supervisor is responsible for:

1. all inventory control and ordering of supplies, reagents, controls, calibrators, equipment, etc.
2. scheduling the preventative maintenance on the lab equipment if this is not done by the section supervisors.
3. scheduling for the lab techs, including scheduling of vacation time, training, in-services and continuing education. Assesses lab workload.
4. most of the budgeting including preparation of the annual budget for lab. Assesses capital equipment needs and includes the next year's capital equipment expenditures in the next year's budget.
5. enforcing lab policies (universal precautions, arrive on time to work, all testing personnel must read and sign the procedure manuals, etc.) on the lab staff including counseling and disciplinary actions on any lab staff that breaks the rules.
6. enrollment and participation in PT, receipt of PT materials, distribution of the PT materials to

the various lab sections, timely completion of the PT testing event and reporting of PT results back to the PT provider.
7. In labs without a QA coordinator, most QA work including corrective actions for PT failure falls on the Lab Supervisor.
8. assists the Lab Director in preparing for inspections and writing Plans of Correction for inspection deficiencies.
9. assisting in writing and reviewing the Lab's policies and procedures.
10. competency testing of the lab staff to include remedial training and/or education.
11. may be required to assist in the hiring of new lab techs (evaluate resumes, interview applicants, etc.)
12. day-to-day, on-site supervision of all testing personnel.
13. assists in troubleshooting for technical problems, analyzer breakdowns, and/or tests out of control, etc.
14. In smaller labs, the Lab Supervisor will typically also do the work of a section supervisor and/or bench level lab tech (i.e. do the day-to-day hands-on testing work of lab as well as the Lab Supervisor work).
15. may be required to be on-call 24 hours a day 7 days a week in case of emergency.

As can be seen from the above list, the Lab Supervisor position requires extensive knowledge of how things work at any given lab. Thus, when recruiting for a vacant Lab Supervisor position the new Lab Supervisor is almost always hired internally and only the section supervisors are considered for promotion to the Lab Supervisor position. Outside hiring is not usually considered unless none of the section supervisors are interested in applying for the Lab Supervisor position. Outside hiring of a Lab Supervisor is very rare in my experience.

In terms of evaluation and competency testing, it is difficult to perform competency testing on the administrative work being done. At most labs I am familiar with, the Lab Supervisor does some hands-on testing. In this capacity, the Lab Supervisor is judged by the same competency testing standards the bench level lab techs are judged by. Otherwise, the evaluation is a largely subjective "judgment call" based on timely completion of paperwork, paperwork completed without errors, attitude, ability to motivate, arrives to work on time, etc.

In terms of promotion, there is no higher position available to the Lab Supervisor of a typical small hospital lab. The next higher position is the Lab Director position which requires a doctoral level degree. The typical small hospital Lab Supervisor has a bachelor's or master's degree and does not qualify for the Lab Director position. Thus, for the typical Lab Supervisor, there is no opportunity for promotion.

Retention is not usually a problem for the Lab Supervisor position. The Lab Supervisor position is usually only vacated by retirement. On the other hand, rapid turnover of the Lab Supervisor position is a warning sign of a troubled clinical lab.

Although I was officially the acting Lab Supervisor once in 29 years, there were several instances where the Lab Supervisor position was occupied, but the person in that position wasn't getting all of the above duties list done. The most critical item on the above list is the ordering of lab supplies and reagents. If the Lab Supervisor has difficulty with this, you will need to help or ask the section supervisors to help.

Several years ago, I was working at a small municipal hospital when the former Lab Supervisor left. The Blood Bank supervisor was promoted into the Lab Supervisor position. There had been little preparation for the turnover, as essentially all positions in that lab were overworked. The new Lab Supervisor didn't have much knowledge of where the Purchase Orders (PO's) and other purchasing documents are kept, how to execute a PO, etc. and also didn't have much experience with general lab inventory.

In the first few months after the Lab Supervisor position changed over, the lab ran out of several different types of reagents and supplies. Some of these were for essential tests. I would get on the phone to the Materials Management Department and beg them to procure the needed reagents and supplies as fast as possible. They would ask me for the PO number, and I'd have to go pouring through the PO manuals since the Lab Supervisor could not find the PO number.

The new Lab Supervisor was having trouble with the inventory and procurement. At this lab, inventory and procurement had always been the responsibility of the Lab Supervisor. Some of the other section supervisors might have had a better grasp on inventory and procurement, but couldn't handle budgeting or personnel issues such as scheduling. It was not possible to hire an outside Lab Supervisor. This is a small hospital lab in the middle of nowhere. Recruitment is extremely difficult, especially for the lab managerial positions.

The decision was made to unofficially split the duties of the Lab Supervisor position. The Lab Supervisor would handle all the budgeting and personnel issues, while the inventory and procurement would be split among the section supervisors. Each section supervisor would have to do the inventory and procurement work for their own section of lab. This arrangement worked out well. The section supervisors didn't mind the extra work.

If this arrangement had not worked out, there would have been two possible paths forward. The Lab Director could take over the inventory and procurement. In that hospital the added work would not have overloaded me, so this is the path I would have chosen. The other possibility is reshuffling one of the other section supervisors into the Lab Supervisor position.

If the Lab Supervisor has trouble with one item on the list of Lab Supervisor duties, follow the same approach. If the Lab Supervisor has trouble with budgeting, delegate off that part of the work to whoever in lab is good with the budgeting. If the Lab Supervisor has trouble with scheduling, delegate that off to whoever in lab is good at scheduling, etc.

If someone is new in the Lab Supervisor position, it is not uncommon for him or her to have trouble with multiple items on the list of Lab Supervisor duties. Assign the section supervisors to help him or her. Give the new Lab Supervisor a few months to try to "grow into" the position. If after a few months the Lab Supervisor is still struggling, you have to think about reshuffling someone else into that position.

As mentioned above inventory control is one of the primary duties of the Lab Supervisor. Inventory control is important in all labs so I will go into detail about this. The basic concepts of inventory control are easy to understand. However, at most hospitals I have worked at, the procurement paperwork must be routed through a complex maze of pathways that is difficult to understand.

Inventory control is the system used to manage inventory. It includes any activity done to check and manage an operation's inventory of goods. Inventory control is a two edged sword. If you do not order enough of an item you will run out. If you order too much of an item you will expire and discard some the item unused. At most hospitals I have worked at, the hospital's administration has been very sensitive about discarding unused items, since it costs the hospital money. You as a laboratory worker will be more concerned about outages as it will prevent you from doing testing.

For most items used in laboratory, you should try to use the shortest dated items first (i.e. First-In-First-Out). This will help to reduce the number of expired items. For example, at one hospital I worked at there was a recurring problem of expired Microbiology agar plates. This was due to shipments of new inventory being put at the front of the refrigerator, resulting in the older inventory being hidden at the back of the refrigerator. I made a rule that all newly received shipments of agar plates should be put at the back of the refrigerator so that the shortest date boxes of agar plates were showing through the refrigerator window.

If your hospital has a computerized inventory system this will make your inventory control much easier. Each item is scanned before it goes into use. The computerized system keeps a running tally of each item and flags you when you run low. In this setting, it is not uncommon for items to be taken out of inventory and put into use without scanning. If this oversight is repeated frequently it will deplete the physical inventory with the computer count showing adequate inventory. Hence the need to count the physical inventory at least monthly, and make correcting entries to the computer count. If significant discrepancies occur between physical inventory and the computer count, you may need to remind the lab staff to always scan items that are being taken out of inventory and put in use.

If your hospital's inventory system is paper-based you will be doing much more work. Most of the hospitals I have worked at have had a paper-based inventory system. In this setting the process of inventory control is as follows: Make a list of all essential items in your area. For each item, the part number or item number and manufacturer's name of the item should be included so as to facilitate easier ordering. For each item on the list, add up the annual usage for the last year. Divide annual usage by 12 to determine monthly usage. Determine a minimum amount of each item you want present at all times (referred to as the Minimum Operating Inventory or "par level"). Each item is reordered as it falls below this level. If local purchase processing takes 2 months, set the "par level" at a 3 month supply. This works for items with an expiration of 3 months or more on arrival. If any critical item repeatedly runs low or runs out, this may indicate you need to check inventory more often and/or raise the par level so as to have a bigger stockpile of the item on hand.

The situation is more difficult with items that have a short date on arrived. This includes all Blood Bank reagents containing red blood cells (checkcells, etc.). These typically have less than 3 weeks shelf life on arrival. You will need to make standing orders for these items, or put them on a contract. A standing order is an order for routine delivery of a fixed amount at regular intervals. A contract between the hospital and the vendor (or any similar legal document such as a Memorandum Of Understanding) will allow the vendor to send items as needed with the hospital paying later.

If your inventory system is paper-based, you will need to count the physical inventory more frequently than if you had a computerized inventory system. A paper-based inventory system does not keep a running count the same way a computerized system does. With a paper-based system I would recommend inventorying all critical items at least weekly or every 2 weeks.

Procurement is the process of acquiring goods and/or services from an outside vendor. All hospitals I am familiar with require all procurements to go through the hospital's procurement office. This office is typical referred to as the Materials Management Office, Supply Chain Office, Medical Supply Office or other similar name.

Older literature indicates that at one time hospitals would allow departments to procure at the departmental level; however, this is apparently an outdated practice, and is no longer done. If you want to procure supplies for your lab, you will need to fill out whatever paperwork your hospital's procurement office wants and the paperwork must be completed to their satisfaction before the purchase proceeds.

At most hospitals I have worked at, the request to purchase an item is submitted to the Procurement Office as a Request For Quotation (RFQ). The Procurement Office then asks vendors to bid on the item. When the bidding is completed the Procurement Office picks the lowest bidder and prepares a Request For Purchase (RFP). The RFP is submitted to lab for the Lab Supervisor's signature. The signed RFP is submitted back to the Procurement Office. The Procurement Office then processes it to a Purchase Order (PO). The PO is transmitted to the vendor that won the bidding. The item is sent from the vendor to the lab. When the item arrives lab inspects the item. If the item is unsatisfactory (damaged, expired, too short date, etc.) lab rejects the item and the item is sent back to the vendor. If the item is satisfactory the lab keeps the item, signs the vendor's invoice and transmits the invoice to the hospital's Procurement Office. The signed invoice is processed into a Receiving Report and submitted to the hospital's Accounting Office for them to make payment for the purchase.

If you run low on an essential item, my advice is to call or e-mail the hospital's procurement office daily to remind them. Ask them to expedite the paperwork. In most instances they will accommodate and expedite the procurement.

If you have a shortage/outage of a critical item, and it is truly an emergency, my best advice is to call the Hospital Administrator and ask him or her to intervene and expedite the procurement process. Be prepared that the typical hospital's procurement office does not like making an emergency procurement, since it overrides their usual procurement process. The procurement office will do as told, but may be upset that you have asked a higher authority to override their usual way of doing things. This option should be a last resort, since you do not want to upset people you will have to work with in the future.

It is imperative to keep a good supply of your lab's essential reagents and supplies. If your supplies and/or reagents run out and patient testing stops, you could get into deep trouble with your regulatory agency.

The procurement rules have been different at every hospital I have worked at. I have spent my entire career working in government hospitals. The procurement rules are typically set by the government operating the hospital (Federal, local, etc.). In most municipal hospitals the procurement is done through the local government. This results in prolonged processing time for purchase requests to process. Processing of purchase requests may be somewhat faster at private hospitals.

If the processing of purchase requests is prolonged, you can compensate by submitting them earlier than you otherwise would. For example, if the procurement process takes 2 months, set the "par level" of all durable products at a 3 month supply. If the procurement processing takes 6 months, keep a 7 month stockpile of all durable items. If processing of purchase requests is prolonged at your hospital, try to have all essential items on Standing Orders or contracts.

Let's use inventory control for blood units as an example. Blood units are one of the most critical items in the lab and no Blood Bank should ever be allowed to run out of blood. The hospitals I have worked at did not draw their own red cell units and obtained all their blood from the Red Cross in weekly or biweekly shipments.

To calculate the amount to order as standing orders (i.e. orders for routine delivery), add up the prior year's usage and divide by 52 to calculate the weekly usage. This is the amount to order if you receive shipments weekly. If the shipments come every 2 weeks, the number to order per shipment is twice the weekly usage. If your annual usage has been going up over the past few years, add in an increment to compensate for the increasing annual usage. If there is significant seasonal variation in blood usage, the ordering should be increased and decreased seasonally to coincide with the variations in usage.

For example, in the municipal hospital where I was working during 2007 the Blood Bank transfused 3100 units of blood. In 2006 the Blood Bank had transfused 2725 units of blood. This means that the number of units transfused increased 13.7% in 2007 compared to 2006. This continued the pattern of year-over-year increases of about 10% seen over the prior several years. The reason for the greater blood utilization is that municipality's population is increasing and aging. There had also been an influx of hematologist/oncologists compared to prior years, with more hematology/oncology patients staying in that municipality for treatment, and not leaving to the nearest large city.

In 2006 Blood Bank was receiving an average of 62.5 units per week (alternating 50 and 75 unit shipments on alternate weeks). This means that Blood Bank was receiving 3250 units from the Red Cross per year.

If utilization continued to increase about 10% per year, the ordering of blood would need to be increased by 10% per year as well. Otherwise, the demand for blood would likely have outstripped the supply for blood sometime toward the end of 2008 or start of 2009. Because Red Cross ships blood in containers of 25 units, Blood Bank prefers to order in increments of 25. My recommendation was that Blood Bank should increase its baseline shipments from the Red Cross to 75 units per week starting November, 2008.

If Blood Bank kept the baseline ordering pattern at an average of 62.5 units per week it would likely have resulted in sporadic shortages. If this happened Blood Bank would have to E-mail the Red Cross and ask them to add on units to the next shipment.

If Blood Bank sets its baseline at 75 per week, Blood Bank may end up with too many units from time to time. In this case Blood Bank can tell Red Cross to decrease the number of units in the next shipment. It is much easier for the Red Cross to decrease the number of units in a shipment as compared to increasing it.

An important concept in inventory control is called Minimum Operating Inventory (MOI) also known as the "par level". The MOI is the minimum number of units of blood that Blood Bank wants on hand before reordering. If Blood Bank falls below the MOI this triggers reordering. Blood Bank asks Red Cross to send more blood, either by sending more units in the next shipment, or sending an unscheduled emergency shipment of blood in addition to the regularly scheduled shipments.

For the remote places where I have worked, I have asked for an MOI of at least 3 weeks supply of blood. Running a high inventory means that you will occasionally expire a unit which you might not have expired if you hadn't run such a high inventory. In remote areas, shipments from the Red Cross can take up to 5 days to arrive. Having an occasional expired unit is infinitely preferable to having Blood Bank run out of blood.

Another possibility is reducing utilization. All hospitals are required by TJC to have a committee which retrospectively reviews blood utilization. This is usually called the Blood Utilization and

Transfusion Review (BUTR) Committee. In my experience only about 2% to 5% of transfusions fall out and are reviewed by the Committee. The Committee finds most of these are appropriate transfusions. Usually only one or two cases a month are considered inappropriate and referred to the respective Department for review. To the best of my knowledge, there has not been significant corrective action against any Physician for inappropriate utilization of blood.

In my experience most hospitals would be able to decrease utilization of blood by a percent or two by giving the BUTR Committee "teeth" to discipline doctors for inappropriate transfusions. However, in my opinion, this would not be well received by the Medical Staff. The number of transfusions prevented would likely be so small that it would not make much difference.

The Lab Supervisor is responsible for ordering more of any item that is in short supply or short dated (near expiration). The Lab Supervisor typically delegates the physical inventorying of lab supplies to the section supervisors. In other words, each of the section supervisors is assigned to count all of the essential items in his or her area to ensure an adequate number remains with adequate remaining shelf life.

Expired reagents and supplies are a CLIA violation and will result in a citation. Discard all expired items unless they are essential. If you must use expired items, immediately order in-date items, document the need to use the expired items, and QC the expired items. As soon as in-date items arrive, discard the expired items. At the next CMS inspection you should be prepared to explain to the inspector why you used expired items.

Infection control is typically mandated on the lab by the hospital's infection control policies and Infection Control Office. The Lab Supervisor is charged with enforcement of all policies on the lab staff including infection control. Infection control is aimed at preventing healthcare associated (i.e. nosocomial) infection. Infection control in lab includes the phlebotomist hand hygiene (handwashing or use of alcohol based hand rub) and proper use of Personal Protective Equipment (PPE) when going from patient to patient drawing blood. The staff should be trained in all types of PPE that may be needed in the course of their work (e.g. N95 respirator mask needed when drawing patients on respiratory precautions).

The Lab Supervisor is also charged with enforcing the lab safety practices. Handling of live cultures and known infectious specimens in lab falls under lab safety practices and not infection control.

Aside from the Lab Supervisor position, I have filled in for other positions as well. I spent a year working in a Veteran's Hospital that had one secretary in the Pathology Department. The days she took leave, I had to type my own reports. At first, it was disconcerting. I would go from looking at slides under the microscope to typing part of the report on the computer, back to looking at slides under the microscope, back to typing more of the report on the computer, etc.

At first, it took me almost 12 hours to examine the slides that would have only taken 8 hours with the secretary present. Within a short time I became more proficient as a typist. I could do both the slide reading and the typing within 8 hours. I would also have to answer the phones while the Secretary was on leave.

At one time or other I have filled in for virtually every other position in lab, except for phlebotomy and testing. On one instance I spent a few hours at the front desk, covering while the front desk secretary left due to a personal emergency. I occasionally have to lift boxes up to the highest levels in the storeroom for techs that are too short or too weak to lift the heavy boxes to the top shelf.

On one occasion, a particularly rainy day, my office got muddy from various people entering with dirty shoes. I called housekeeping but they were busy mopping up all the other mud in the hospital. After the working day was over, I ended up mopping my own office.

Chapter 20 - Section supervisor qualifications, duties, responsibilities, promotion and retention

The section supervisors are more or less the equivalent of the "General Supervisor" in a high complexity testing lab as defined under CLIA. The qualifications for a general supervisor of a high complexity testing lab are given at 42 CFR § 493.1461. To summarize the general supervisor must possess a current license issued by the State in which the laboratory is located, if such licensing is required. There are several permutations of educational and training requirements that would be acceptable:

1. Qualified as a lab director or else
2. Qualified as a technical supervisor or else
3. Doctor of medicine, doctor of osteopathy, or doctor of podiatric medicine licensed to practice in the State in which the laboratory is located or have earned a doctoral, master's, or bachelor's degree in a chemical, physical, biological or clinical laboratory science, or medical technology and have at least 1 year of laboratory training or experience or else
4. Qualified as testing personnel and have at least 2 years of laboratory training or experience or else
5. Grandfathered under older rules.

In the typical hospital lab, the section supervisors are all lab techs with many years experience. They started out as bench level techs and worked their way up to the section supervisor position over the course of many years. The section supervisors are typically responsible for:

1. All inventory control and ordering of supplies, reagents, controls, calibrators, equipment, etc. for their section of lab.
2. Scheduling the preventative maintenance on the equipment for their section of lab.
3. Enforcing lab policies (universal precautions, arrive on time to work, all testing personnel must read and sign the procedure manuals, etc.) on the lab staff in their section including counseling and disciplinary actions on any lab staff that breaks the rules.
4. Timely completion of the PT testing.
5. Prepare their section of lab for inspections.
6. Assisting in writing and reviewing the policies and procedures for their section of lab.
7. Orientation, supervision and competency testing of the lab staff in their section to include remedial training and/or education.
8. Assists in troubleshooting for technical problems, analyzer breakdowns, and/or tests out of control, etc. for their section of lab. Must be accessible on-site at all times testing is performed to resolve technical problems.
9. Day-to-day hands-on testing work of lab as well as the section supervisor work.
10. Assess the workload and staffing of their section of lab.

In my experience, it is very rare for a lab tech to be hired into a section supervisor position without first working many years in the same lab. As can be seen from the above list, the duties require some knowledge of how things work at that particular lab. A lab tech should have enough knowledge and experience to carry out the above list of duties in order to move up to a section supervisor position. If not, that lab tech should not be promoted into a section supervisor position.

As you can see from the above list, there is considerable overlap between the duties of a section supervisor and the duties of a lab supervisor. Each section supervisor is in effect acting as a lab supervisor for his or her section of lab. This helps to spread the administrative work of lab on several people so that no one is overloaded with administrative work.

This arrangement can fall apart in two ways. As documented in the prior chapter, the lab supervisor may not get his or her share of the lab's administrative work done in which case it falls on the section supervisors. The other way things can fall apart is when the section supervisors do not do their share of the lab's administrative work, in which case it all falls on the lab supervisor such that the lab supervisor feels overloaded.

The lab supervisor is responsible for ensuring that all the section supervisors carry out the duties listed above. I have only seen one instance in which the section supervisors as a whole did not do as much administrative work as was expected of them. This occurred at a small community hospital lab in the middle of nowhere, with no way to hire more lab techs or any administrative staff for lab. This particular Lab Supervisor was doing bench level work, section supervisor work in chemistry, and also the lab supervisor work. The other section supervisors were not doing much of the administrative work listed above, and it was all falling on the Lab Supervisor. The Lab Supervisor was not being assertive in requiring all the section supervisors to carry out the duties listed above. As a result, the Lab Supervisor felt overwhelmed by the administrative work, and was threatening to resign from that lab if not relieved.

In this circumstance, I called a series of meetings with the Lab Supervisor and section supervisors and reminded all the section supervisors of the duties of their positions and informed them that going forward they would be expected to carry their fair share of the lab's administrative work. I informed the Lab Supervisor that she had my backing to enforce this. In private, I advised the Lab Supervisor to be more assertive when assigning the sections supervisors their fair share of the lab's administrative workload. Going forward, if any section supervisor does not complete the work assigned he or she will be called for a closed-door counseling session with write-ups.

In terms of evaluation and competency testing, it is difficult to perform competency testing on the administrative work being done. At all labs I am familiar with, the section supervisors all double as hands-on testing personnel. In this capacity, the section supervisors are judged by the same competency testing standards the bench level lab techs are judged by.

In terms of promotion the next higher position is the Lab Supervisor position. In my experience the Lab Supervisor position is usually only vacated by retirement and in most labs the order of succession is not worked out in advance. When the Lab Supervisor position is vacated most of the section supervisors will be interested in promotion. Only one section supervisor can be promoted to the Lab Supervisor position. You must be prepared to give something of value to the section supervisors who applied for the Lab Supervisor position but were passed up.

In my experience retention of section supervisors is not difficult. They tend to be older, typically above age 50, and tend to remain in the same position until retirement or until promoted to the Lab Supervisor position.

Chapter 21 – Pathologist hiring, orientation, competency testing, promotion, retention and retirement

CLIA considers a Pathologist to be a technical supervisor in anatomic and/or clinical pathology. Under CLIA a Pathologist is required to be an MD or DO licensed to practice medicine or osteopathy in the State in which the laboratory is located. If the Pathologist is doing both anatomic and clinical pathology the Pathologist must be certified in both anatomic and clinical pathology by the American Board of Pathology or the American Osteopathic Board of Pathology or possess equivalent qualifications. If doing only anatomic or clinical pathology, only that board certification (or equivalent) is required. The reference is 42 CFR § 493.1449.

In my experience Pathologist hiring is even more difficult than lab tech hiring. For most of my 29 year career in Pathology and Lab Medicine I have been solo. The hospital where I was working at the time had hired Pathologists twice, once in 2000 and again in 2008. There were no other Pathologists in that municipality so hiring by word of mouth was not an option. Advertisements were placed in the Pathology journals – CAP Today, AJCP and Laboratory Medicine. In 2008 advertisements were also placed online.

In both instances there was only one applicant. In each instance the applicant was vetted by the usual state licensure process and hospital privileging process. The applicant's credentials were verified, and the applicant was licensed and privileged.

The Pathologist hired in 2000 was Dr. B. He started work in August, 2000. Immediately after staring work Dr. B began arguing with everyone in the lab. He argued with the Lab Supervisor as to whether the Lab Supervisor or the Pathologist has more authority in lab. These arguments occurred on a daily basis in public areas within the lab. He argued loudly and daily with the histotechs about the quality of the slides. After 2 months of this, Dr. B. resigned and went back where he came from.

The Pathologist hired in 2008 was Dr. W. Immediately after starting work, Dr. W. began having problems of such a nature that the hospital Medical Director mandated that Dr. W. should see the hospital Psychiatrist. The hospital Psychiatrist said that Dr. W. could not work and needed to take sick leave. The problem is that Dr. W. just stared work, and does not have any sick leave saved up. Dr. W. left on unpaid leave time, and never returned.

When it comes to Pathologist hiring, I am batting zero. This is why I was solo for so many years. You may want to take my Pathologist hiring recommendations above with a grain of salt due to my dismal track record. In my part of the world, there is no oversupply of pathologists. I am aware of anecdotal evidence to suggest a large oversupply of Pathologists in the continental US, with significant Pathologist unemployment and underemployment. If you want to, you can sign a petition at the following website asking to reduce the number of Pathology training positions in the US:

http://www.ipetitions.com/petition/oversupply-of-pathologists-in-the-us

Other than the above, I have not had experience with Pathologist hiring. In reading the literature, and discussing this subject with other Pathologists, the typical hiring process is largely subjective. Some Pathology groups will set absolute rules, such as the applicant must be Board Certified to be considered for hiring. The applicant cannot have more than 1 malpractice claim recorded at NPDB. Any applicant with 2 or more malpractice claims and/or other derogatory information recorded at NPDB (involuntary loss of licensure, criminal convictions, etc.) is excluded from consideration for hiring. The typical small hospital will not be as restrictive as a large group in a large city. In any event, if you hire a pathologist with a spotty track record you will need to monitor his or her performance closely, especially when he or she is new on the job.

In terms of orientation, a Pathologist should only need orientation to the particulars of the new lab where he or she will be working. The computer system tends to be the most troublesome feature for a new Pathologist. If you are using a computer system the new Pathologist is not used to, it may take a great deal of orientation. Other particulars such as work flow may vary slightly from one lab to the next. The menu of immunostains available also varies from lab to lab and may take some getting used to. However, tissue diagnosis is the same everywhere, and should not require orientation.

In terms of promotion, the next higher position in lab is the Lab Director position. The Lab Director position is typically only vacated by retirement. As the current Lab Director ages, the Lab Director work will increasingly be delegated to the second most senior Pathologist in the group (i.e. second only to the Lab Director in the number of years worked).

Usually, by the time of retirement, a Lab Director will be delegating off most of his or her duties to the second most senior Pathologist. Oftentimes this person will be officially designated as lab's second in command. Thus, it is usually easy for the second most senior Pathologist to move up to the Lab Director position when it is vacated.

In some instances the second most senior Pathologist will not want the Lab Director position, and/or wants to work exclusively in Anatomic Pathology. In this case, the delegation of the Lab Director work and later the promotion to the Lab Director position will be offered to the third, then fourth, then fifth, etc. most senior Pathologist in the group. My advice is that if you are offered this, do not pass it up. Since the Lab Director position is typically vacated only by retirement, it is likely to be many years before the position comes open again.

Most of the hospitals I have worked at have been cash strapped, making retention difficult. Retention, including Pathologist retention, faces the issues of stagnant salaries, salaries set by the hospital which lab cannot raise, elimination of bonuses, limited benefits, etc.

If the hospital offers annual increments, it is imperative that you as Lab Director complete the paperwork for the Pathologists' increments in a timely manner. If this paperwork is delayed they will likely not receive their increments for that year. These increments will be seen as automatic by the Pathologists. If you fail to give out the annual increments, this will be seen by the affected Pathologists as a huge affront.

Without much to offer in the way of financial incentives for retention, the best you can do as Lab Director is to ensure a nice, happy working environment where everyone is as friendly as possible. There are numerous points to mention is this regard. In my experience it is best to allow every position in lab as much autonomy as possible. The Pathologists can function independently, so allow them complete autonomy. If you micromanage, and take away their autonomy, it will cause resentment. If a Pathologist makes a suggestion for improvement to the lab, take that suggestion seriously. In the majority of situations, treat the Pathologists as equals, not subordinates.

As Lab Director you will supervise anatomic pathology and cytopathology. This is a little different than directing the clinical lab in that you are supervising other physicians. It also differs in that the interpretations of a slide are very subjective, whereas the results turned out by an analyzer are cut and dry – the test is either positive or negative, or else it generates a number, with no subjective interpretation. Thus, evaluating the performance of a Pathologist and/or Cytopathologist is harder than evaluating the performance of a lab tech.

The best advice I can give is as follows. All anatomic pathology and cytopathology diagnoses are interpretive opinions. No one can claim his or her opinion is the gold standard. In my experience, there is a huge amount of variation in slide interpretation among different pathologists. You must be very tolerant of every other pathologist's interpretation.

Before you begin Pathologist performance evaluation, you must decide what criteria to measure, and what constitutes outstanding work, passing, and failing for these criteria. Some labs mandate a 10% lookback on the slides signed out by each Pathologist in the group. There is a small allowable rate of error. In most of these labs a "major error" rate of 1% is allowed. However, even the definition of a major error is subjective.

I have seen biopsy cases so difficult that a group of nine pathologists split three ways – 4 wanted a malignant diagnosis, 4 wanted a benign diagnosis and one was noncommittal. The case was sent out in consultation. The consultants equivocated and recommended re-biopsy. Which if any of this group made a major error in interpretation?

In my experience most practices do not do retrospective review of the pathology and cytology slides. In these labs, the evaluation of the pathologists is based on other criteria such as complaints received and rates of revised (corrected) diagnoses. Even this is problematic, as one patient can file multiple unjustified complaints on a Pathologist. Pathology cases tend to be amended after the fact to add results of outside tests. If the computer adds these cases to the list of revised cases, it will make the rate of revision look much worse than it otherwise would be.

Other possible evaluation criteria such as correlation with outside consultation, frozen section correlation to permanent section, cytology correlation to histology, etc. are fraught with the same problems of subjectivity. The bottom line is that when dealing with subjective interpretations, there is no gold standard. All performance measurements are relative.

Completely subjective measures of performance evaluation should be avoided. My advice is to never act on a group's "gut feeling" toward one particular pathologist. Keep the evaluations as objective as possible and avoid acting on personal likes and dislikes within the group. Avoid making decisions based on hearsay. If anyone in the Pathology group has anything negative to say about another in the group, the accuser must produce the paperwork or else retract the accusation.

Most people think of competence as being all-or-none, like a light switch which can only be in the off or the on position. In reality there is a continuum or spectrum ranging from perfect competence to perfect incompetence with infinite possibilities in between. In my experience there are a few warning signs:

1. The practitioner is practicing beyond the usual age of retirement for the specialty. For Pathology the usual retirement age is 66 or 67.
2. The practitioner has medical problems, especially medical problems that would compromise cognition or vision. The practitioner may try to hide these problems and not inform co-workers or management.
3. The practitioner would like to retire, but is compelled to continue working for financial reasons.
4. The practitioner is out of touch with the latest developments in the specialty, uses outdated terminology, and only has the minimum Continuing Medical Education (CME) to meet

licensure requirements.
5. Multiple instances in a short time of the practitioner making a diagnosis on a slide that is completely different from all other Pathologists looking at the same slide.
6. The practitioner progressively slows down, getting less and less work done in an 8 hour day. As a result more and more work is delegated to the younger Pathologists. This work slowdown runs its course over many years, such that few people will notice until it is in a very advanced state. You will look back over the past several years, and wonder how this practitioner got away with doing so little work for so many years.

Of the above warning signs, number 5 is the most important. It indicates loss of skills and abilities. The CMS defines competency as the ability of personnel to apply their skill, knowledge, and experience to perform their duties correctly. Implied but not stated is that loss of these abilities indicates incompetence. I have also seen incompetence defined as "too many mistakes too fast".

The Joint Commission (TJC) requires Ongoing Professional Practice Evaluation (OPPE) for all physicians at least every 6 months. Annual review is not frequent enough to be "ongoing". Virtually all hospitals in the US are TJC certified. If you are Lab Director of a hospital lab you will have to fill out an OPPE form for each Pathologist at least every 6 months. If you are Lab Director of an outpatient lab that is not TJC certified, you are not required to fill out OPPE forms.

A Focused Professional Practice Evaluation (FPPE) is similar but only occurs when there is a triggering event. Triggers include a Pathologist arrives new to your hospital, an existing Pathologist applies for increased privileges, and/or a Pathologist has made one or more mistakes significant enough to trigger an FPPE. An FPPE is a one-time event which does not recur. Otherwise an FPPE is similar to an OPPE.

The OPPE form typically has fill in the blank boxes and/or checkboxes for workload, timeliness and competency. After completing the OPPE form you will need to check a box for overall grading as "pass" or "fail". See the form on the next page.

MY LAB					MY PROCEDURE MANUAL		
Ongoing Practitioner Performance Evaluation (OPPE) Form							
Provider:				**ID #:**		**Department:** Pathology	
Status:				**Department Chairman:**			
Specialty: Pathology							

Indicator	Most Current 6-mo. Period				6-month Thresholds		
	1H 2020	2H 2020	1H 2021	2H 2021	Exceeds	Meets	Below
Number of Cases - Pathology							
Number of Cases - Cytology							
Number of Cases - Autopsies							
Percent major disagreement at retrospective review					0%	< 1%	1% or more
Correlation of Outside Consultation with Pathologist's Diagnosis					> 95%	95%	< 95%
Surgical Pathology Report completed w/in 2 days					> 97%	97%	< 97%
Cytology Report completed w/in 3 days of receipt of specimen					> 97%	97%	< 97%
Validated Patient Complaints					0	1-3	> 3
Validated Staff Complaints					0	1-3	> 3

Overall Grade	Pass	Fail	Signature of practitioner	Signature of Department Chair
1H 2020				
2H 2020				
1H 2021				
2H 2021				

I have seen cases where the workload is zero for a particular specimen type. In general, no action can be taken against the practitioner for low or nonexistent workload. If the turnaround time is prolonged, the usual result is a brief motivational talk with the Pathologist involved.

The TJC mandates that you evaluate competency, but has no specific requirement on how to measure it. In some institutions it is measured by retrospective review of cases. However this is not mandatory, and other performance measures can be chosen such as complaints received and rates of revised (corrected) diagnoses.

If your lab is doing retrospective review of cases and finds one or more Pathologist with the percent of cases having reviewer disagreement exceeding the allowable threshold, this will trigger close scrutiny. Look at the slides for the cases that have fallen out to referee them. After reviewing these cases, refer any discrepant cases back to the original signing Pathologist. Ask the original signing Pathologist to reconsider his or her diagnosis and consider issuing an amended pathology report.

If the original signing Pathologist does not reconsider, but you and the reviewing Pathologist feel strongly about the case, you will need to have the case reviewed further. If you are in a large group, show the slides to the entire group and vote on the diagnosis. A simple majority vote wins. If you are in a small group, send the case out to a subspecialist for refereeing.

A few minor disagreements are common; nothing further needs to be done. If one or more major disagreement is identified, you will need to call that Pathologist into your office and have a long talk. Ask how this happened and how it can be prevented in the future. Suggest to that Pathologist that you are always open for consultations, and can review any case(s) that Pathologist wants reviewed.

If this is an isolated instance, nothing further needs to be done. If it recurs, there are a number of options to consider. At first the approach should be educational. Mandate some education, training, seminars, etc. in that Pathologist's areas of weakness. If this solves the problem, nothing further needs to be done.

If the problem continues, you may need to assign that Pathologist a proctor to review some or all of that Pathologist's cases before sign-out. You are in effect demoting an Attending level physician to a Fellowship level, but this may be necessary given the circumstances. If the Pathologist is having medical problems, request that Pathologist to submit medical clearance from his or her physician. If that Pathologist is still in the probationary period, extend the probationary period if possible.

If the problem is resolved by any of the above means, no further action needs to be taken. If the excessive rate of major discrepancies continues, you are going to have to call that Pathologist in for a long series of talks about retirement. Give a retirement pep talk: You are really going to love retirement, it is so much fun to be retired. I retired from Pathology to Lab Director work and love it. You can spend more time with your grandchildren.

The needs of the patient take priority over the needs of this Pathologist. If you can't talk this Pathologist into retirement and the Pathologist still has an excessive rate of major discrepancies, the next step is to take the matter to the hospital Medical Director. The Medical Director will likely not have much understanding of pathology and the situation may require quite a bit of explaining. You may have to meet more than once with the Medical Director to adequately explain the situation. Provide copies of all the documents related to the retrospective reviews, major discrepancies, etc. to the Medical Director.

Any seasoned Medical Director will have prior experience dealing with physician performance issues, and will have a good idea of what to do. The Medical Director will call in that Pathologist for a very unpleasant series of meetings. You as Lab Director will likely have to sit in on the majority of these meetings.

The hospital Medical Director can force a retirement, typically on threat of summary suspension of clinical privileges. The Medical Director will not be bluffing. I have seen at least one case in which the hospital Medial Director actually did follow through on the threat of summary suspension for a Pathologist that refused retirement. This is a horrible way for an elderly Pathologist to end his or her career but in some cases it can't be avoided.

Doing this to a colleague can be heartbreaking, especially if you have worked with that Pathologist for many years. It will make you feel like Judas, the betrayer, but it is necessary given the circumstances.

I will give the example of Dr. S. an elderly Pathologist I was working with at my first job after graduating training in 1996. Dr. S. was born around 1923. He had three wives, two divorces, and a total of 8 children (3 children with his first wife, 3 children with his second wife, and 2 children with his third wife). He had lost all his savings to divorce, alimony and child support.

He had no savings for retirement and for financial reasons continued working as a Pathologist into his late 70s. Sometime in 1999 he had an episode of acute angle glaucoma in his right eye. He went out on sick leave for a few weeks. There was some debate as to whether he should be allowed to return to work. He had some loss of vision in the right eye, correctable to about 20/60. The ophthalmologist did not know the visual acuity necessary to be a Pathologist. The literature does not state any minimum visual acuity for working as a Pathologist.

While Dr. S. was out on leave his situation was discussed a number of times between the Pathologists and Lab Director. I was in a Pathologist position, and had no strong feelings either way as to whether he should or should not be allowed to return. The Lab Director for that hospital had worked with Dr. S. for many years and was a close friend. The decision was made to allow Dr. S. to return to work.

Dr. S. wanted to keep working, and was allowed to keep working. In the subsequent 6 months he made significant mis-steps. One involved a mastectomy for carcinoma. He correctly called the breast lesion as an infiltrating ductal carcinoma. He called one lymph node positive for metastatic carcinoma. The patient was referred to a different hospital for chemotherapy. As is the usual practice, the pathologists at the referral hospital reviewed the case. They called the lymph node negative for carcinoma.

This same lymph node slide has been looked at by over a dozen Pathologists and all Pathologists except for Dr. S. have called that lymph node negative for metastatic carcinoma. The block was recut and stained with immunos, and over a dozen pathologists called the immuno slides negative for metastatic carcinoma.

Dr. S. had two other mis-steps in the first 6 months after his episode of acute angle glaucoma. In one of these he mistook an endocervical adenocarcinoma in-situ for adenoma malignum. In the other, he mistook a reactive lymph node for lymphoma.

Dr. S. was forced to retire from his Pathologist position. He was around 78 years old at the time. He subsequently got a desk job as a Lab Director in a different state. He worked as a Lab Director for another 8 years until he got Parkinson's disease and became wheelchair-bound. The story as I have been told is this practitioner had Parkinson's disease for many years. He tried to hide his condition from co-workers and did not inform co-workers he was on medication for Parkinson's disease. When he became wheelchair-bound he could no longer hide his condition from co-workers. He was around 86 years old when this happened. He wanted to continue working, but was forced to retire from that Lab Director position because he could no longer carry out the duties of the job position.

The point of this story is that there are people in this world who will continue to work until well after it is obvious that they can no longer do the job. Such a person has no insight into their own condition and will continue working until forced to stop. Your mission is to help them to retire. They may not like it, but at this point retirement is in their best interest and in your best interest as well.

The above story is an extreme example of a retirement done the wrong way by the retiree. Most Pathologist retirements I have seen have been done more or less the right way. The right way to retire, as I see it, is a gradual cutting back on work to match the slow declines in cognitive function and vision due to aging.

When I started my first job after graduating training in 1996 the Lab Director at that hospital was in his mid 60s. He was the sharpest Pathologist I had ever seen. Over the course of the next few years, he would lose some of his brilliance but was still very sharp. He retired from tissue exams in the year 2000 while in his late 60s. At that time he retained several Lab Directorships, including one at a major hospital lab.

He continued losing sharpness over the ensuing years. He retired from the hospital Lab Director position in 2005 while in his mid 70s. He retained Lab Directorships at a few small clinics. These were very easy desk jobs that consisted of coming in a few times a month to sign papers for a few hours.

At present, he is an extremely elderly, frail gentleman in his late-80s, almost completely lacking the sharpness and energy he had 24 years prior. He has cut back to one small clinic Lab Directorship. He would like to retire from that position, but the clinic can't find a replacement.

This story, of a slow cutting back of one's work, is typical of a Pathologist's retirement. Less common is the situation where one stops work completely when one becomes eligible for Social Security retirement, currently the 66th birthday. I have known a few Pathologists who took this approach, ending their career abruptly, like a door slammed shut on their 66th birthday.

Chapter 22 – How to go through the inspection process

    A. How to pick an inspecting agency and prepare for the inspection

In the US all clinical labs fall under CLIA. For labs doing moderate and/or high complexity testing, the CMS requires inspections to ensure compliance with the CLIA regulations. Each lab will have one inspection shortly after applying for CMS certification (or equivalent) and at least biennially thereafter. Inspections are carried out by the CMS, or any inspecting agency with deemed status. The CMS will call its visit to your lab a "survey" but everyone else calls it an "inspection".

The deemed status inspecting agencies include CAP, COLA and TJC. The States of New York and

Washington also have deemed status. These accrediting organizations have been "deemed" by CMS as having standards and inspections that meet or exceed the Medicare/Medicaid Conditions of Participation (CoP). Labs inspected by the "deemed status" inspecting agencies are not subject to the CMS inspection and certification process since they are assumed to already meet minimum Medicare and Medicaid requirements. After successful completion of the inspection a CMS Certificate of Compliance, CAP Certificate of Accreditation, or similar documentation is issued. This certification is necessary to bill Medicare, Medicaid and most private insurance companies.

The difficulty level in passing an inspection from any of the inspecting agencies is roughly the same. The deemed status inspecting agencies must meet CLIA requirements at a minimum but can also add their own requirements. Hence CMS is probably the easiest, most minimal inspection to pass. For small labs with little staffing, CMS inspections are likely to be the best choice. For larger labs with more staffing, consider CAP inspections which are seen as more prestigious.

Some insurers will only reimburse to labs accredited by CAP. Before you pick your inspecting agency, make sure you discuss with your billing department as to what the local insurance companies require for reimbursement.

The FDA and AABB only inspect Blood Bank, not the entire lab. The AABB does not have "deemed status" with the FDA such that if you sign up for AABB inspections you will still get FDA inspections. Elect for FDA inspections alone if you are heading up a small lab with limited resources. If you are in a large Blood Bank with a great deal of staff, consider adding AABB inspections for the prestige. The process of preparation, inspection and remediation of deficiencies is the same for FDA and AABB inspections as for the general lab inspections described below.

To prepare for the inspection, go through your lab the way the inspector would. Look at all the procedure manuals. Are the manuals complete? Is there a procedure for every test done in-house? Are all procedures formatted properly with the current version signed by the Lab Director? For CAP inspections, were the manuals signed by the Lab Director within the last 2 years? Have the staff signed all procedures? Is the table of contents complete with accurate page numbers? Have all comments and written corrections been addressed and incorporated into the procedures?

Look at your lab's proficiency testing. The inspectors will generally only look back at the last 2 years of data. Is the lab enrolled in PT for every regulated analyte tested? Are the attestation sheets signed? How many failures did you have in the last 2 years? Do all PT failures have an acceptable corrective action?

Go through the lab general documents and each of the sections – chemistry, hematology, Blood Bank, urinalysis, etc. Look through the procedure manuals, QC logs, temperature monitoring logs, preventive maintenance logs, competency testing records, etc. as if you were an inspector. Was QC done on all days when patient testing was done? Was the QC acceptable or a corrective action done before patient testing was done? Are the temperature monitoring logs complete with no instances of the temperature range being exceeded? Do the PM logs have checks in all checkboxes in the appropriate time frame? Do all lab testing personnel have competency testing forms filled out within the acceptable time frame? This does not have to be as formal as a "mock inspection" or self-inspection, but should at least cover the basics.

In the hospitals I have worked at, the lab staff personnel files are stored in the hospital-wide Human Resources (HR) department, and only the competency testing forms are stored in lab. Contact your HR department and ensure that someone in the HR department will be available on the day of inspection to produce the personnel files to the inspector. Ask the HR department to review the lab staff personnel files in advance of the inspection to ensure that all licenses are current, all diplomas are present, etc.

The inspector may ask to see documentation delegating the authority for the General Supervisor, Technical Supervisor, Testing Personnel, etc. This requirement is typically met by showing the inspector the position description for the personnel in lab. In most hospitals these positions are referred to as "Lab Supervisor", "Section Supervisor", "Lab Tech", etc. and in my experience few labs use the CLIA terminology for these positions. As long as the position description lists duties meeting the CLIA requirements for "General Supervisor", "Technical Supervisor", etc. this should satisfy the inspector.

In advance of the inspection make sure the position descriptions in your lab list the CLIA duties specified for these positions. Ask HR to check all lab staff's file folders to make sure the position descriptions are present. For example, if you put down "Dr. Dauterman" as Lab Director and Clinical Consultant on your form CMS-209, you must ensure the position descriptions for Lab Director and Clinical Consultant are present in my file folder in the HR office, and these position descriptions must list the duties specified for these positions under CLIA. It is possible to specify additional duties, but the CLIA duties must be specified as a minimum.

The inspectors will likely want to see some or all incident reports involving lab. In most hospitals, the only copy of an incident report form is kept in the Risk Manager's Office. When you receive notice of the pending inspection, inform the Risk Manager's Office and ensure someone will be available on the day of inspection to produce the lab's incident report forms to the inspectors if requested. Do the same for any other documents stored outside of lab that could be subject to inspection.

The lab Quality Assurance program will be scrutinized closely in any inspection. Make sure that the documents are up to date. For each QA indicator, there should be data in the folder for each month up to the most recent month. Any QA failures should have corrective action documented.

Lab safety will be part of any inspection. Make sure all hazardous chemicals are locked in the appropriate storage areas (fire cabinet, corrosives cabinet, etc.) Make sure all fire extinguishers, emergency eyewashes and emergency showers are working and have current certification stickers. Make sure the emergency exits are not obstructed and open properly. Make sure there is a procedure for hazardous chemical spills and all staff are familiar with this procedure, etc.

If you have put any new analyzers into service since the last biennial inspection, the verification work is likely to be inspected. Have the folder with the verification work available for review. If you have created any new IQCP since the last biennial inspection these new IQCP will likely come under scrutiny.

There have been rare instances when an inspector has asked to see the prior biennial inspection citations and corrective action. This usually only occurs when you get a new inspector that has not inspected you before. In one instance a veteran inspector asked to see the prior inspection citations which he himself had written 2 years before. He admitted he lost the original in a hard drive crash; he had not made a backup copy and needed to see our copy. Keep the prior biennial inspection citations and corrective action available for the next inspection. Review the prior biennial inspection citations and corrective actions to ensure there has been follow-through on the corrective actions and no recurrences of the problems.

This will give you some idea if you are ready or not for the inspection. If you are ready, then it is just a matter of keeping things in order in the time left before the inspection. If there is still much work to be done, you will be staying late, or very late at work trying to get it all caught up before the inspection. In this regard, it is important to start the preparation early. Start the preparation as many months in advance as possible. You do not want to run out of time such that the inspectors arrive before the lab's preparations are complete.

You may or may not be informed in advance of the date of inspection. In any event, you will know the general time frame of the inspection. The inspectors will typically send you paperwork that should be filled out and returned prior to the start of the inspection. This typically includes CMS form 209. See pages 5 to 7 for instructions on filling out CMS form 209. Receiving this paperwork indicates the inspection is imminent, typically within the next 2 months.

To briefly summarize, the checklist of items that are likely to be inspected are:

1. Quality Control (QC) logs
2. Proficiency Testing (PT)
3. Lab safety (fire exits, use of PPE, etc.)
4. Preventive Maintenance (PM) logs
5. Personnel records/competency testing
6. Procedure manuals
7. Adequate stocks of reagents and supplies
8. Prior biennial inspection citations and corrective action
9. The lab Quality Assurance (QA) program
10. Incident Reports (IR) involving lab
11. Temperature monitoring logs
12. Verification work for any new analyzers
13. Newly created IQCP
14. Expiration dates of reagents and supplies

In my experience the two most common citations involve expired reagents/supplies and storage of excessive amounts of paper records in lab. While preparing for the inspection, assign each section supervisor to inventory their section for expired reagents/supplies. These expired reagents/supplies must be replaced with in-date reagents/supplies by the time of the inspection. If there are numerous boxes of paper records being stored in lab, check which records are old enough to be shredded. Shred any boxes of documents that are beyond the required retention time. If you have many boxes of documents that are too recent to shred, you can send them to off-site storage as long as they are easily retrievable from that storage and safe from destruction. Make sure any boxes of records present in lab are off the floor and not blocking fire exits.

First impressions are important. If the inspectors come into your lab and find it dirty, with boxes of records stacked up to the ceiling, they will not think too highly of your lab. This could result in a citation in and of itself. Try to keep the number of boxes of records to a minimum. Try to have the lab cleaned to the extent possible. Usually the hospital Housekeeping Department is called in during the run-up to the inspection to give lab a thorough cleaning. In most labs I have worked at, the lab gets its floors waxed once every 2 years in the run-up to the inspection. If the floors have not been waxed in years, this will go a long way toward making the lab look cleaner.

At any inspection, the burden is on you to produce all paperwork requested. If the inspector asks for paperwork and you cannot produce it the inspector will assume the work was not done and you will be cited. You will then need to send copies of that paperwork to the inspector after the inspection is over. Producing duplicate copies of documents is cumbersome and time consuming. Hence it is in your best interest to keep all documents organized in a manner that is easily retrievable so that all documents can be produced on a moment's notice.

Here is a tip that a CMS inspector once gave me. The inspector is only allowed to ask for the last 2 years of lab documentation, which should correspond to the documentation since the last inspection. However, if you leave lab QC manuals sitting out that are more than 2 years old, the inspector is allowed to look at them. If you had a QC failure 3 years ago, and the inspector missed it on the last inspection, the only way it could be caught is if you leave the manual in plain sight at the next inspection. Thus when preparing for the inspection, try to only leave the last 2 years of documentation in plain sight. Keep the older documentation locked in a cabinet where it can't be seen, but can be retrieved if necessary.

Another caveat is that hospital-wide inspectors can visit lab. In an educational course regarding hospital-wide inspections, the CMS inspector said that when going through a hospital-wide inspection he will stop in each department including lab and ask the staff in that department about the QAPI indicators for their area, how incident reports are routed, etc. If the staff are not able to answer, this is cited as a deficiency on the hospital-wide inspection. Make sure that all lab staff are aware of the lab's

QAPI indicators, how an incident report routes, etc. since they could be asked during an inspection.

For the most part hospital-wide inspectors don't inspect lab. Your lab has already been inspected by CMS or a deemed agency and found to be acceptable. Everything in your lab that is covered under CLIA has passed a lab-specific inspection. The typical hospital-wide inspector has very little lab-specific training and is very unlikely to question the findings of a lab-specific inspector. Thus, hospital-wide inspectors will typically avoid the lab entirely, or only pay a very cursory visit to look for deficiencies of the following:

1. Lab safety (physical plant) such as fire extinguishers, SDS binders, fire exits, no blocking of egress, toxic/flammable chemical storage, etc.
2. Blood Bank notification of units recalled by Red Cross. This does not fall under CLIA. The FDA mandates this, and it typically gets inspected by hospital-wide inspectors.
3. Hospital-wide QA activities involving lab.
4. The flow of specimens to lab and the reporting of test results from lab back to the rest of the hospital, clinics, etc.

> B. The day of the inspection

In general, routine biennial inspections are unannounced. However, they are typically timed to coincide with the expiration of an existing CMS Certificate of Compliance (or equivalent). For new labs the inspection is typically conducted within 90 days of the application for certification (or equivalent). Either way, you will know the time frame of the inspection within a few months but will not typically know the exact day.

The inspectors will typically arrive before the start of the work day. They will show you their ID badges and typically give you a copy of the letter directing them to inspect your lab. They will typically want a brief meeting with the Hospital Administrator before starting the inspection. The inspectors will need office space on the day of inspection. The lab breakroom is usually given over to the inspectors for their use on the day of the inspection. Sometimes the Lab Secretary's Office is used for this purpose. Make sure to have a large breakfast and lunch served. At the minimum, you do not want the inspectors to be hungry during the inspection.

The inspection typically starts with a meeting for introductions and discussion of the work at hand. The inspection work typically starts immediately after this introductory meeting concludes. The inspectors will look through all your documentation, make observations of your lab, check expiration dates on your supplies and reagents, interview your staff, ask your staff if the supplies and equipment are adequate, etc. They may or may not watch the lab techs do the testing. They may or may not follow specimens as they are processed through your lab. They may take a quick tour of other parts of the hospital – morgue, fingerstick glucose testing in other wards, the computer center, etc. If patient testing is spread across multiple sites, they will likely inspect all sites performing patient testing. The inspection must include an assessment of lab safety. The inspectors will check your fire extinguishers, emergency exits, emergency eyewashes, emergency showers, storage of chemicals in the fire cabinet, etc.

At the end of the inspection you and the hospital administrator will be called for the summation meeting. This meeting is sometimes referred to as an "exit interview". In this meeting the inspectors will recite their list of findings. Many of these will be recommendations. A recommendation is a suggestion as to how to improve your lab. You are not obligated to follow the recommendations; you can continue doing things the same way if you want.

In regard to the recommendations, inspections are very useful. Outside lab experts are coming to your lab and looking at how your lab does things. Their input is valuable. The inspectors are likely to be as current as possible on the latest developments in the lab field, and their recommendations should be taken seriously.

A citation is a finding that you are obligated to correct in order to continue being certified by the inspecting agency. Almost all labs will get a few small citations on any given inspection. From what I have heard, the inspectors feel obligated to give at least one citation so as to justify their inspection. In a CMS inspection the citations are divided into three levels of deficiency. I will discuss these at length later in this chapter. In increasing order of severity they are:

1. standard level deficiency
2. condition level deficiency
3. immediate jeopardy

Pay close attention to everything the inspectors say in the exit interview. You will need to respond to the citations. Make sure you are very clear on the citations. If you don't understand a citation, ask for further clarification. For any complex citation, I would ask the inspectors for suggestions on how to correct the citation.

In the exit interview, the inspectors will rattle off a list of findings. It is important to maintain your composure in this meeting and be as nice as possible. The inspectors may give off a long list of things you have done wrong, but it is not a personal attack. They are just doing their jobs. Avoid arguments with the CMS inspectors. If you disagree with the inspectors on a finding, it may be best to approach them after the meeting is over to discuss that particular finding further. I am aware of one physician Nursing Home Director who was fired for getting into an argument with CMS inspectors at the exit interview.

After the end of the inspection you will receive a copy of the inspection paperwork with the list of citations. The inspection citations will typically be handwritten at this point. The CMS inspectors will then go back to their main office, the form 2567 will be typed and then mailed to your lab.

Your lab will need to prepare a response to each citation, usually within 10 days of receiving them. The timer starts ticking when you receive the typed form 2567 in the mail. This typically arrives 2 to 3 weeks after the inspection is over, allowing you more time to work on the plan of correction. You may or may not receive an accompanying letter with the following verbatim from CMS on how to make a plan of correction.

> The acceptable evidence of correction that you must provide to CMS must include at a minimum:
>
> 1. documentation showing what corrective action(s) have been taken for patients found to have been affected by the deficient practice;
> 2. an explanation of how the laboratory has identified other patients having the potential to be affected by the same deficient practice and what corrective action(s) has been taken;
> 3. a description of the measures that have been put into place or systemic changes made to

ensure that the deficient practice does not recur;
4. a description of how the corrective actions are being monitored to ensure the deficient practice does not recur.

Although this is the verbatim from CMS, there is much more to making a Plan of Correction than the skeletal outline given above. If you followed the instructions from CMS given above, and did no further work, the CMS inspectors would almost certainly reject your Plan of Correction when you send it in to the CMS. I will go in great detail below about how to make a passable Plan of Correction.

In theory, the Lab Supervisor is responsible for all corrective actions in Lab, including responses to inspection citations. In reality, the Lab Supervisor and Lab Director write the responses together.

Re-inspections are additional inspections in between the biennial inspections. If your lab is inspected by CMS and found to have condition level deficiencies or immediate jeopardy, you are almost guaranteed to have re-inspections before the next biennial inspection. I have never seen the CAP conduct re-inspections. The CAP literature equates a re-inspection with the next biennial inspection. Thus it is doubtful the CAP ever carries out additional inspections between the biennial inspections.

A re-inspection is conducted to ensure continued compliance with a plan of correction made after a biennial inspection. A re-inspection is handled somewhat differently than a biennial inspection. At a re-inspection the inspector can only ask to see something cited at the prior inspection, or related to the ensuing plan of correction. The inspector is not allowed to ask for anything else but can cite anything obvious that he or she sees.

The way this is handled in the typical lab is that on the day of the re-inspection, the inspector is assigned the lab breakroom as the inspector's office space. The inspector is told that the Lab Supervisor and/or other lab staff have been assigned to retrieve whatever documents the inspector wants, while the inspector waits in the breakroom. We would prefer if the inspector does not leave the breakroom. As a result, the inspector will not be able to give any additional citations beyond those already on the prior form 2567.

Complaint inspections only occur if your inspecting agency has received a complaint about your lab. Complaint investigations can come at any time and are unannounced. Thus it is imperative to keep your lab up to standards at all times, since it is possible for inspectors to arrive unannounced at any time.

C. How to fill out CMS form 2567 and write a Plan of Correction

You will typically receive handwritten inspection notes on the day of inspection. The typed inspection report will come back a few weeks to a few months later.

I have seen several instances where the inspector said at the exit interview that he or she was going to cite something but the form 2567 came back without the citation. This typically means the inspector reviewed the findings later and determined that the findings could not be cited (no rules or regulations violated). I have seen a few instances where inspection citations appeared on the form 2567 but were not discussed at the exit interview. When I asked the inspector about this, I was told that this was an oversight. The inspector forgot to mention the citations at the exit interview, but a later review of the handwritten notes while typing the form 2567 reminded the inspector about the citation. Be prepared that there could be some surprises on the form 2567 when it arrives back to your lab.

Here is an example of the form you will receive if inspected by the CMS and found to have citations. This is form CMS-2567 Statement of Deficiencies and Plan of Correction:

DEPARTMENT OF HEALTH AND HUMAN SERVICES CENTERS FOR MEDICARE & MEDICAID SERVICES				PRINTED: FORM APPROVED OMB NO. 0938-0391
STATEMENT OF DEFICIENCIES AND PLAN OF CORRECTION	(X1) PROVIDER/SUPPLIER/CLIA IDENTIFICATION NUMBER:	(X2) MULTIPLE CONSTRUCTION A. BUILDING B. WING		(X3) DATE SURVEY COMPLETED
NAME OF PROVIDER OR SUPPLIER		STREET ADDRESS, CITY, STATE, ZIP CODE		
(X4) ID PREFIX TAG	SUMMARY STATEMENT OF DEFICIENCIES (EACH DEFICIENCY MUST BE PRECEDED BY FULL REGULATORY OR LSC IDENTIFYING INFORMATION)	ID PREFIX TAG	PROVIDER'S PLAN OF CORRECTION (EACH CORRECTIVE ACTION SHOULD BE CROSS-REFERENCED TO THE APPROPRIATE DEFICIENCY)	(X5) COMPLETION DATE
K 029 SS=F	NFPA 101 LIFE SAFETY CODE STANDARD One hour fire rated construction (with ¾ hour fire-rated doors) or an approved automatic fire extinguishing system in accordance with 8.4.1 and/or 19.3.5.4 protects hazardous areas. When the approved automatic fire extinguishing system option is used, the areas are separated from other spaces by smoke resisting partitions and doors. Doors are self-closing and non-rated or field-applied protective plates that do not exceed 48 inches from the bottom of the door are permitted. 19.3.2.1	K 029	The facility checked all exit doors and verified all were working as required. The door in on A wing was adjusted and is working properly. It will continue to be audited on a monthly basis by the Maintenance Department. Maintenance and the Administrator will be responsible for oversight.	

In the above example, the facility has been cited for violating the fire code because one fire door is not working properly. The left column under the header "Summary Statement of Deficiencies" should contain a description of the problem written in plain language. The inspector should have explained the citation to you at the exit interview. If you are not clear on the citation, you should be able to call the inspector at the inspector's office and ask for more explanation of the deficiency.

As with all corrective actions, the plan of correction must state how the lab has fixed the problem or plans to fix the problem, This could involve buying new equipment, new supplies, additional training and education for the lab staff, or could involve changing the lab's policies, procedures and/or processes (i.e. a "systemic change" meaning the lab is changing the way it does things). I have seen literature indicating that serious problems require systemic change, and anything less is an unacceptable "band-aid fix". There must be a time frame for completing the corrective action, preferably within 60 days but not to exceed 12 months from the last day of the inspection.

The corrective action must include a plan to monitor the situation to ensure there are no future recurrences of the problem. This often entails adding the cited problem area to the monthly quality assurance reviews. I have seen literature indicating it is mandatory to include all serious problems in the lab's quality assurance program.

This particular citation does not have the potential to affect patient lab results. In this situation it is sufficient to put down a statement that patients were not adversely affected. I will go into extensive detail below on how to handle citations where patient results may have been affected.

In the CMS literature there is no requirement for naming the person who is responsible for making the corrections and ensuring that there are no recurrences of the problem. If you are going to name the responsible party in the Plan of Correction, it is best to designate that person by title (e.g. Lab Director) and not by name (e.g. Dr. Dauterman). If the position changes over (e.g. I retire) all of the form 2567 responses that name me would have to be changed to reflect the name of the new Lab Director.

In the example above, the citation is relatively minor and easy to fix. The facility fixed the fire door in question and verified that all fire doors were working. The facility will continue to monitor the fire doors on a monthly basis to make sure that they keep working. The response was typed into the right column under the header "Provider's Plan of Correction". The date of completion of the corrective action is the date when you fixed the problem or expect to have the problem fixed. This is put in the far right column under the header "Completion Date". The monitoring to prevent recurrence must go on indefinitely and does not end on the completion date.

If there are multiple citations, repeat the same process for each citation. If your lab received a large number of citations, writing the responses can seem like a daunting task. If you look at the big picture, you may get overwhelmed. Try to look at it one citation at a time. Each plan of correction may be a single small step, but if you put all the steps together you will get through the process of writing the plans of correction.

If you have difficulty writing a response to one or more citation, you are allowed to call in consultants, call for advice from the supervisors of surrounding labs, etc. You will become more proficient at writing corrective actions the more you do it. After you have been through several inspections, writing the corrective actions will seem routine and unexciting.

The fire door citation in the example above typifies a very minor citation for a lab. It is an example of a "standard level deficiency". This is the lowest of the three levels of deficiency. This level of deficiency occurs when the lab violates a standard but there is no risk of patient harm and the deficiency does not limit the lab's ability to furnish safe and effective services. In the example above, the fire door citation does not relate to the lab testing per se. The inspectors pay particular attention to details related to the health and safety of the employees, such that this type of citation is very common.

Note that the above corrective action fulfills the minimum criteria set by CMS. The CMS inspectors will be checking your responses against the following four requirements. If these requirements are met your corrective action is likely to be accepted as is. If these requirements are not met your corrective action is likely to be rejected, with a request for you to do more work on the responses:

1. documentation showing what corrective action(s) have been taken for patients found to have been affected by the deficient practice;
2. an explanation of how the laboratory has identified other patients having the potential to be affected by the same deficient practice and what corrective action(s) has been taken;
3. a description of the measures that have been put into place or systemic changes made to ensure that the deficient practice does not recur;
4. a description of how the corrective actions are being monitored to ensure the deficient practice does not recur.

Here is another example of form CMS-2567 Statement of Deficiencies and Plan of Correction:

				PRINTED: ▮▮▮ FORM APPROVED OMB NO. 0938-0391
OF HEALTH AND HUMAN SERVICES FOR MEDICARE & MEDICAID SERVICES				
OF DEFICIENCIES OF CORRECTION	(X1) PROVIDER/SUPPLIER/CLIA IDENTIFICATION NUMBER: ▮▮▮	(X2) MULTIPLE CONSTRUCTION A. BUILDING _____ B. WING _____		(X3) DATE SURVEY COMPLETED ▮
NAME OF PROVIDER OR SUPPLIER ▮▮▮		STREET ADDRESS, CITY, STATE, ZIP CODE ▮▮▮		
(X4) ID PREFIX TAG	SUMMARY STATEMENT OF DEFICIENCIES (EACH DEFICIENCY MUST BE PRECEDED BY FULL REGULATORY OR LSC IDENTIFYING INFORMATION)	ID PREFIX TAG	PROVIDER'S PLAN OF CORRECTION (EACH CORRECTIVE ACTION SHOULD BE CROSS-REFERENCED TO THE APPROPRIATE DEFICIENCY)	(X5) COMPLETION DATE
D6000	493.1403 LABORATORY DIRECTOR The laboratory must have a director who meets the qualification requirements of §493.1405 of this subpart and provides overall management and direction in accordance with §493.1407 of this subpart. This CONDITION is not met as evidenced by: Based on interviews with hospital administration, on August 29, 2011, and an Attorney General memo attached to an Independent Contractor Agreement for Medical Director of Laboratory Services, and review of the routine re-certification survey conducted in June, 2010, the laboratory has failed to assign a director who meets the qualification requirements of §493.1405 of this subpart and provides overall management and direction in accordance with §493.1407 of this subpart. Findings include;	D6000		

This citation is for a lab that left the Lab Director position vacant for more than one year. Per CLIA, the Lab Director position can only be left vacant for 30 days. From talking with the CMS inspectors, they consider this to be the single worst offense a lab can commit.

In the case of this lab, CMS gave the lab a type of citation called a "condition level deficiency". This is the middle of the three levels of deficiency. It means that the lab was not meeting the conditions for participating in Medicare. Condition level deficiencies limit the lab's ability to furnish safe and effective services but do not represent an immediate threat to the patients.

In the case of the vacant Lab Director citation given above, the CMS additionally gave an Immediate Jeopardy citation to this lab's hospital. This is the highest of the three levels of deficiency. An Immediate Jeopardy citation means that the CMS feels the situation is a serious and immediate risk to the life and/or safety of the patients at that hospital.

The process of corrective action is the same. The lab made a plan to hire a Lab Director and followed through on hiring a Lab Director. They hired me. This is the lab that I was hired to "turnaround" in August, 2013. My presence at that lab mitigated the greatest deficiency, and I worked very hard to correct the other problems in that lab. In the subsequent CMS inspection in December, 2013 this lab had only two minor citations.

The point is not that I fly in like Superman to fix up labs. The point is that all corrective actions follow the same process, from the most minor citation (one stuck fire door) to the worst possible citation for a lab (no Lab Director for more than a year).

In both examples of form 2567 given above, the stuck fire door and the vacant Lab Director position, there was no potential for patient harm. In other words, these deficiencies did not adversely affect patient care. If there was a potential for patient harm the Plan of Correction would need additional work. You would need to issue corrected reports for any erroneous test results and determine if the change in test results would have made a difference in patient care. You are required to inform CMS of the findings, even if you don't like what you find.

I will give an example of how this works using the nonexistent test serum radon levels and its mythical association with lung cancer. Let's say your lab was found at a CMS inspection to be out of control for serum radon levels and turning out results too low. You have done 1000 tests in the time serum radon levels were out of control. You get the test back into control, retest these 1000 specimens and find they were all reported too low. You have to issue a corrected report for each of these 1000 specimens. Even worse, 100 were originally false negatives. They were reported as negative, but on retest are above the action level (i.e. positive).

CLIA requires that you promptly notify the person ordering the test and, if applicable, the individual using the test results of reporting errors. The reference for this is 42 CFR § 493.1291. This is interpreted as requiring a phone call to the provider to inform him or her of the change in test results.

Your lab will be making 1000 phone calls to inform the providers of the corrected test results. The providers in question will be unhappy to find that they have received erroneous test results. For 100 of those patients, you will be correcting the report from negative to positive. The providers will be even more upset in this circumstance, as it will change the clinical approach to the patient.

You are required to identify any patients that could potentially have been harmed, document that there was no harm to those patients or try to mitigate the harm to the extent possible. The way that most people interpret this is that you only have to follow up on the 100 patients that had false negative tests. You do not need to follow up the other 900 that had a slight change in test result, but are still negative. This means that you are going to be pulling 100 charts from medical records and reviewing them all to make sure that none of the patients got lung cancer.

The effort described so far (1000 retests, 1000 corrected reports, 1000 phone calls, 100 chart reviews) is a huge amount of work. It would have been much easier to keep the serum radon levels in control in the first place. Hence, this is why it is so important to make sure your techs never turn out test results unless controls are in for that run or day. The cleanup afterward can involve a huge amount of work, and is a huge headache.

It gets worse from there. Let's say you pull the 100 charts from medical records and find that 3 of these patients developed lung cancer within two years of the false negative serum radon levels. Two of these three patients have passed away from lung cancer. The patient population is older, and lung cancer is so common in the elderly that if you pick 100 older people and follow them for two years it is not unlikely that 3 of them will get lung cancer.

The problem is that in this case, the 3 that got lung cancer had a false negative serum radon level from your lab in the two years before the lung cancer diagnosis. If you had turned out a positive serum radon level, these 3 patients might have gotten worked up for lung cancer, and it might have been caught earlier. The CMS inspectors are likely to interpret this as serious patient harm or patient fatalities from the testing in your lab. You have just taken a huge step toward regulatory closure of your lab.

The temptation is to try to cover up the bad outcomes. Keep in mind that as a physician you have an ethical obligation to the patient, not to the hospital that employs you. If your lab is under regulatory scrutiny, the CMS inspectors will be watching you very carefully. They will likely come unannounced, interview your staff privately, and go through your medical records department as they see fit. You will likely get caught if you try to conceal information from the CMS inspectors. If you get caught concealing information, that is another big step towards regulatory closure of your lab and now the CMS inspectors will start thinking about banning you. Thus it is in your best interest to self-report any untoward information you uncover. Let the chips fall where they may and take your lumps.

After you complete all the responses, mail the CMS form 2567 back to the inspecting agency. Include all relevant documentation, such as copies of revised procedures, invoices for newly purchased equipment, examples of corrected test reports, results of chart reviews, etc. These separate pages should be marked with the citation number (for example D6000 in the above Lab Director citation) so that they are easier for the inspectors to cross-reference to the form 2567. The responses can be mailed, FAXed or scanned and E-mailed back to the inspecting agency.

The form 2567 and responses are due back 10 days after you receive the form in the mail. While working on the responses, it is not uncommon to run out of time and/or find that the corrections take longer than the 10 days allowed for submitting the responses. For any citations with incomplete work put down a statement as to how the lab is attempting to correct the problem, identify and correct any possible adverse patient effects. For citations with incomplete work, put down the expected completion date. For citations with complete work, put down the corrective action and the date the work was completed. As mentioned above, the time frame for completing the corrective action is preferably within 60 days but not to exceed 12 months from the last day of the inspection.

If the citations are few and small, the inspecting agency will likely accept the responses, and you will then receive your notice of renewal. If your lab is having multiple small problems, your responses will be scrutinized more carefully. One or more of the initial responses may be rejected in which case you have to modify the rejected responses and send them in again.

If your facility is having significant problems, you may be asked to file a formal Plan of Correction (PoC). When making a PoC you have to respond to all the deficiencies in form 2567. In addition, you will be expected to examine your lab's methods, processes, and/or systems to identify what is not working or not consistent with current regulations. In other words, you are expected to re-think the whole way your lab does business and conducts its operations. Needless to say CMS only mandates this on a lab if it thinks there is something seriously wrong with that lab.

You will need to send your PoC in to CMS in addition to the form 2567. The PoC is due 24 days after you are requested to prepare it. Both the PoC and the form 2567 are subject to multiple rounds of revision, so as to meet CMS approval.

The next higher level of CMS oversight on a lab involves a directed Plan of Correction. The difference between the PoC described above and a directed PoC is that CMS mandates a directed PoC on you. You do not have much input in a directed PoC. This generally happens to a lab that proves incapable of making its own PoC.

Avoid the temptation to put little effort into making your own PoC simply because CMS will do it for you. You are much better off making your own PoC since you will have more control over the process. If CMS has to make a directed PoC for you, it is likely to be much more onerous.

Here is an example of a form you can use if you ever get requested to make a Plan of Correction:

Plan of Correction Form					
Provider Name:				**Phone:**	
Provider Contact for follow-up:				**Fax:**	
				Email:	
Address:			**Provider NPI #:**	**Date:**	
Finding (State the Problem)	**Corrective Action Steps** (How will this problem be corrected?)	**What systems changes will be made to ensure this situation and others like it do not occur again?**		**Responsible Party**	**Time Line**
					Implementation Date:
					Implementation Date:
					Implementation Date:
					Implementation Date:

Accepted _____ Not Accepted _____ Date _____ Initials _____ Revision Due _____

In some situations a lab may be asked to file a Credible Allegation of Compliance (CAoC) with CMS. The CAoC is very similar to a PoC with a few minor differences. The CAoC is typically used for more serious citations (condition level deficiencies or Immediate Jeopardy deficiencies) while the PoC is more often used for minor citations (standard level deficiencies). The corrections must be completed by the day of signing of a CAoC whereas with a PoC it is acceptable to list future dates for completion of the corrections. If there are no Immediate Jeopardy citations, the CAoC is due 45 days from the last day of inspection. If the lab has one or more Immediate Jeopardy citations, the CAoC is due 23 days from the last day of inspection. Otherwise a CAoC and a PoC are similar.

The next higher level of CMS oversight involves a series of re-inspections on a lab. These re-inspections are typically done to ensure enforcement of a PoC or CAoC; hence a PoC or CAoC is typically in place before the re-inspections begin. The lab without a Lab Director referred to above had at least 3 re-inspections between its August, 2012 biennial inspection and the next biennial inspection 2 years later. In this situation, the CMS is sending personnel on-site to the lab similar to what the lab is lacking. However, this is not a regulatory takeover of the lab in the conventional sense. The CMS can't station Lab Directors permanently at a lab, and the CMS will expect a lab to correct its problems on its own.

If all the above fails to correct the problems in a lab, CMS has the authority to close down a lab. This is done by revocation of the CMS Certificate of Compliance. In theory a lab could continue to operate if its Certificate of Compliance is revoked. The lab wouldn't be able to bill Medicare or Medicaid and most private insurance would not reimburse. Any lab that could not bill would quickly become financially nonviable. I am not aware of any lab that has ever lasted any time at all without a Certificate of Compliance or equivalent. Thus I use the term "regulatory closure" as synonymous with revocation of the Certificate of Compliance.

I am aware of regulatory closure of only one lab in my 29 years experience in Pathology and Lab Medicine. It was a small clinic lab located about 125 miles from the municipality where I was living at the time. This lab was supposedly caught "sink testing". Sink testing is a type of fraud in which the specimen is not tested; the specimen is discarded down a sink (hence the term "sink testing"), and a fraudulent lab report is generated. This fraudulent lab report typically indicates the patient has a normal test result, since normal lab results typically get little suspicion from the clinician.

This lab got caught because it was generating reports in which the time of the reporting was before the time of collection. An astute clinician noticed this and made a complaint to the CMS. The CMS inspector came unannounced to this lab, and found that the lab did not have reagents or equipment to do testing, but had still turned out test results earlier on the day of inspection. The regulatory closure for this lab was immediate and happened on the spot when the sink testing was discovered.

To summarize, the possible outcomes of a CMS inspection are:

1. No citations. A Certificate of Compliance is issued without having to fill out form 2567
2. Few minor citations. The lab fills out form 2567 and it is accepted without revisions
3. Several minor citations. The form 2567 is accepted after one or more revisions
4. Significant citations. The lab is required to submit a Plan of Correction (PoC)
5. CMS makes a directed PoC for the lab
6. Severe citations. The lab is required to submit a Credible Allegation of Compliance (CAoC)
7. PoC or CAoC with one or more re-inspections.
8. Regulatory closure. (i.e. revocation of the CMS Certificate of Compliance).

In my experience, more than two rounds of modifying the form 2567 responses is unusual, having to file a Plan of Correction is rare and re-inspections are very rare. After your responses are accepted, you will get your notice of renewal from the CMS. This is followed by a bill. Always ensure this bill is paid in a timely manner. After you have paid the bill to CMS they will send your Certificate of Compliance.

The deemed status inspecting agencies use other accrediting documents such as a CAP Certificate of Accreditation. Regardless of the inspecting agency, the certificate is good for two years from the date of issue. Your next regularly scheduled inspection will be in 2 years time. You can be inspected sooner than that if the inspecting agency receives one or more complaints about your lab.

If CMS can't complete an inspection by the time your existing Certificate of Compliance expires, they will grant an administrative extension of the old certificate. The CMS has limited numbers of inspectors, and has difficulty making travel arrangements to the most remote areas. In my experience working in remote areas, the biennial inspections can occur months after the old Certificate of Compliance has expired necessitating multiple administrative extensions of the old certificate. Once the biennial inspection is completed, the next Certificate of Compliance is set to expire 2 years after the old certificate had expired. The same problem does not usually occur in the continental US.

D. Testing your abilities to make a Plan of Correction

As a Lab Director writing Plans of Correction is an important part of your work. I will conclude this chapter with two Plan of Correction writing tests. The first **TEST** is a portion of the CMS form 2567 from one of my recent CMS inspections:

D5551	493.1271(a)(1)(f) IMMUNOHEMATOLOGY	D5551		
540H 550H	The laboratory must perform ABO grouping, D(Rho) typing, unexpected antibody detection, antibody identification, and compatibility testing by following the manufacturer's instructions, if provided, and as applicable, 21 CFR 606.151(a) through (e). The laboratory must determine ABO group by concurrently testing unknown red cells with, at a minimum, anti-A and anti-B grouping reagents. For confirmation of ABO group, the unknown serum must be tested with known A1 and B red cells. The laboratory must determine the D(Rho) type by testing unknown red cells with anti-D (anti-Rho) blood typing reagent. The laboratory must document all control procedures performed, as specified in this section.			

FORM CMS-2567(02-99) Previous Versions Obsolete   Event ID: ▓▓▓   Facility ID: ▓▓▓   If continuation sheet Page 6 of 10

D5551	Continued From page 6	D5551		

	This STANDARD is not met as evidenced by: Based on review of current director approved procedure and interview with a general supervisor on ▓▓▓ it was determined that the laboratory failed to follow compatibility testing procedures for patients with current positive antibody screens and/or patients with a history of a positive antibody screen. Findings include;
	
	   1. Director approved laboratory procedure BB210.01 states that phenotyping of donor units will be performed by the reference lab the performs the antibody identification on the recipient. The reference lab is supposed to send units that have phenotyped negative for the corresponding antibody identified in the recipient.
	   2. Per interview with a general supervisor, this is not being followed. Recipients with positive antibody screens are given blood that is crossmatch compatible by Anti-human globulin cross-match.
	   3. A recipient with a low titer antibody and/or a donor unit with a week expression of the corresponding antigen may not react in in-vitro compatibility testing, but may cause an increase in titer in the recipient and shorten the life of the transfused red blood cells, and/or cause a delayed transfusion reaction.			

The Blood Bank has been cited for transfusing crossmatched blood to patients with unexpected antibodies without typing the donor units for the corresponding antigen. This is a standard level citation which could affect patient care.

The circumstances surrounding this citation are as follows. This is a small hospital lab Blood Bank with a relatively low volume, about 100 units transfused a month. There are about 6 patients a year with unexpected antibodies. The workup for the unexpected antibodies is sent out to the regional Blood Bank. If a request is made to transfuse a patient with an unexpected antibody, the small hospital Blood Bank is supposed to call the regional Blood Bank and ask them to send donor units negative for the corresponding antigen, and do the crossmatch using the specimen sent for antibody identification.

In reality what was happening is that the doctors involved would not wait for the antigen negative unit to come from the regional Blood Bank. The doctors were demanding immediate transfusion, and signing the emergency release forms to release crossmatched donor units from the local Blood Bank that had not been antigen typed. The donor unit antigen typing was not done after the fact. How would you respond to this citation?

The **ANSWER** to the citation could take one of two possible forms. First, enforce a rule that transfusion for patients with an unexpected antibody has to wait for the antigen negative blood to arrive from the regional Blood Bank. Second, start doing the donor unit antigen typing on-site.

This particular small hospital Blood Bank was very remote from the regional Blood Bank such that it would take 2 days or more for any units to arrive after being requested. Thus the first choice is not an option. Pick the second choice, starting antigen typing on-site.

In this case, the decision was made to continue sending the antibody identification to the regional Blood Bank. Once the results were received from the regional Blood Bank, the small hospital Blood Bank would be able to type donor units for the corresponding antigen.

Next, review the past 2 years of unexpected antibody data. The unexpected antibodies at this Blood Bank were all from the Rh, Duffy, Kell, Kidd and Lewis systems. Submit a request for purchase for these antisera to your hospital's purchasing department along with all the paperwork needed to generate a Purchase Order. When contacting the vendors, make sure the antisera they send will have the longest shelf life possible. You will be doing this typing only 6 times a year, and hardly using any of the antisera. The majority of what you order will expire.

Next write a procedure for the antigen typing. This is a common Blood Bank procedure and can be downloaded from the internet. Call a meeting of all the Blood Bank techs to inform them of the new procedure and if necessary show them how to do the procedure. Make sure they are aware that all patients with unexpected antibodies are to receive crossmatched donor units typed as negative for the corresponding antigen.

While reviewing the prior 2 years of unexpected antibody data from the files, there were 12 patients identified with unexpected antibodies. Most of them were pre-natal screens, and not transfused. Only 2 patients with unexpected antibodies were transfused. Pull the charts for those two patients, and review the charts to make sure there was no evidence of a hemolytic transfusion reaction.

You only need to review the past 2 years of data. Anything prior to that would predate the prior biennial CMS inspection. You are only responsible for events occurring since the most recent biennial CMS inspection two years ago.

Once you have that work done, you can write the Plan of Correction. Here is my Plan of Correction for the citation given above:

D5551) The lab has ordered antisera for typing of the relevant minor red blood cell antigens. A procedure has been written for typing of donor units for the minor red blood cell antigens. All Blood Bank staff have been informed of the new procedure, and the requirement to type donor units before crossmatching to a patient with known unexpected antibody or history of unexpected antibody at Blood Bank. The Blood Bank files have been reviewed for the past 2 years. There were 2 patients with a positive antibody screen or history of a positive antibody screen that received crossmatched blood without donor antigen typing. Review of the charts for these 2 patients reveals no evidence of harm to the patient. There were no hemolytic transfusion reactions.

This was typed into the right-hand column of form 2567, and sent in to the CMS along with copies of the vendor quote and Purchase Order for the antisera, and the procedure for antigen typing. The CMS accepted this response on the first try, without requiring any reworking.

If you are going to send your worksheets in to the CMS, be very careful to black out the patient names or other patient identifiers. Failure to black out patient information on documents sent in to the CMS is a HIPAA violation, and will get you into deeper trouble than the original citation.

For the above citation, here are examples of responses you do not want to put down on form 2567 and why they will get rejected if you do:

Response	Why it will get rejected by the CMS inspectors
The BUTR Committee will meet and discuss the patients with an unexpected antibody or history of an unexpected antibody that were transfused with crossmatched blood without typing the unit for the corresponding antigen.	Too vague. No concrete plan of action is offered. The CMS expects you to fix the problem, and get it fixed as soon as possible, not have a series of meetings that may or may not accomplish anything.
From now on, all patients with an unexpected antibody or history of unexpected antibody will only be transfused with crossmatched units typed as negative for the corresponding antigen.	No effort has been made to identify the patients that may have been harmed by the practice.
The lab staff will receive an in-service on typing blood for the minor red blood cell antigens. The situation will be monitored by the Lab Director.	Too vague. It does not specifically state that all patients with an unexpected antibody or history of unexpected antibody will only be transfused with crossmatched units typed as negative for the corresponding antigen.
The lab techs involved will be disciplined.	This assumes wrongdoing on the part of the lab techs. The CMS will look at the situation as a "system" problem. In other words, the lab's whole way of doing things in this situation is wrong; it is not just the lab techs' fault.

The second Plan of Correction writing **TEST** is the second citation from one of my recent CMS inspections.

D5411
320M
	This STANDARD is not met as evidenced by:
	
	493.1252(a) TEST SYSTEMS, EQUIPMENT, INSTRUMENTS, REAGENT
	
	Test systems must be selected by the laboratory. The testing must be performed following the manufacturer's instructions and in a manner that provides test results within the laboratory's stated performance specifications for each test system as determined under §493.1253.
	
	This STANDARD is not met as evidenced by: Based on observation and interview with testing personnel on ▮▮▮▮▮▮▮▮▮ it was determined that the laboratory failed to have in place the appropriate procedure for the urinalysis methodology being used at the time of the survey. Findings included:
	
	    1. The manufacturer's package insert being used as the urinalysis dip-stick (macroscopic analysis) procedure was for Siemens Multistix.
	    2. The manufacturer's dip-stick in use at the time of the survey was Accutest URS10.
	    3. Testing personnel confirmed that there was no procedure in place for the manufacturer Accutest URS10.
		D5411

This involves the procedure for dipstick urinalysis. The vendor supplying lab had switched dipsticks from one manufacturer to another. The testing was the same, the interpretation was the same, everything about these dipsticks was the same except for the name on the container. Since everything about these dipsticks is identical I am assuming one is the generic and the other is the brand name for the same dipstick. However the name on the container changed. My lab had the name of the old manufacturer written into the procedure manual. The inspector caught this and gave us the citation above. How would you handle this?

ANSWER: This is a trick question. Dipstick urinalysis is a waived test. Waived tests do not need a procedure manual. All that is required for a waived test is that the manufacturer's package insert has to be available at the place and time of testing. The dipsticks in question arrived from the manufacturer with the package insert stuffed into the same cardboard tube as the dipsticks. The package insert was still present in the same tube as the dipsticks at the time of the CMS inspection. Thus we should never have been cited.

CMS inspectors are human, they make mistakes just like everybody else. My lab does testing of all three complexity levels: waived testing, moderate complexity testing and high complexity testing. Even though the urine dipsticks sit right next to high complexity testing equipment, urine dipstick is still a waived test. The CMS inspector got confused, and mistook dipstick urinalysis for a higher complexity test or otherwise would not have written us the citation above.

The question is how to respond to this mistaken citation. If you confront the CMS inspector head on, about 90% of the time they will admit they made a mistake and back down. The rest of the time, you will have just made an enemy that you can't afford to make. Thus in this situation, I played along, and make a corrective action as if urine dipstick is a moderate complexity test which it is not, it is a waived test.

Here is my approach to the Plan of Correction. The citation is a standard level citation. The two different tests have the same interpretation meaning that lab could not have turned out erroneous results for urine dipstick. Hence there is no risk of patient harm, no need to retest specimens and no need to track down patient charts. I added the name of the new manufacturer and new dipstick into the dipstick urinalysis procedure, signed and dated this change to the procedure manual. I did not strike the name of the old manufacturer and old dipstick from the procedure manual, in case the vendor ever switched us back to the old dipstick.

I added the package insert for the new dipstick into the procedure manual. I did not remove the package insert for the old dipstick from the procedure manual, for the same reason as given above, in case the vendor ever switched us back to the old dipstick. I wrote the following for the Plan of Correction:

D5411) The urinalysis manual has been updated to reflect that either Accutest URS10 or Siemens Multistix may be used. The package insert for Accutest URS10 has been added to the procedure manual. The method of testing and interpretation are the same for both types of urine dipstick such that there was no risk of patient harm.

The Plan of Correction was typed into the right hand column of form 2567 and sent in to CMS. The CMS inspector accepted it the first try without requiring modifications. The entire time, the inspector never realized her mistake of requiring a procedure manual for a waived test.

It is possible to protest any of your citations. The only time I will protest a mistaken citation is if the Plan of Correction would entail significant outlays such as new equipment or new hires. The above Plan of Correction required writing in the procedure manual, and putting the package insert in the procedure manual. The package insert would have been discarded anyhow when the product was used up. Thus it did not cost anything to play along and make a Plan of Correction for this mistaken citation.

Vendor substitutions of one product for another happen occasionally. It usually means that the vendor was unable to obtain the exact same product you asked for. The vendor is supposed to ask permission from your lab beforehand for the switch. In this case, the vendor did not ask lab for permission to switch, and we found out when we got cited by the CMS. This should prompt a stern phone call to that vendor to remind them they are required to ask permission for a switch. This is also a good example of why you don't want to write the manufacturer's name into a procedure unless you have to.

One final tip is that the CMS can only cite current noncompliance and cannot cite a problem if it is not ongoing at the time of inspection. If your lab had a problem in the past, resolved the problem, and the inspectors ask you about this problem, show all the associated paperwork to the inspectors – the steps taken to fix the problem, monitoring to ensure the problem does not recur, the fix has been sustainable without recurrence of the problem, etc. In this situation, the inspectors would only be able to cite you if they believed the problem is likely to recur. This is a judgment call on the part of the inspectors but in most situations they will not issue a citation. On the other hand, if your lab has a problem, is trying to fix the problem, and it is not fixed by the time of the inspection or has recurred at the time of the inspection, you can be relatively confident that you are going to get a citation for this problem.

Chapter 23 – Regulatory scrutiny syndrome

As a Lab Director, it is important that you keep your lab up to standards to the extent possible. I have noticed that once a lab has a bad inspection, the next time the inspectors come, they conduct a much more thorough inspection. This has the potential to put a lab on a downhill course that I refer to as "Regulatory Scrutiny Syndrome".

In the typical small hospital lab inspection CMS sends one inspector for one day. There is no way that one person can look over all the lab's documents in one day. In the typical small hospital lab, there are multiple sections (Blood Bank, hematology, chemistry, etc.). Each section will have hundreds of pages of procedure manuals. The quality assurance and proficiency testing may also run into the hundreds of pages for each section. Even a small hospital lab will have thousands of pages of documents. The inspector will only have time to look at a small sampling of the documents subject to review, due to the time constraints of the inspection.

If the inspector finds something seriously wrong, the findings will be documented. The next time this lab is inspected, it is likely there will be more than one inspector coming, and these inspectors are likely to stay for more than one day.

The typical small hospital lab is likely to have a few skeletons in the closet. Maybe a failed proficiency test but not two consecutive. Maybe several procedures are not well written, etc. This will likely not be noticed by one inspector on a one day inspection. However a team of inspectors given multiple days to inspect are not as subject to time constraints and can look at much more.

This team of inspectors is likely to find a great deal more wrong with the lab than was found at the initial inspection. The lab gets worse citations in the second inspection, and any subsequent inspection will involve even more inspectors staying for even more time and doing an even more thorough inspection.

In this manner, the lab ends up in a self-reinforcing cycle of more regulatory scrutiny leading to more problems found leading to even more regulatory scrutiny. I refer to this as Regulatory Scrutiny Syndrome. This is likely what happened to the municipal hospital that hired me in August, 2013 to "turnaround" its lab.

Once a lab starts on this downhill course it is very hard to pull up from this. In my experience it is more difficult to fix a lab with major problems than it is to start a whole new lab. In many cases it is less expensive to start a whole new lab than to fix up a lab with problems. Thus, many labs going down this slippery slope will voluntarily close down and cease to exist as a going concern. As a Lab Director, it is imperative that you should keep your lab up to standards at all times to the extent possible. You do not want to go down this slippery slope; it will lead to very unpleasant places.

A good part of my 29 years in Pathology and Lab Medicine has been spent at two municipal hospitals that were both struggling financially. In the first of these the supply and reagent shortages caused repeated citations on the inspections. It was a struggle to keep the lab up to par. One becomes very proficient at writing corrective actions when one works at such a hospital.

The second municipal hospital I worked at hired me in August, 2013 to "turnaround" a lab that had numerous citations for multiple problems. This lab had a PoC in place with CMS and 2 re-inspections following its August, 2012 regular biennial inspection. The turnaround was completed quickly. By the time of the December, 2013 re-inspection all the citations from the prior biennial inspection were corrected and only 2 additional minor citations were uncovered.

In my experience it is possible for a lab to pull back from the brink up until it gets regulatory closure.

The second municipal hospital lab referenced above was very close to regulatory closure when I was hired.

As a Lab Director, lab "turnaround" is a dangerous profession. You are being hired by a lab that has a good chance of voluntarily closing down in the near term. Even worse, the federal government has a rule on the book, the reference is 42 U.S.C. § 263a(i)(3), stating that the Lab Director of any lab that has regulatory closure will not be allowed to own or operate a lab for the following 2 years.

If you are Lab Director of a lab that has regulatory closure, your name will go onto Medicare's "blacklist" of banned providers. CMS refers to this as the Medicare Exclusion Database (MED). Although it is supposed to be for only 2 years, once that 2 years is up you will have a difficult time getting your name off of the Medicare "blacklist" of banned providers.

I have spent a good part of my career as a lab "turnaround" specialist. In that time, I have been successful in pulling labs back from the brink. None of the labs I have directed has had regulatory closure. Thus, I have never been on the "banned" list.

The only Lab Director I know of that has been on the "banned" list is the director for the lab doing sink testing referenced in a prior chapter. That Lab Director never worked again in the field, in effect forced into retirement by the closure of his lab and by the Medicare ban which prevented him from getting work elsewhere. It took him an extended length of time for him to get his name off of the "banned" list. Even after he was off the "banned" list no one would hire him. The "banned" list acts as a de facto "blacklist" whereby no one in the field will ever hire anyone that has ever been on the "banned" list.

From what I have been told, the only other offense that will result in the immediate regulatory closure of a laboratory is intentionally cheating on proficiency testing. I am not aware of any lab closed for this offense. At every lab I head, I am very careful to make sure that the lab techs perform the PT correctly. The CMS has never questioned the veracity of the PT testing at any lab I headed.

I am aware of a few labs caught doing something irregular with the PT testing that the CMS inspector objected to, such as accidentally performing duplicate testing on a PT specimen. For example, one lab tech doesn't know that another lab tech has already tested the PT specimen. The PT specimen is tested again, and both results are filed in the PT workbook. In all these cases, the lab was given the benefit of the doubt and cited for the offense without regulatory closure.

If you are considering working as a Lab Director at a lab with problems, speak privately with the CMS inspectors assigned to that lab. If the Lab Director position has been vacant for some time, as it tends to be at a deeply troubled lab, the CMS inspectors will be glad to see you come. Their job is to regulate labs; and they don't like having to shut labs down. Ask the CMS inspectors if the CMS intends to carry out regulatory closure on that lab. Ask for an unwritten agreement that if you take the position, they would inform you if regulatory closure ever becomes imminent for that lab. If regulatory closure becomes inevitable, my advice is to voluntarily close the affected part, or all, of that lab before the lab has regulatory closure. You want to avoid the Medicare "blacklist" as it tends to be a career ender.

If you are working in a lab that is starting to have problems (i.e. starting to have PT failures, etc.), your lab will come under increasing regulatory scrutiny. If the regulators tell you they are getting ready to send you a "cease testing" letter my advice is that you should voluntarily discontinue in-house testing for that analyte and send the test out rather than risk a "cease testing" letter. A "cease testing" letter typically comes with sanctions including loss of your ability to bill Medicare or Medicaid for 6 months.

My advice is to always do exactly as the regulators tell you. If they send you a "cease testing" letter you must immediately stop testing that analyte at all labs covered under the CLIA number referenced.

If the regulators tell you they are getting ready to revoke your CMS certificate (i.e. perform regulatory closure on your lab) my advice is that you should voluntarily shut down that part, or all, of your lab before that decision is handed down. If your lab has regulatory closure before you can voluntarily close it down, you will be added to the Medicare "blacklist" as described above.

Chapter 24 – How to avoid HIPAA pitfalls

The Health Insurance Portability and Accountability Act of 1996 (known in the business as "HIPAA") regulates the release of Protected Health Information (PHI). PHI is defined as any individually identifiable health information. Using this definition, all lab results are PHI.

PHI can only be released in the following situations: to facilitate treatment, payment or health care operations, when consent has been granted by the patient, as required by law (i.e. under subpoena), when required for law enforcement, disclosure of communicable disease to the Public Health Department, research, government functions including disclosure of prisoner's lab results to a correctional facility, disclosure to the military, workers' compensation, etc. In most circumstances HIPAA requires covered entities to respond to requests for PHI within 30 days. In my experience most labs treat such requests as urgent, and will make the decision to release or not release the information the same working day.

HIPAA requires the hospital to take a number of actions such as designating a Privacy Official, training the workforce on HIPAA compliance, documenting the training, making a notice of privacy practices and giving the notice to all patients, making sure all policies and procedures comply with HIPAA, etc.

The hospital takes care of almost everything on this list. The lab's HIPAA training and documentation of training are typically done by the hospital's HIPAA office, not the lab. The HIPAA privacy rule requires training only once and it must be for "each new member of the work force within a reasonable period of time after the person joins". In my experience most hospitals require HIPAA training on hiring and annually thereafter for all hospital employees. If any lab employee becomes delinquent in the annual HIPAA training, the HIPAA Compliance Office will inform lab. Lab should then mandate the employee to attend the HIPAA training the next time it is offered.

The typical hospital lab is only responsible for making sure its own policies and procedures are HIPAA compliant, and that all lab staff comply with HIPAA. As with all other lab policies and procedures enforcement is the responsibility of the Lab Supervisor.

In the typical hospital lab, the HIPAA policies and procedures involve password security (no sharing of passwords), physical security (no patient information is allowed on laptops or other removable devices), no patient information in clear view of the front desk or drawing areas, no Web surfing at work, and no unauthorized downloads or programs on lab computers. When stepping away from the computer always lock or turn off the computer. Lab staff should not discuss patient information outside of the testing areas of lab. No unauthorized visitors are allowed in the testing areas of lab. Lab staff can only relay lab results to the known providers of that hospital. Requests for test results coming from unknown persons are referred to the Lab Secretary or hospital Medical Records Department.

With HIPAA there are basically only two types of mistakes you can make. First, you can give out PHI when you should not have. Second, you can withhold PHI when you should have given it out.

In my experience, labs are very tight-lipped. I have never seen a lab make the mistake of giving out PHI when it should not have. I have seen a number of instances of labs failing to give out PHI when they should have.

Failure to appropriately release PHI typically results from a request by an unknown doctor in a distant city asking for one patient's lab results. Many labs will require a consent form signed by the patient, and will refuse to give out the information until a consent form signed by the patient is FAXed back. Under HIPAA, all the lab has to do is verify the requesting doctor is legitimate and is treating the patient in question, and then the test results can be given out.

Prior to February 6, 2014 all PHI except for lab results could be requested by the patient under HIPAA. HIPAA made an exception for lab results and CLIA prohibited labs from giving test results directly to the patient.

On February 6, 2014 a final rule was issued in the Federal Register modifying both CLIA and HIPAA to specify that upon the request of a patient (or the patient's personal representative), laboratories may provide the patient, the patient's personal representative, or a person designated by the patient with copies of that patient's completed test reports. The reference is the Federal Register, volume 79, issue number 25, pages 7290-7316.

This change solves many problems for labs but brings up the issue of how labs will handle this direct release of results to patients. Since all PHI can be requested by the patient under HIPAA and there is no longer an exception for lab results, all labs in the US must be prepared to produce a copy of the patient test results upon patient request. Most hospital labs that I am familiar with will refer all such patient requests to the hospital's Medical Records Department. This should meet regulatory requirements. Furthermore, it puts the onus on the Medical Records Department for checking the patient's ID, making the patient sign the release form, etc.

My advice is that if you are going to release results directly to patients, ask the hospital Medical Records Department for their PHI release procedures and forms, and copy those over to lab. An example release form is given on the next page.

MY LAB   MY PROCEDURE MANUAL
AUTHORIZATION TO DISCLOSE PROTECTED HEALTH INFORMATION

Patient's Name			Patient's Social Security #
Street Address			Patient's Date of Birth / /
City	State	ZIP	Patient's Phone # ( ) -

I authorize MY LAB to disclose the above-named individual's Protected Health Information (PHI) as described below. (Identify lab test by name and date if known. Indicate "all lab tests" if all lab results are being requested).

I understand that this information may include, when applicable, information relating to sexually transmitted disease, Human Immunodeficiency Virus (HIV Infection or AIDS) and any other communicable disease (as permitted by 42 CFR Part 2). This information may be disclosed to and used by the following person and/or organization:

Name of person and/or organization authorized to receive the lab test results.

Street Address

City, State, ZIP

Phone Number ( ) -	Fax Number ( ) -

This disclosure is for the following purpose(s):

I understand that if I give permission, I have the right to change my mind and revoke it. This must be in writing to MY LAB. I also understand that any uses or disclosures already made with my permission cannot be taken back.

If I give permission and then revoke it, MY LAB is held harmless from any resulting damages including my loss of health care eligibility and/or coverage, and for any resulting monetary losses on the part of any health care entity involved.

Unless otherwise revoked, this authorization will expire on the following date, event or condition. (If I fail to specify an expiration date, event or condition, this authorization will expire one year from the signature date.)

Date, event or condition of expiration:

I understand that authorizing the disclosure of these lab test results is voluntary. I also understand that I may refuse to sign this authorization and that my refusal to sign will not affect my ability to obtain treatment, payment for services, or eligibility for benefits unless the information is necessary to demonstrate that I meet eligibility or enrollment criteria.

By signing this Authorization, I understand that any disclosure of information carries with it the potential for an unauthorized re-disclosure and the information may not be protected by federal privacy rules. I further understand I may request a copy of this signed Authorization. I understand that I should seek interpretation with my provider, and that MY LAB is not able to provide medical advice or prescriptions.

Legal Representative's Name (If applicable)	Legal Representative's Relationship to Individual (A Power of Attorney may be requested.)
Signature of Patient or Legal Representative	Date / /
Signature of Witness	Date / /

The typical PHI release procedure is as follows. First, check one or more photo IDs to make sure you are dealing with the right person. If anyone comes in place of the patient ask to see the photo ID and documentation proving the relationship to the patient (medical power of attorney, marriage certificate, civil union, domestic partnership, etc.). Make a xerox copy of the photo ID and any other documents used to release the test results. Fill out the release form, print a copy of the patient's test results, give the printout to the patient or representative, and ask the patient or representative to sign for the release of the lab results. The completed release form with attached copy of the photo ID and all other associated documents is filed in a secure area of lab. A copy of the completed release form and all associated documentation goes to the Medical Records Department.

At the time, most people felt this change would likely increase the lab's direct contact with patients. In my experience most hospital labs refer all external requests for lab results to the hospital's Medical Records Department. Thus, there has been no increase in lab's direct patient contact.

In my 29 years experience in Pathology and Lab Medicine, I have had only very rare contact with patients. There have been only a few instances in which a primary care physician did not understand the significance of a lab result and referred the patient to me. I limited myself to explaining the significance of that result only, and referred the patient back to the primary doctor for all other matters. Regardless of the changes in CLIA and HIPAA I have not been giving out general medical consults, nor prescriptions, nor has any other Lab Director I am familiar with.

Chapter 25 – How to interact with the legal profession

As a Lab Director there are two ways you could get called into court. The first is that your lab could be sued over test results produced in your lab. This would be a malpractice suit, and you would be a party to the suit. This has never happened in my experience. In my 29 years in Pathology and Lab Medicine, no lab I have ever worked for has ever been sued over the lab results generated. Nor to the best of my knowledge has any other lab in any municipality where I have ever lived. I assume that the process would be similar to that described below, with the exception that you are a party to the suit, not a disinterested bystander.

Much more commonly, you will be called as an expert witness to testify in a case in which you are not a party to the lawsuit, but the testing was done in your lab. The most common situations are paternity testing and testing for Driving Under the Influence (DUI). In these cases you are not a party to the lawsuit. In a DUI trial the parties to the lawsuit are the DUI driver (the Defendant) and the Attorney General's (AG's) Office (i.e. the Prosecutor). You are a disinterested party called in to testify on questions related to the alcohol testing done in your laboratory.

In my career I have worked at two municipal hospitals. In both municipalities, the procedure for DUI states that if a suspicious driver is stopped, the police do a field sobriety test and/or breath test. If the driver fails either or both tests, the driver is taken to the municipal hospital lab for the blood test. The testing is done in Lab. The entire DUI case turns on the outcome of this testing, and you will occasionally be called into court to testify that the Lab did the testing properly. This happens about once every year or two at the typical municipal hospital.

If you receive this call of duty from the Attorney General's (AG's) Office it will be in the form of a subpoena. This is literally an invitation you can't refuse. If you fail to show up for this scheduled court appearance you could be jailed. The subpoena will show up in the form of a Sheriff or other law enforcement officer coming into your lab and asking for you by name. Try not to have a heart attack when a uniformed law enforcement officer shows up in lab and asks for you by name. The law enforcement officer will hand you the subpoena and ask you to sign for receipt.

Most hospitals' administrative manuals require that you inform the hospital legal department and/or risk manager immediately if you receive a subpoena. Call them and inform them of the subpoena. The hospital's legal department and/or risk manager should be able to give you all the advice you need.

Like all patient test results, alcohol results are covered by HIPAA and are confidential. In this case, you have a legal mandate in the form of a subpoena requesting the information. HIPAA allows for disclosure of the confidential information in this circumstance. Be careful to only disclose the information to the Prosecutor, Defendant's Attorney or any court official with a reasonable need to know. Do not disclose the alcohol results to anyone that does not need to know as part of the court proceeding.

Most hospital administrative manuals state that you will need the permission of the hospital's legal department and/or risk manager to release any test results outside the hospital. In almost all circumstances they will approve of the release of information requested by the subpoena. If they disapprove, they will send the hospital's attorney into court to try to "quash" the subpoena.

Next, call the Prosecutor whose name appears on the subpoena. Ask the Prosecutor the details of the case such as the date of the testing and name of the Defendant. Look up the testing records for that Defendant, and the relevant QC. In particular make sure the controls were in for the alcohol testing on that day of testing. Make a note of the dates of calibration immediately prior to and after the Defendant's testing.

Make copies of the alcohol test results, the quality control documentation for the alcohol testing and chain of custody form. Once you have the hospital's permission for external release of this information, provide the copies to the Prosecutor and Defendant's Attorney. You will be asked to provide your resume or Curriculum Vita (CV) to both the Prosecutor and the Defendant's Attorney.

Make sure your CV lists all your qualifications. This includes not only Anatomic Pathology and Clinical Pathology Board Certification (if applicable), but also sub-specialty training, other training, publications, books written, etc. The Prosecutor and Defendant's Attorney will review your CV. The Prosecutor will almost never object to your credentials. If you are Board Certified, the Defendant's Attorney will not likely question your credentials.

The Defendant's Attorney would rather not have you at the trail, and rarely will question your credentials in the long-shot hope of getting you disqualified as an expert witness. If the Defendant's Attorney objects to your credentials, your credentials will be presented to the Judge before the trail starts. The Prosecutor will inform the Judge that you are Board Certified, and this is the highest training possible in a clinical lab. The Judge will almost certainly admit you as an expert witness.

The decision on admitting you to court as an expert witness has to be made before the trail starts. You will be informed of this decision in advance of the trail. There should be no objections to your credentials during the trail. As noted below, the Defendant's Attorney may question your credentials at the trial, but can't make an outright objection to your credentials at the trial since this matter has been settled in advance of the trial.

The majority of the time there will be no objections to your credentials. If the Defendant's Attorney does not object to your credentials before the trail starts, the Defendant's Attorney has accepted you as an expert witness.

As an expert witness you should be available to both the Prosecutor and the Defendant's Attorney. Answer phone calls and meet with either side as requested. You can set the schedule to your own convenience. You do not need to have the Prosecutor on the phone call when talking with the Defendant's Attorney, and vice versa. You do not need to have the Prosecutor present to meet with the Defendant's Attorney, and vice versa. You are an independent expert, not beholden to either side of the trial.

It is not uncommon to get phone calls from both the Defendant's Attorney and Prosecutor before the case comes to trial. The lawyers won't be very familiar with lab testing and will phrase the questions in general terms: "Was the lab testing good?" "Was there a problem with the lab testing?".

You may or may not be called for depositions. A deposition is a formal meeting between the Prosecutor and the Defendant's Attorney. If you are called into a deposition you will be given the oath. Be very careful to answer truthfully while under oath. The deposition will be recorded and later transcribed.

By the time of the deposition, both the Prosecutor and the Defendant's Attorney should have copies of the chain of custody form. They are usually satisfied with the chain of custody form, and you will not be questioned much on it. You will typically be asked a few general questions about the testing for that particular DUI case. Was the testing good? Was there a problem with the testing?

Some time later, you may be asked to sign a transcript of the deposition. Always check the transcript very carefully for transcription errors. You can't change your testimony after the fact. However, there are usually transcription errors to correct, since the transcriptionist is usually a legal secretary with little to no medical knowledge.

If it is a first offense DUI with no injuries, it will likely get settled by plea bargain and you won't be called for depositions or called into court. If the case is a vehicular homicide with DUI there is less chance of a plea bargain and it is much more likely you will be called for depositions and the case will go to trial. A case of DUI with injuries but no fatalities falls somewhere in between. If the case goes to court, you will be notified of the court date.

You will need to take one or more days off from work to do the court testifying. In both municipal hospitals I worked at this was allowed to be administrative leave with pay. Since the request was coming from a different agency of the same municipality, the hospital could not ask you to use your own annual leave (vacation time) to do the testifying.

You have to sit in court all day waiting for your turn to testify. Since the Prosecutor does not know the exact order of the cases in advance, you have to come early and wait all day for the case to come up.

No talking is permitted in the seating area inside the courtroom. Everyone has to turn off their cellphones and pagers. You have to go outside to talk. As a result, the courtroom will be quieter than any library you have ever been in. The room is completely silent except for the Judge, lawyers and the defendants quietly talking at the front of this large room. It can be a struggle to stay awake all day under these conditions. It is embarrassing to have your name called and be caught sleeping in the seating area of the courtroom.

Bring a copy of all relevant paperwork with you to the trial. Read it all so as to prepare yourself for the testimony. If there have been depositions, read the transcripts from end to end. This will help you to remember all the details. It will also make good reading material as you struggle to stay awake all day in this silent room.

Eventually, the case in question comes before the court and then your name is called as an expert witness. You will be directed to the witness stand. It is really a chair, not a stand, you will be seated in front of the jury during your testimony. Next, they administer the oath. You will be told to place one hand on a bible and will be asked something to the effect "Do you swear to tell the truth, the whole truth, and nothing but the truth?". The only acceptable answer is "I do".

Next, you are introduced to the jury as an expert witness. There may be a short recitation of your credentials. Your testimony begins with the Prosecutor asking you to present your findings. This is known as the direct examination. When and where was the testing done? What was the outcome of the test? Was the Defendant intoxicated?

Answer the questions truthfully and to the best of your abilities. Speak clearly. Some courts do not have a microphone in which case you have to speak loudly enough to be heard in the furthest back row of the courtroom. Keep all explanations in layman's terms. In most jurisdictions, the minimum qualification for a juror is high school graduation or equivalent. Your explanations should be simple enough for a high school senior to understand. Do not give extraneous information unrelated to the question that was asked. If a fact is important, one side or the other will eventually ask you about it.

After the Prosecutor is done questioning you, the Defendant's Attorney will question you. This is known as the cross-examination. The Defendant's Attorney will try to cast doubt on the case in any way possible. The evidence is stacked against the Defendant, otherwise the case would not have been prosecuted. In most cases, the Defendant's Attorney knows that he or she is playing a losing hand, and is usually desperate to win the case any way possible.

Be prepared that the Defendant's Attorney will try to attack your credentials as an expert witness. You will be peppered with questions like "What are you qualifications? ", "Are you sure you're qualified to be an expert witness?", "How long have you been an expert witness?"

My assessment: If you are Board Certified in Clinical Pathology, that is all you need. You are an expert in lab testing, and the case turns on the lab test for alcohol. Given the context of this case you really are an expert, even if this is the first time you have served as an expert witness.

Do not take this questioning by the Defendant's Attorney personally. The Defendant's Attorney is just doing his or her job, trying every maneuver possible to get the Defendant acquitted. At this stage of the questioning, the important point is to stay calm and stay focused on the testimony at hand. Do not get into an argument with the Defendant's Attorney. If you get into an argument while on the witness stand, it will only serve to discredit you, which will play into the hands of the Defendant's Attorney. Stay focused on the testimony at hand and do not lose your concentration.

Next the Defendant's Attorney will try to question the testing: "Are you really sure the test is positive?", "How do you determine a positive test in your lab"?, "Did your lab follow the correct chain of custody?"

My assessment: Answer the questions honestly and to the best of your abilities. Remember that you are under oath. If you get caught lying under oath, the consequences would be devastating to your career. In most cases the answers are straightforward "Yes, the test is positive," "Yes, we followed the correct chain of custody".

If there was a problem with the test, such as the controls were out on that day of testing, you have to inform the court at this point. Since you had previously been on the phone and/or in depositions with both the Defendant's Attorney and the Prosecutor, there should be no surprises in your testimony.

If you say something different in the trail compared to the prior depositions, phone calls, etc. you should explain why you changed your mind. If there are discrepancies between your prior testimony and the testimony on the day of trial, the Defendant's Attorney will notice and point out every last discrepancy to the jury. The Defendant's Attorney is looking to discredit you. If you repeatedly change your mind, you will be helping the Defendant's Attorney to discredit you.

Keep in mind that you are an expert in Lab only. The Defendant's Attorney may ask you questions that are beyond your area of expertise. If this happens do not answer the question and state that your area of expertise is limited to Lab. If the Defendant's Attorney asks inappropriate questions or makes a personal attack such as "you are unqualified" the Prosecutor will object.

If you do not know the answer to any question, state that you do not know. It is very unlikely for the Prosecutor to ask you a question you can't answer. The Prosecutor needs your testimony to help win the case. Thus the Prosecutor is not looking to discredit you. The Defendant's Attorney is more likely to ask a question that you are unable to answer. The Defendant's Attorney is hoping that you will answer a question beyond your area of expertise, or beyond your possible range of knowledge. If you fall into this trap, the Defendant's Attorney will discredit you with the intent of discrediting your testimony.

After the Defendant's Attorney is done questioning you the court is then open to all questions. This is basically a free-for-all in which both the Prosecutor and the Defendant's Attorney can ask you anything they want. Both attorneys are under pressure and making questions on-the-fly at this point. Be prepared for some bizarre questions, especially from the Defendant's Attorney. Take your time answering the questions, and avoid feeling pressured to answer quickly. If one side asks an inappropriate question, the other side will object.

After this round of questioning is done you will be excused from the witness stand. The typical DUI trial lasts only a day or two. You will not be informed of the results (conviction, acquittal or last-minute plea bargain). If you are curious you can find out by calling the Prosecutor's Office a few days later.

I am a golfer and from time to time meet some of the Prosecutors from the AG's office while golfing. As we sit in the clubhouse after the golf game we chat about topical matters, I bring up the issue of DUI. They tell me that the plea bargain offered for first offense DUI with no injuries is so lenient you have to be crazy to turn down the offer. Very few people contest a first offense DUI. That is why I am only called in once every year or two to testify. Very few people get a second offense DUI, higher number DUI offense, or DUI with injuries and/or fatalities. Those that do likely have a serious drug and/or alcohol problem, and for them the jail time is really drug/alcohol rehab time.

There are exceptions to the general rules given above. In one case I was called to testify in a DUI with injuries trial that resulted from a two vehicle accident occurring during the late night hours in February, 2015. Both drivers were brought into the hospital's Emergency Room. One tested positive for alcohol, the other was negative. The alcohol testing was ordered as medical alcohol testing, not legal alcohol testing (i.e. there were no chain of custody forms used). The sober driver was injured in the crash but the injuries were not life-threatening. The drunk driver was arrested and prosecuted.

The case came to trial in January, 2016. I was subpoenaed along with the lab's night shift phlebotomist and lab tech. There was only one phlebotomist and one lab tech working the night shift at that hospital, such that the lab's entire night shift and I were called into court. In advance of the testimony the Prosecutor said she would try to have the hospital personnel testify first, so that we would finish quickly. When we arrived in court, instead of going first our case was repeatedly postponed due to more urgent matters going before the court. The lab staff and I were made to wait on a court bench for three working days waiting to testify. As a result, the lab's night shift schedule had to be rearranged on-the-fly since the night shift personnel were not able to sleep during the day. It is not possible to work all night, testify all day and work again all night for 3 consecutive days.

Everyone in lab thought this case was a lost cause for the prosecution, since there was no chain of custody form for the alcohol testing. This case was not that serious since there were no fatalities involved in the DUI. However, the prosecution persevered, playing this losing hand until the bitter end. As a result lab had to commit critical staff members to sitting on a court bench idled for 3 working days waiting to testify. When called to the witness stand my testimony only took about 30 minutes. During my testimony, it was obvious that the Prosecutor was desperate to win, and the Defendant's Attorney seemed more confident.

After the court proceeding was over, I asked the Hospital's Attorney to inform the local AG's office that the court proceeding had disrupted the hospital lab's operations by drawing in the entire night shift for 3 consecutive days. The Hospital's Attorney said that she would speak to the AG's office to make sure they do a better job of scheduling witness time in the event of future DUI cases.

Several months later the response came back from the local AG's office as follows: Some delays are unavoidable and/or unpredictable. Most delays are outside the prosecutor's control. You have the right to ask the witness coordinator or the prosecutor why you are having to wait. If an emergency happens and you have to leave court, try to inform the prosecutor before leaving. Try to be understanding if the prosecutor provides a valid reason for the delay. Bring your laptop, the court library has wifi.

You can limit your wait time by being honest and realistic about your availability, being responsive when the prosecutor tries to contact you and providing current contact information to the prosecutor. Ask to be notified as soon as the trial/hearing date is set. Plan accordingly and arrive on time.

Typical excusable causes for court delays include: An unexpected legal issue arises during or after the previous witness's testimony. Cross-examination takes significantly longer than expected. The defense makes a last-minute objection to your testimony or an exhibit that will be used during your testimony. The judge orders that you arrive at a certain time, not knowing how long the previous witness will take. The judge decides to handle some other cases on the docket before you testify.

The following types of delays are unacceptable and should be reported as a complaint to the chief prosecutor at the AG's office: The prosecutor or witness coordinator tells you to be there much earlier than you will be needed. The prosecutor changes the order of witnesses at the last minute. The prosecutor has not informed the court that you are waiting outside. The prosecutor is unprepared and unsure whether he or she will need you to testify. The prosecutor is not respectful of your time.

These responses came back to me at the same time the AG's office handled a different complaint from a different Physician. Sometime in 2016, a Pediatrician had been repeatedly harassed by a defense attorney and the defense attorney's hired investigator in regards to an unrelated case. The AG's office handed down an expert witness "bill of rights" responding to the Pediatrician's complaint at the same time they responded to my complaint about the 3 days wasted in court on the DUI case. This expert witness "bill of rights" was given to all physicians in the same municipality and applies to all physician expert witness testimony in this small town.

The local AG's office determined that an expert witness has the right to refuse to meet with or receive phone calls from the defense attorney. If you meet with the defense attorney, you can set the time, date and place of the meeting to your own convenience. You have the right to have the prosecutor and/or your own attorney present. You have the right to end the meeting anytime you want and walk out. If you meet with the defense attorney, it is best to meet in a conference room in the hospital. That way it is easier to walk out if the defense attorney becomes obnoxious. It is not a good idea to meet with the defense attorney in your office. If you have to walk out from a meeting in your office, this would leave the defense attorney unattended in your office. If you are not under subpoena, you can refuse to answer questions and refuse to produce documents to the defense attorney.

The reference for the above responses by the AG's office is "CHC Forensics" written by Betsy Weintraub and Shannon Foley in 2016.

The process for testifying in a paternity testing case is similar to the DUI cases described above. In my 29 years in Pathology and Lab Medicine I have been called to testify in paternity testing cases 4 times. This comes out to once in about 7 years.

In a paternity testing case the alleged father is the Defendant and the municipal Department of Social Services (or similar agency) is the Plaintiff. The case is a civil lawsuit, not a criminal trial. The rules of evidence are different for a civil lawsuit as opposed to a criminal trial. The different rules of evidence make a significant difference to the lawyers involved in the case; however for you as an expert witness this will not make much difference.

Here is a brief summary of the process. A child is born to an unmarried woman. If the paternity is undisputed the mother and father sign the birth certificate. If the paternity is disputed the mother contacts the municipal agency that handles child support. In most municipalities this is known as the Department of Social Services. Other possible names include the Department of Human Services, Local Child Support Agency, etc.

The Department of Social Services serves papers on the alleged father. The alleged father will need to hire an attorney at this point. The case will go to court and the Judge will issue a court order requiring paternity testing.

Specimens must be collected from the alleged father, the mother and child for testing. For lab testing purposes, the court order is accepted as equivalent to a Physician's orders for testing. The specimens are usually collected at the local municipal hospital lab and sent to a reference lab for testing. The results come back to the municipal hospital lab and are transmitted to the court.

If your lab does paternity testing, or collects the specimens used for paternity testing, it is imperative that your lab should require at least two valid photo IDs of the alleged father that comes in for testing. Your lab should make copies of the photo IDs presented by the alleged father at the time of specimen collection.

Paternity testing is currently done by genetic testing. Testing by blood groups is obsolete. The genetic testing used in this type of case is much more complicated than the alcohol testing in a DUI case. Neither the Plaintiff's Attorney nor the Defendant's Attorney will have much understanding of the testing and will need you to explain the testing to them, the jurors and the Judge.

The proceedings follow the same layout as for the DUI trial described above. You will receive a subpoena. Drop a copy of the subpoena with the hospital's legal department and/or risk manager. The subpoena will likely be followed by one or more phone calls from the Plaintiff's Attorney and Defendant's Attorney. You may or may not be called in for depositions.

Make additional copies of the two or more valid photo IDs that the alleged father had produced to your lab on the day of testing. These copies should be provided to both the Plaintiff's Attorney and the Defendant's Attorney.

In a paternity testing case, the Defendant's Attorney will oftentimes question whether you have done the paternity testing on the right person. The Defendant's Attorney may make the claim that someone else, not the alleged father, had come in for the testing. Hence the need for at least two valid photo IDs of the person who showed up for paternity testing. Otherwise, the process is similar to the DUI cases described above.

Paternity cases are frequently settled prior to trial. If the genetic testing conclusively proves paternity, the Defendant will oftentimes acquiesce, and admit paternity. This obviates the need for a trial. If the case goes to trail, the procedure is the same for direct examination, cross-examination, and free-for-all questioning.

At the trial, you will be under oath. Answer the questions truthfully and to the best of your abilities. Keep all explanations in layman's terms. In most jurisdictions, the minimum qualification for a juror is high school graduation or equivalent. Your explanations should be simple enough for a high school senior to understand. Since the testing for a paternity case is more complex than the alcohol testing in a DUI case, it is much more difficult to explain this in simple layman's terms.

There is one final point to make. In both DUI cases and paternity testing cases the prosecuting attorney is an official of the municipality where you live. If you are Lab Director of the municipal hospital you too are an official of the same municipality. Even so, an expert witness is supposed to be an unbiased, disinterested party to the legal proceeding. Do not put any "spin" or bias on your testimony so as to favor the prosecution. Let the chips fall where they may.

Chapter 26 – How to be a waived test Lab Director and a PPM Lab Director

CLIA does not specifically state the qualifications to be a Lab Director for waived testing. Since the qualifications are not stated, essentially anyone can be a waived testing Lab Director. It is my understanding that the majority of waived testing Lab Directors are physicians (can be of any specialty and does not require a Pathologist) followed by nurses, lab techs and high school graduates.

Waived testing is commonly referred to as "Point Of Care (POC) testing". I consider that to be a misnomer, and prefer the term "waived test". By definition a waived test is so simple that a high school graduate can do the test with little risk of making a mistake if the manufacturer's instructions are followed. The significance of the test is typically low, such that erroneous results are unlikely to make a difference in patient outcome.

In contradistinction, POC testing is done at the patient's bedside. The hand-held devices used for this bedside testing are oftentimes able to perform moderate and/or high complexity testing. Thus, POC testing and waived testing are not synonymous.

CMS requires that any testing facility that does waived testing needs to have a Certificate of Waiver if it does not already have a Certificate of Compliance or Certificate of PPM. In other words if you have no CMS certificates (i.e. not doing any lab tests at all) and you want to add waived testing you need a Certificate of Waiver from CMS. If you are already have a lab doing PPM, moderate and/or high complexity testing and have a Certificate of PPM or Certificate of Compliance, you do not need an additional certificate from CMS in order to add waived testing.

If you need a Certificate of Waiver, you must apply for and receive it before starting the waived testing. When doing the testing you are obligated to follow the manufacturer's instructions. You are required to pay the fee for the Certificate of Waiver and required to notify the CMS within 30 days of any changes in ownership, name, location or Lab Director for the lab.

Other than the above requirements these tests are "waived" meaning that CMS waives all other testing requirements. You do not have to do verification, calibration, calibration verification, determine Analytical Measurement Range (AMR), write a procedure manual, etc. You can assign high school graduates as testing personnel, the requirement for a lab tech degree is waived. There is no need for training and competency testing for the personnel doing the test; these are waived as well.

The requirements for quality control and quality assurance are waived. However, the manufacturer's instructions typically require you to run controls on each day of testing. Even though CLIA doesn't require controls, you will in most cases still be running controls because CLIA requires you to follow the manufacturer's instructions.

As far as I can tell, daily QC is not always necessary for waived testing. I have seen at least one urine dipstick manufacturer's package insert that read "run QC tests per your laboratory procedures" and with use of new lots, new shipments of reagents, and on opening a new tube of reagent strips. This urinalysis dipstick testing was the only test being done at a small clinic with a Certificate of Waiver. The clinic procedures called for QC once a week on Mondays, no daily QC, and no QC on every day of use. Since a small clinic with a Certificate of Waiver will almost never be inspected by CMS, we will probably never know if this would pass muster in a CMS inspection.

There have been several instances in my career where I have been asked to take on the Lab Directorship for waived testing, since no one else wanted the Lab Directorship. For an example, a Family Practice doctor wanted to do waived fingerstick glucose and urine dipstick testing in his office. This Family Practice doctor felt completely out of place doing anything with lab testing. He felt that he has absolutely no knowledge or understanding of lab, and couldn't handle the Lab Directorship of waived testing. He had an Internist, two Pediatricians and some nurses working for him in his small clinic, but none of them wanted the Lab Directorship or felt that they could handle it. I was called and asked to serve as Lab Director for this facility.

A waived testing Lab Directorship does not count towards the maximum of 5 Lab Directorships that CLIA allows. I took on the Lab Directorship of this waived testing, since no one else wanted it and the testing was felt to be essential to that particular outpatient clinic.

The application was sent in to CMS using form CMS-116 Application for CLIA Certification. The CMS processed the application and send a bill with some associated paperwork. Once the bill was paid, the Certificate of Waiver came back a few weeks later. In my experience, CMS issuance of a Certificate of Waiver is a knee-jerk reflex whereby to the best of my knowledge they have never turned down an application for a Certificate of Waiver. As soon as you receive the Certificate of Waiver, you can begin testing.

The caveat here is that this exchange of paperwork through the mail could take up to 2 months. Always apply for a CMS certificate at least 2 months before you need it, otherwise you may have to delay the start of patient testing while you wait for the certificate to arrive. Do not send in the application more than 6 months before you plan to begin testing, since CMS will expect testing to start within 6 months of issuing a certificate.

As Lab Director for this lab, your responsibilities include making sure the staff write the results for the controls in the control log, the testing is only done when the controls are in, the staff follow the manufacturer's instructions and do not use expired reagents and/or expired test kits.

The first day testing is started, come out to the lab for a few hours at the start of business to show them how to operate the test equipment and how to write control results in a control log. Bring several blank copies of control log sheets with you when you come and drop these off at the waived testing site. Observe them doing the testing a few times to make sure they are following the manufacturer's instructions.

It should be made very clear to the testing personnel that they should never release test results if the controls are out. Instruct them that if the controls are out, they are to call the hospital lab for help, and someone will be dispatched to help them. In my experience, I have never seen a waived test repeatedly fail controls when the manufacturer's instructions are being followed.

If you receive this call of duty to come back to the small outpatient lab due to failed controls, it almost certainly means they are performing the test improperly. When you come, the main thing you will be looking for is whether they are following the instructions. Other possibilities include something wrong with the controls (outdated controls, hemolyzed controls, etc.). For disposable test kits, check the date of opening and expiration date on the test kit and reagents. Check the storage conditions (too hot or cold) for the waived testing supplies and equipment. Check the lab room temperature to make sure it is within the manufacturer's instructions for temperature of testing. Glucose meters and other similar equipment can wear out over time, and may need to be maintenanced or replaced.

Once you have the waived testing up and running, it should not require more than about an hour a month of work on your part. I usually make the trip to these waived testing sites on Saturday mornings. This is mainly because my hospital lab job requires me to be on site weekdays from 8AM to 5PM.

In your trips to the waived testing clinic you will mainly be checking that they are following the manufacturer's instructions, keeping the package insert readily available at the time and place of testing, running controls in accordance with the manufacturer's instructions, maintaining the control log, and all the controls are in. Make sure they are writing the opening date on all test kits and reagents, as some types of test kits and reagents have a shorter expiration date after opening. Make sure they are properly disposing of expired test kits and reagents without ever using expired test kits and reagents.

Make sure they are preparing the patient as needed (overnight fasting, etc.), using the correct collection devices, proper collection techniques, labeling samples properly, following universal precautions, reporting results properly (if results are handwritten make sure they are legible), calling all critical values, reporting significant infectious diseases to Public Health, and retaining test records for the required length of time. Make sure they are properly disposing of used test kits and specimens in red bag biohazard trash.

If they are doing testing daily they should become familiar with the testing procedure very quickly. If they are not doing the test very often, they may need an occasional refresher.

It is possible to intentionally modify an existing test, be it waived, moderate complexity or high complexity. Any test so modified automatically becomes a high complexity test. This would be particularly problematic at a waived testing site. The waived testing site is not doing any of the quality control and quality assurance work associated with moderate and high complexity testing. Thus, you must be very careful that no one at the waived testing site intentionally modifies the test.

My advice on this issue is that you should never intentionally modify a test, even a high complexity test in the main part of the hospital lab. If you do so, you will essentially become the manufacturer for your new test, responsible for all sorts of work such as determining the linearity, AMR, reference range, etc. Avoid modifying tests, unless you like to do a huge amount of work that isn't really necessary.

There is one big caveat here. You can add more waived testing onto a Certificate of Waiver but you cannot add moderate or high complexity testing. Some analyzers are capable of both waived testing and more complex testing. Be very careful when adding tests to these types of equipment.

For example an Abbot I-stat can do glucose and chemistries as a waived test. However, if you add on BNP to the same Abbot I-stat the BNP testing is moderate complexity. In other words this one piece of equipment will be doing testing of two different levels of complexity. If you do this, you will have exceeded the scope of a Certificate of Waiver. You now need a Certificate of Compliance for the moderate complexity testing being done on that same piece of equipment.

I have known at least one small clinic to get itself into trouble this way, by adding on testing that was beyond the scope of its Certificate of Waiver. If you are Lab Director of any lab doing moderate complexity testing and that lab only has a Certificate of Waiver you will be in deep trouble with the CMS inspectors when they find out about it. If you have a Lab Directorship at a small clinic doing waived testing, make sure it is very clear to them that they need your approval before adding any tests.

A waived testing lab is not subject to routine CMS inspections, but you have to allow the inspectors to come if they want to. In my experience, when the CMS inspectors are in town, they stick to the moderate and/or high complexity testing labs, and bypass all the small clinics with Certificates of Waiver. If they do stop by a waived testing site, the inspection typically lasts less than an hour. The CMS inspectors will check your control log for a few minutes, spend half an hour making sure that your staff are following the manufacturer's instructions properly, spend a few minutes checking the expiration dates of the supplies and reagents, and then the inspectors move on.

When I first started in Pathology and Lab Medicine there were very few waived tests. At present, there is a long list of waived tests. In my opinion waived testing is taking over, and the future of lab testing seems to be heading towards all or nearly all waived testing.

In circumstances where I have to add a new test that cannot go onto existing equipment in my lab, I try to add a waived test if available, in preference to adding a moderate or high complexity test. Even though the hospital labs I run have Certificates of Compliance, I preferentially add waived tests since a waived test is so much easier to deal with from a regulatory perspective.

Provider Performed Microscopy (PPM) is much more common in the outpatient setting than in a hospital lab. CMS requires that any testing facility that does PPM needs to have a Certificate of PPM if it does not already have a Certificate of Compliance. In other words if you have an outpatient lab with a Certificate of Waiver (i.e. doing waived tests only) and you want to add PPM you need an additional certificate from CMS. If you are already doing moderate and/or high complexity testing and have a Certificate of Compliance, you do not need an additional certificate from CMS in order to add PPM.

The Lab Director of a PPM lab can be a physician of any specialty, dentist or a midlevel practitioner (nurse midwife, nurse practitioner, or physician assistant) licensed in the State where the testing is done. In this regard, the standards are higher than the standards for waived testing but lower than the standards for moderate complexity testing. However, CMS considers PPM to be a subset of moderate complexity testing.

The qualification for the testing personnel is the same as the qualification for the Lab Director (physician, dentist or midlevel practitioner licensed in the State where the testing is done). Hence, in almost every PPM test site I am aware of, the Lab Director is the same as the person doing the testing.

The list of PPM tests is wet mounts, KOH preps, pinworm exams, fern test, post-coital direct qualitative examinations of mucous, urinalysis with microscopic exam with or without dipstick, fecal leukocyte examination, semen analysis and nasal smears for eosinophils.

The PPM test site must have a procedure manual. The PPM provider should not need training on how to do the test. If the provider has not had training during their education on how to do the test, the provider should not be doing the test.

Proficiency testing is required for all PPM tests. Each PPM provider must have competency testing at least semiannually the first year of employment and annually thereafter for each PPM procedure done by that provider. The CMS rules for competency testing are the same for PPM providers as for lab techs. Thus, PPM provider competency testing is done in the same manner as lab tech competency testing. PPM provider competency testing could be carried out by retrospective review of the PPM slides, assigning PT material as unknown PPM slides for review, etc. The documentation typically involves using forms that have been modified from lab tech competency testing forms.

In this setting, controls consist of example positive and negative slides to compare the patient specimen to. Correlation would be possible by showing 20 unknown slides to different PPM providers and correlating the results. I have never seen correlation done for PPM testing.

The remainder of lab quality control is not applicable to PPM testing. There is no such thing as PPM calibration, verification of calibration, reportable range, AMR or linearity. The test consists of a provider looking down a microscope at a specimen that the provider has collected.

There is a normal range for each test (negative for pinworms, negative for nasal eosinophils, etc.). The concept of a critical result (panic value) is not applicable since the provider does not need to call himself or herself to inform himself or herself of the result.

I am the Lab Director for a mobile PPM lab aboard a van used for Public Health outreach. This is a satellite operation of the hospital where I work, but it requires a different CLIA certificate because the testing is done off-site from the hospital. No one else wanted this Lab Directorship so it was assigned to me. Lab Directorship of a PPM lab counts toward your limit of 5 lab directorships.

Chapter 27 - How to start a new lab from nothing

There are two ways a large lab can start. It can grow from a small lab or it can be built as a large lab from the beginning.

In my 29 years experience in Pathology and Lab Medicine, I have only once helped in the founding of a large lab. This lab was built in a small municipality where I lived for several years. Here is the story.

Some years ago a pharmacist founded his own company, selling pharmaceuticals to the small to mid-size clinics in this small town. Although ostensibly a pharmaceutical company it was really more of a general medical merchandise store. This small town lacked medical suppliers, and the pharmacist-businessman stepped in to fill the vacuum. His company sold everything from orthotics to pharmaceuticals to waived testing kits.

The pharmacist-businessman was very experienced in pharmacy and CMS regulations pertaining to pharmacy. He was also surprisingly knowledgeable about lab and CMS regulations pertaining to lab.

He had approached several small doctor's offices and clinics offering to supply them with all sorts of medical merchandise including waived testing kits. In some instances the doctors would say that they wanted waived tests, but they did not feel they could handle the Lab Directorship or the regulatory aspects of the testing.

The pharmacist-businessman made the following deal with the doctors. The pharmacist-businessman will fill out the CMS forms with the doctor's name as Lab Director for the waived testing. The CMS certificate will come with that doctor's name on it as the Lab Director. However, the pharmacist-businessman will do all the Lab Director work, to include educating the staff, checking the control logs for completeness, CLIA compliance, etc.

This arrangement is entirely legitimate. Under CLIA the Lab Director of waived testing labs can delegate the entirety of the Lab Directorship to someone else, and do no work whatsoever.

This pharmacist-businessman got about 20 clinics to sign up for his waived testing program. Before this waived testing program started, there was only one lab in this town. It was the local satellite lab of a Regional Reference Lab. The Regional Reference Lab was very unhappy when a competitor set up shop in a town that lab formerly had a monopoly on.

This pharmaceutical company was supplying waived testing kits, equipment and supplies for almost all testing that could be done as a waived test. This includes electrolytes, glucose, lipid panel, complete metabolic profile, etc.

However, at the time there was no waived testing for CBCs. The first waived CBC test was not cleared by the FDA until 2017, several years after this story takes place. At the time of this story, all CBC testing was moderate complexity. The pharmaceutical company would have to collect up all the CBC specimens and send them to the Regional Reference Lab they were in competition with. No businessman anywhere likes to send work to the competition; it means that you do not make money and your competition makes money instead.

This pharmacist-businessman decided that it would make good business sense to set up his own lab to do the CBC testing, instead of sending the CBCs to the competition. Since this was moderate complexity testing, he needed a Pathologist to be Lab Director.

At the time, I was the only civilian pathologist in this small town. When I received the call from this pharmacist-businessman, I told him that I was the Lab Director of the municipal hospital in this small town. I'd have to check if it would be a conflict of interest before taking the outside position on.

The municipal hospital only did inpatient testing. The municipality's procurement code was so convoluted that if outpatients wanted lab testing at the municipal hospital, they would have to fill out a great deal of paperwork before being drawn. The pharmacist-businessman's waived testing and the Regional Reference Lab both had a streamlined process of collecting specimens. No outpatient testing was going to the hospital.

The municipal hospital does not do outpatient testing, and the proposed outside lab will do no inpatient testing. Hence, they are not in competition. The municipal hospital lab isn't going to be doing any direct business with the proposed outside lab.

I spoke to the Municipal Hospital Administrator, relaying the request for me to help with setting up the outside lab. As far as I can tell, it is not conflicted with my job at the municipal hospital.

The Municipal Hospital Administrator said that I could take on the project provided that I was still committed to doing the municipal hospital work Monday to Friday 8AM to 5PM. The outside work could be done on weekends and/or after hours.

CLIA sets a limit of 5 lab directorships per person. I was not reaching my limit on lab directorships at this time, so this limit did not stand in my way of taking on another position.

I called back the pharmacist-businessman and told him that I can take the position, and help him set up CBC testing. The analyzer was put in a warehouse that also housed pharmaceuticals. He placed the advertisements for lab staff, and I evaluated the resumes. I followed the procedure to install a new analyzer as outlined in a prior chapter.

The pharmacist-businessman was responsible for putting in place the computer system, billing, reporting and administrative mechanisms for the new lab. This was relatively easy since the computer, billing system, etc. for lab were an extension of the existing systems for the pharmacy. The lab's malpractice insurance was "piggybacked" onto the existing pharmacy malpractice policy. For all intents and purposes, this lab was created as an extension "piggybacked" onto the existing pharmacy.

A new lab must apply for and receive CMS certification (or equivalent from a deemed status inspecting agency) before starting patient testing. Your choice of inspecting agency may be dictated by the medical insurance companies you are planning to do business with. If you are planning to be inspected by CMS, use CMS form 116 Application for CLIA Certification. The CMS will issue a Certificate of Registration if the lab will perform any moderate and/or high complexity testing. A Certificate of Registration is temporary and will be changed to a Certificate of Compliance after the lab's first inspection. If the lab is only doing waived testing, a Certificate of Waiver is issued. If the lab is only doing PPM testing with or without waived testing, a Certificate of PPM is issued.

Issuing a new CMS Certificate could take up to 2 months. Always apply for a CMS certificate at least 2 months before you need it, otherwise you may have to delay the start of patient testing while you wait for the certificate to arrive. Do not send in the application more than 6 months before you plan to begin testing, since CMS will expect testing to start within 6 months of issuing a certificate.

Things went very well for this new lab. A year later, the pharmacist-businessman decided to add a chemistry analyzer to his lab. The cost of testing for chemistries is lower for moderate complexity than waived testing. The throughput is much higher for moderate complexity chemistry testing. Some of the clinics that were doing the waived testing were having staffing problems, and didn't want to commit the staff time to waived testing. It is much faster to draw a tube of blood, and make someone else test it.

The year after the CBC analyzer went live, I helped put the chemistry analyzer into service. The following year, the pharmacist-businessman wanted to add microbiology testing in-house. He was sending all microbiology testing to his competitors, the Regional Reference Lab. As mentioned above, nobody likes to send paying work to the competition. Furthermore, by this time the relationship between the pharmacist-businessman and the Regional Reference Lab had soured, as I will detail in the next chapter.

The microbiology equipment needs to have a hood with exhaust. However, the lab was housed in a warehouse that was primarily intended for pharmaceuticals. The microbiology equipment could not be set up in that warehouse. If it was, the exhaust from the microbiology hood could contaminate the area where the pharmaceutical supply techs were working. The lab would have to be set up in a different building in order to accommodate the microbiology hood. Medical office building space was selected that had a ventilating system capable of accommodating the microbiology exhaust ducts.

This is an example of why you have to be careful when choosing new equipment to purchase. As I mentioned in the chapter on putting a new analyzer into commission, you have to be very careful that a new piece of equipment will fit into the space allotted and will not have any unusual requirements such as special water supply, special electricity supply, etc. that would exceed the resources available in the lab where the equipment is to be located.

In this case, the situation was unavoidable. It was not possible to put a microbiology hood into that pharmacy warehouse. Two years prior, when the CBC analyzer was put into that warehouse, nobody knew that the lab would be very successful and grow so rapidly. If anyone had foreseen that the lab would expand so rapidly, the CBC analyzer would have gotten its own office space, not a pharmacy warehouse.

The problem is that the CBC analyzers and chemistry analyzers would have to be physically moved from their current location. There is supposedly a small risk that moving equipment can damage it, or otherwise cause it to become inaccurate.

The typical procedure used when moving a piece of equipment is to split 20 samples and run one split before the move. After moving the instrument, run QC. If the instrument fails QC after relocation, perform corrective action. If it passes QC, run the 20 split samples again. Correlate the analyzer results from the old site to the analyzer results at the new site. I would also recommend recalibrating and running calibration verification after the move.

Two years after its start this lab is offering CBCs, microbiology, and chemistry testing on site. Over the course of the next 3 years this lab would add coagulation testing, urinalysis, etc. on site so as to become more of a full service lab. It does not offer anatomic pathology or blood banking in-house. The volume of testing did not justify this.

This lab was built over the course of 5 years, constructed one analyzer at a time. I consider it one of my greatest accomplishments, almost as difficult as the 2013 "turnaround" of a troubled lab described in a prior chapter.

For most of my career I have had one main job working 8AM to 5PM weekdays at a hospital lab and a series of simultaneous side jobs. If you are thinking about taking on this sort of part-time side job, you must be very careful to ensure it is not a conflict of interest with your main job. You must also clarify in advance the time commitment. In the above example, I was very careful to ensure that there was no conflict of interest between the two employers. The original agreement was that I would commit 2 hours per month at the part-time side job.

As the outside lab grew in size and added testing, my time commitment grew over the years. On February 27, 2007 I sent a letter to the pharmacist-businessman stating that we initially agreed to 2 hours per month but the work has been much more. I documented my time commitment for the most recent few months.

I was being frequently called and requested to come to the outside lab during the working hours, usually to review peripheral blood smears or sign papers. However, it is not a good idea for me to leave the hospital lab during the working hours as there are constant problems at the hospital lab (Blood Bank, frozen sections, etc.) and these problems would come up unexpectedly during the day. It is against regulations for me to be clocked-in at the hospital lab and working somewhere else. Most of the outside lab's work could wait until after 5PM. I requested that for anything urgent, the outside lab should have a courier drive the slides and paperwork from the outside lab to the hospital lab for me to do the work at the hospital lab. The routine work can wait for me to come after 5PM.

My primary position takes priority over the part-time side job. I told the outside lab the time conflicts with my primary position must be reduced or I would not be able to continue on in my position as Lab Director of the outside lab. This situation was resolved amicably and I retained this part-time side job for several more years until I moved out of that municipality.

In my 29 years experience in Pathology and Lab Medicine I have only once seen an entirely new hospital built in the community where I lived. It was a 130 bed hospital. The construction of its lab was contracted out a firm in a large city. I was not directly involved with the construction of this lab. From the time the new hospital received an occupancy permit (i.e. was deemed structurally safe for entry/occupancy) until it opened was only about 4 months. I am guessing that the construction of its lab must have seemed quite rushed.

The process of building the new hospital's lab would be similar to that described above for the outpatient lab with two major differences. The first major difference is that there is no existing computer system, billing system, administrative mechanisms, etc. to "piggyback" onto. These all must be created from nothing and put in place before the lab opens. The staff would all be newly hired, and would all need extensive training on how to use the computer, how to do billing, etc. before the lab opens.

The other major difference is that all the analyzers would be getting put into the same lab at the same time. Time and space constraints would be much more of an issue in this setting. You would have a deadline for finishing this work and would likely be very time-pressured. If you miss your deadline you will delay the opening of the entire hospital, and everyone else at that hospital will be very upset about the delays.

You may be given some input into the floor plan and floor space allocation for the new lab. The floor plan tends to be a matter of personal preference. My advice is to always ask for at least 20% more floor space than is initially needed. You want to start out with some vacant space available in lab in case you have to put in additional equipment later on.

Each analyzer being installed would follow the procedure for putting a new analyzer into commission given in a prior chapter. There would likely be multiple Service Reps, Lab Directors and lab techs working as multiple teams with each team assigned to set up one or a few analyzers. There would likely be an overall Lab Director supervising the various teams setting up the analyzers. That overall Lab Director would have to pay particular attention to space constraints and time constraints given so much work being done in a limited area and limited time.

Chapter 28 – Lab Director ethics

As a Lab Director, you are expected to uphold the same code of ethics as any other medical professional. The medical code of ethics dates back to Hippocrates and enumerates certain basic rights that patients have. Patients have a right to autonomy (the right to make their own decisions), beneficence (always act in the patient's best interest) and non-maleficence (avoid harm to the patient). The distribution of medical care must be fair and just.

Some lab organizations have created their own codes of ethics. These tend to stipulate additional requirements such as duty to the profession, duty to the community, commitment to excellence, dedication to competence, showing compassion and respect to the patient, continuing medical education, maintaining confidentiality, respect human rights, etc.

In my experience the vast majority of Lab Directors follow the above ethical codes to the letter. I have only seen a few instances of a Lab Director deviating from what I though was acceptable ethical conduct. The first story involves the same pharmacist-businessman and Regional Reference Lab as referenced in the chapter above. The Regional Reference Lab had a small satellite lab in the small town where I lived. It was mainly a draw station with most of the testing being sent to the big city where that lab had its headquarters.

The businessman-pharmacist and the Regional Reference Lab were competitors. From the start they did not get along, and their relationship would further sour over time.

A few years after setting up the main lab described in the prior chapter the pharmacist-businessman asked me to take on the Lab Directorship for a mid-size outpatient clinic. The clinic was doing a few moderate complexity tests on point of care testing equipment, so they needed a Pathologist to be Lab Director. I said yes I could take on that position; it would not be a conflict of interest with any of the other positions I held.

I knew before taking on this Lab Director position that the clinic lab had formerly done business with the Regional Reference Lab. I assumed that there was nothing wrong with the switch of that clinic from one lab to another.

About a month later, one of the Lab Directors from the Regional Reference Lab called me. This Lab Director made an allegation that the pharmacist-businessman had gotten the clinic to switch labs based on offering lower prices for testing. I said there is nothing wrong with that. America is a capitalist country; that is perfectly legal.

The Regional Reference Lab Director made allegations that there had been an improper inducement for the clinic to switch to the pharmacist-businessman's lab. I said that I was not party to the negotiations between the clinic and the pharmacist-businessman. I am just an employee and do not have ownership interest in the business; thus I do not sit in the closed door meetings. I said I'd ask the pharmacist-businessman if there had been any improprieties.

The Regional Reference Lab Director said that the transaction amounted to "bribery" and threatened legal action. I said that the statutory definition of bribery is an improper inducement to a government official to influence the government official in the discharge of his or her duty. Neither the clinic owners nor the pharmacist-businessman are government officials, nor do they conduct business directly with the government. Hence this cannot be bribery.

The Regional Reference Lab Director then threatened to sue alleging breach of contract. He alleged that an improper inducement had caused the clinic to break its contract with the Regional Reference Lab.

I said that my lawyer is Mr.____. You can serve the lawsuit papers on my lawyer. Be advised that if you sue me, I will counter-sue you alleging harassment and monopolistic business practices. If you lose the lawsuit you will have to pay me for wasting my time. I will charge you something punitive, like $500 per hour, for wasting my time.

The phone call ended at this point and I immediately called the pharmacist-businessman, followed by a phone call to my private attorney. The pharmacist-businessman denied wrongdoing and claimed that there was no improper inducement.

My attorney called the pharmacist-businessman's attorney. The pharmacist-businessman's attorney had been party to the negotiations, and said there was no inappropriate inducement. I took this at face value. Contrary to popular opinion, in my experience one lawyer will not lie to another lawyer. Instead, they refuse to answer the question if giving a true answer would be against their best interests. I later talked to the clinic owners, and they also said there was no improper inducement.

My attorney told me that I was right, and the Lab Director from the Regional Reference Lab could get in deep trouble for making such a phone call. The phone call could be construed as harassment and/or intimidation. However, without any way to document the contents of the call, it would be my word against his word. The Regional Reference Lab should have had its lawyer contact the pharmacist-businessman's lawyer. The call should not have been made from Lab Director to Lab Director.

My private attorney sent a letter to the Regional Reference Lab attorney complaining about the Lab Director's phone call and instructing the Regional Reference Lab not to call me anymore. The letter further instructed the Regional Reference Lab to send all correspondence to my attorney and/or the pharmacist-businessman's attorney. I did not hear further from the Regional Reference Lab. They did not take any legal action that I am aware of (i.e. they were bluffing).

My attorney wanted to send a letter directly to the Lab Director of the Regional Reference Lab. This proposed letter would inform the Regional Reference Lab Director that his actions were dishonest, unethical and probably also illegal and warn him against slander and liable. Slander and liable are defined as making false statements with the intent of causing damage. I told my lawyer not to send a letter directly to the Regional Reference Lab Director. The letter to the Regional Reference Lab attorney is sufficient. The Regional Reference Lab can handle the matter internally.

The take home points here are:

1. Always know as much as possible about a job position before taking it. In this case, I knew

almost nothing about the clinic Lab Director position when I took it.
2. Let the lawyers do the lawyer work. Do not overstep the bounds of your office or perform work in areas where you have no expertise.
3. Lab can be a cutthroat business, just like any other business.
4. When two competitors go to war, try to stay out of the fight to the extent you can.
5. Always do the right thing. If you know you're in the right, you cannot be intimidated by threats of legal action.
6. Some of the basic principles of ethics include "Do not say or do anything to another person that you wouldn't want said or done to you", "Do not say or do anything that you would not want to be public knowledge". The Regional Reference Lab Director said things to me that he probably wouldn't want anyone else saying to him.

The following story relates to the sale of a laboratory that occurred in 1995 in a municipality that I would later live in. I was not living in that municipality at the time and this entire story is composed of second and third hand accounts. Rumor and hearsay are defined as circulating stories that cannot be substantiated.

Sometime in the 1970s a businessman-Lab Director founded his own lab in a small municipality in the middle of nowhere. In 1995 he sold this lab to the same Regional Reference Lab discussed above. The sale price was reportedly $3,500,000. The terms of the sale were that the Regional Reference Lab gets all the equipment on-site, and the businessman-Lab Director gets to stay on as Lab Director of that lab after the sale. The Regional Reference Lab thinks that they were buying all of the equipment on-site at that lab.

After the sale is completed, the Regional Reference Lab found out that some of the equipment on-site was leased. In other words, the businessman-Lab Director did not own some of this equipment and could not sell it. The amount that the Regional Reference Lab overpaid was about $1,500,000 out of the $3,500,000 purchase price.

My assessment of the story so far: There is a Latin saying "caveat emptor". It translates as "let the buyer beware". It is used as a legal term to imply that the buyer has the legal obligation to do due diligence, and properly investigate the situation before entering into the purchase. If this story is true, it means that the Regional Reference Lab did not do its due diligence before entering into the purchase agreement. Equipment leases are usual and customary in the lab business, and the Regional Reference Lab should have done its homework better before going ahead with this purchase.

Supposedly, at this stage of the game, the Regional Reference Lab demands the return of $1,500,000 from the businessman-Lab Director. The businessman-Lab Director refuses. The Regional Reference lab retains an attorney that sends letters to the businessman-Lab Director threatening a lawsuit if the disputed monies are not returned. The businessman-Lab Director then tells the Regional Reference Lab that if they sue the businessman-Lab Director, he will quit as Lab Director of that lab.

My assessment of the story so far: This is not unreasonable. It would not make sense to keep working for a company that is suing you.

The threat of the Lab Director quitting sends the Regional Reference Lab scrambling to find another Lab Director for that lab. The position requires someone on-site, it can't be done remotely. No other Pathologist lives anywhere near that small municipality. Lab Directors are extremely hard to find, especially for such a remote municipality.

The head of the Regional Reference Lab called in his subordinate Pathologists one-by-one and asked if they would voluntarily move to this remote municipality for a while until this is sorted out. They all refused. The head of the Regional Reference Lab then called in the lower ranking Pathologists and told them that he might send one of them to this remote municipality involuntarily. They all said that they would quit their jobs rather than move to this small municipality.

At this point, the Regional Reference Lab knows that it is caught in the proverbial "deal with the devil". The term "deal with the devil" is used metaphorically to describe a deal from which one would like to extricate oneself, but is unable to do so.

The Regional Reference Lab has to keep doing business with the businessman-Lab Director. If he quits as Lab Director at the lab in question, there would be no replacement. The Lab Director position would go vacant. Any lab without a Lab Director would be quickly shut down by the regulators, in this case, CMS. If this lab got shut down by the regulators, the Regional Reference Lab would lose the entire amount of money it put into the purchase. Supposedly, the matter is later settled with the businessman-Lab Director agreeing to pay back a much smaller amount than the $1,500,000 disputed amount.

As mentioned at the start of this story, it is entirely composed of unsubstantiated rumor and hearsay. There were other, similar unsubstantiated stories circulating about this businessman-Lab Director. If any of these stories were true, it would imply he had cheated most of the entities he had ever done business with. The only tangible evidence was the 2003 routine annual audit of the municipal hospital by the Public Auditor. The Public Auditor caught this businessman-Lab Director working in a consultant position for the hospital without the prerequisite paperwork in place. This audit was public record and appeared on the Public Auditor's website.

The Public Auditor couldn't figure out how anyone could get into a paid position at the municipal hospital without the employment paperwork being in place. My reading of the this is that the municipal hospital had very poor accounting controls; and the businessman-Lab Director was friends with the Hospital Administrator such that the Administrator had appointed the businessman-Lab Director to a hospital position without making the businessman-Lab Director fill out the appropriate paperwork.

The businessman-Lab Director should have known better. One of the basic principles of ethics is "don't say or do anything that you wouldn't want to be public knowledge". After the audit, the businessman-Lab Director was required to fill out all of that hospital's extensive pre-employment paperwork in order to maintain his job position. This episode brought unwanted scrutiny from the Public Auditor on the municipal hospital and the businessman-Lab Director.

Let's think about my ethics in repeating such a story. The story is educational and entertaining (beneficence). I haven't mentioned any of the parties by name, so there is no real damage done (non-maleficence). I can tell my stories to anybody I want (autonomy). I am willing to tell my stories equally to everybody in the whole world (fair and just distribution).

In a situation where you have not substantiated a story, do not repeat the story and/or do not repeat the names of the parties involved. If you repeat the names of the parties involved in the story you will make enemies of all the parties involved and you could get sued for slander and/or liable.

For the purpose of this chapter, the main question is how to deal with someone like the businessman-Lab Director referenced above, during the time when he had multiple unsubstantiated stories circulating alleging unethical conduct. This is a judgment call, and each person must decide on their own what to do in this circumstance. The best I can do is give advice. In general, I will ignore any stories that are unsubstantiated and will not repeat any such stories, not even to ask the person in question if the stories are true. If the stories are unsubstantiated, I do not shy away from doing business with that person. I will do business with such a person the same as for everyone else.

My advice is to avoid doing business with anyone under an ethical cloud. If there is substance to any allegation of unethical conduct (e.g. a municipal hospital's annual audit reveals that the Lab Director is working in a paid position without the prerequisite paperwork in place. The audit with detailed findings was made public knowledge on the Public Auditor's website), I try to avoid doing business with that person. If there is no other vendor and I am obligated to transact with that person, I will be very careful to check all details of all proposed transactions. In private I will ask my lawyer to go over the documentation in more detail than the cursory review of the typical proposed contract. Once the arrangement is in place, I ask the accounts payable personnel in private to carefully scrutinize any bills coming from that person.

Chapter 29 – Lab Director leadership skills and how to deal with conflict in the clinical laboratory

There is a saying that rich and powerful people are judged by how they treat the people below them. As a Lab Director you will be the most powerful person in Lab and also likely the wealthiest. In many ways, you will be judged by how you interact with the rank and file employees in Lab.

The following story is made up of rumors circulating among the residents and attending Pathologists at the time of my training. Therefore, this entire story can be assumed to be fictitious, but it illustrates important points.

For the purposes of this story, one of the hospitals I trained at is called "Hospital A". The Lab Director for Hospital A had been present at the founding of the hospital in 1957. He set up the Pathology Department as a group which he owned. This was a brilliant move, and played in his favor for decades to come. I will refer to his pathology group as "Slavedriver Pathology Group" for the purposes of this story.

When I started training in 1991 at Hospital A the group had 7 Pathologists. The Lab Director was a very elderly gentleman by then in his early 80s. He was doing very little work, and delegating almost everything to the younger pathologists. He had been encouraged to retire, but refused to do so. He could not be forced to retire since he owned the group.

He had a reputation as a "slavedriver" assigning as much work as possible to the other 6 Pathologists in the group. They were his direct employees and he could force them to work as hard as possible. Since he owned the group, he stood to profit from this. The money that was not paid in salary added to his profit. Exploitation is defined as forcing people to work as hard as possible for as little pay imaginable.

This Lab Director also overworked the histotechs, secretaries and all other positions under his control. The way he did this was by intentionally leaving positions vacant. This lab had allotted slots for 11 pathologists but the slavedriver Lab Director did not want to do any hiring. Instead he wanted to make the existing Pathologists work harder. He did the same with all other job positions under his control. The result was poor morale and high turnover of essentially all positions in this lab.

Sometime in 1993 Hospital A acquired another hospital which I will call "Hospital B" for the purposes of this story. Hospital B is a nearby mid-size to large hospital with 4 pathologists. The plan was that the

Pathology Departments for the two hospitals would be merged. The Lab Director of Hospital A wanted to lay off 2 of the 4 Hospital B Pathologists and centralize the Pathology services at Hospital A.

All the other pathologists objected to layoffs. The other Hospital A pathologists are already working like slaves, and the added work from Hospital B would send their workload into the stratosphere. The Hospital B pathologists object because they don't want to get laid off. The slavedriver Lab Director dug in his heels. He is going to lay off 2 of the Hospital B pathologists, and tells the other Pathologists they will have to tow the line because they are all just employees. This resulted in a series of arguments between the slavedriver Lab Director and the other pathologists. These arguments progressively worsened over time as the merger date approached.

About this time, the 6 Hospital A employee pathologists and the 4 Hospital B pathologists began having closed door meetings. The slavedriver Lab Director was not invited to these meetings. His absence from meetings was unusual since he headed the department. I did not sit on those closed door meetings. Later I found out that the pathologists were meeting to plan the ouster of the slavedriver Lab Director and form their own pathology group.

The 6 employee Pathologists from Hospital A and the 4 Pathologists from Hospital B approached the Hospital Administration of both hospitals. Both hospitals administrations and all pathologists met in one big meeting. The Pathologists threatened to resign en-mass. All ten will quit if there is any attempt to lay off any Pathologist, and force the other Pathologists to take monstrous workloads. The slavedriver Lab Director is called into this meeting. He again digs in his heels. He will lay off some Pathologists and make the others work harder. He figures that since he owns the group, he is untouchable. He is wrong.

Both hospital administrations involved know that their entire Pathology Departments are getting ready to resign en-mass. They cannot allow this to happen. If events play out this way their hospitals will be seriously damaged. The administrations of both hospitals help to unseat the slavedriver Lab Director.

The mechanics of his unseating are as follows. The 6 employee Pathologists from Hospital A and all 4 Pathologists from Hospital B form their own group. For the purposes of this story I will call this "Mutiny Pathology Group". Needless to say, the slavedriver Lab Director is not invited to join Mutiny Pathology Group. Both Hospital A and Hospital B revoke their contracts with Slavedriver Pathology Group and hire Mutiny Pathology Group on the same day.

Two weeks later, the slavedriver Lab Director shuffles off into retirement. Everyone in the department is glad to see him go. Not one person misses him.

I was not involved in the mutiny at Hospital A, and kept my distance from the proceedings. I was a pathology resident at the time. The trainees were seen as very low ranking and expected to be seen but not heard. The pathology residents had no say in the events that played out.

The Pathology residents were "out of the loop" meaning we were excluded from all decision making and informational meetings among the attending Pathologists. Since there was never any official briefing, this entire story is based on rumors circulating at the time. The lack of official information encouraged wild speculation among the residents on the events that were transpiring. More than 20 years later I would send a copy of this book to my former Residency Program Director, now retired. He claims this story is inaccurate. This points out the need for transparency within Pathology groups and clinical labs since you don't want inaccurate stories circulating.

The Lab Director for Hospital A was a slavedriver for the pathology residents. The other residents and I did essentially 100% gross exams, working from 7AM to 6PM, working like we really were slaves, until this Lab Director was forced out. The other pathology residents all hated this Lab Director. I figured that the heavy workload was a rite of passage, similar to a "hazing" at a college fraternity. All these years later, I have no ill will to the slavedriver Lab Director, and figured that I learned a huge amount about gross exams working those long hours in his lab.

This sequence of events in which rank and file employees unite to throw off a cruel boss very closely resembles the Mutiny on the Bounty. The Mutiny on the Bounty really did happen. It took place in the year 1789. I have seen at least three similar mutinies in my 29 year career, the most spectacular of which is given above. The other two mutinies involved administrative removal of lab supervisory personnel that were universally disliked by their subordinates.

The three lab mutinies I have seen occurred in different labs years apart from each other and thousands of miles away from each other. In each instance, I was not Lab Director, but instead in the Pathologist position or Pathology Resident position. In each instance, my job position did not require me to take any administrative action, and I kept my distance from the proceeding. Do not get involved in this type of situation unless you are required to. In my experience the pathway to mutiny involves:

1. An authoritarian supervisor with an attitude of "I am the boss". Typically a perfectionist with an expectation that everything should be done his or her way.
2. Seasoned rank and file employees that are not going to put up with the supervisor. The employees are good at what they do and they know it. They resent the dominating supervisor.
3. Slow buildup of resentment. The relationship between the supervisor and the employees deteriorates over time. The lab techs may begin to act passive aggressive, intentionally making mistakes to upset the supervisor. The supervisor being authoritarian, responds the only way he or she knows how – by repeatedly chewing out the lab techs.
4. The situation deteriorates further and faster. The lab techs increasingly feel that the supervisor is unapproachable and/or they don't want to have anything to do with the supervisor. The supervisor acts increasingly authoritarian as control slips away. The lab techs and supervisor will typically start reciprocal write-ups on each other at this stage if they haven't already done so.
5. The triggering event. In the story above it was the proposed layoffs. In the second mutiny I have seen, the supervisor asked the employees to pay out of pocket for tickets to a fundraiser dinner for a charitable organization that the supervisor headed. In the third mutiny I have seen, the triggering event was the supervisor withheld annual increments for a number of employees.
6. Open rebellion. The lab techs refuse to take orders from the supervisor and typically threaten a mass walk-out. At this stage, there are loud arguments in public areas. The parties involved have come to hate each other and will not conceal their hatred of the other party. There is likely going to be a huge number of write-ups between the parties involved.

As noted above, the triggering event can be very petty, but is causes the situation to explode. If you see the laboratory going down the pathway leading to mutiny, you must try to stop this at the earliest stage possible. In my experience, the further a lab goes down the pathway to mutiny, the harder it is to pull back from the brink and the more likely it is to run to completion. In other words, if you see conflict building between the lab supervisor, and/or any of the section supervisors and/or the bench level lab techs you should try to resolve that conflict as soon as it becomes apparent. Do not wait for the situation to get out of hand.

You will be doing negotiation between the Lab Supervisor and the rank and file employees. You will be the go-between for the Lab Supervisor and the lab techs who feel that they cannot communicate with the Lab Supervisor. Meet privately with the Lab Supervisor and meet privately with the lab techs to discuss the situation. What do they want from each other? What can you offer to either party?

Try to defuse the situation to the extent you can. Bring all parties into one big meeting, and try to make peace. Offer whatever appeasements you can without offending any of the parties at the table. Be as diplomatic as possible. In this meeting, try to concentrate on points in common and do not dwell on the differences between the Lab Supervisor and the lab techs. It will take more than one meeting to patch up the differences. Hopefully, this first meeting can prevent things from getting worse.

It is imperative that you should be impartial. Do not take sides. You are an authority figure in much the same way that the Lab Supervisor is an authority figure; however, you must resist the temptation to join the battle on the side of the Lab Supervisor. Likewise, do not join the battle on the side of the lab techs.

I have seen a few instances where a series of meetings between the Lab Supervisor and lab techs probably prevented a mutiny. In the other cases, the mutiny ran to completion. Much of the problem relates to the personalities involved. You cannot change other people's personalities. If the Lab Supervisor is going down the pathway to mutiny, you must try to reshuffle the Lab Supervisor into a different position. Usually you can switch that person into a section supervisor position, and switch one of the section supervisors into the Lab Supervisor position.

I have never had a Lab under my command go into a full scale mutiny. If it happened, I would be on the phone to the Hospital Administrator telling the Administrator that the Lab Supervisor has to be removed immediately or the lab is going to stop functioning.

I have told these stories to many people and most do not believe they really count as mutinies. The definition of a mutiny is that it is an agreement among multiple individuals to stop following authority. There is no requirement that the action has to take place aboard a ship, and no requirement that the mutineers have to be military. Thus the stories given above really are mutinies in which multiple Pathologists agree to stop following orders from the slavedriver Lab Director and multiple lab techs agree to stop following orders from their despised Lab Supervisor.

The point of these stories is that you always have to be nice to your subordinates. You cannot take their place in doing their work. You need them more than they need you. Never berate or speak disrespectfully of anyone, even if they are not present at the time. Never criticize unless absolutely necessary. Even then, the counseling should be carried out behind closed doors and phrased in a constructive manner. Be quick to thank employees for a job well done. Try to find something that the lab staff excel at, and give them awards at least twice a year. Give awards for all goals met. Be sincere in your praise when handing out the awards.

As Lab Director, these leadership skills are important. In my experience the most important aspect of leadership is your ability to relate to the people around you. A good leader is a team player and gets along with all co-workers. Try to be on friendly terms with all co-workers. The lab staff all have their own hopes and aspirations. Do your best to help them advance professionally (encourage continuing education and training). Encourage the personal development and career aspirations of the lab staff.

As a leader, a few basic qualities are necessary. A leader must be honest. If others can't trust you, they will not follow you. A leader should have a positive attitude, and lead by example. A leader should be confident, but should also know his or her limits. Always project a positive attitude, but don't "sugar coat" the situation by reporting things as being better than they really are. A leader should act in the best interest of the organization, be selfless and committed to the good of all. A good leader will be committed to excellence in the organization. A good leader is accountable and will admit to making mistakes. A good leader will never cover up his or her own mistakes and will not try to blame others.

A leader will plan and act proactively. Oftentimes, plans do not turn out as expected. A good leader will be able to rearrange plans on the fly based on the changing situation and will not act as if all plans are inflexible and unchanging. You should be able to handle unexpected situations. This may require creativity and intuition.

As a leader you must be able to communicate the organization's policies, decisions and changes to all employees you supervise. There should be open lines of communication and an open door to your office.

You as Lab Director should be dependable, so as to earn the trust and confidence of those around you. As a leader, your goal is to contribute as much as you can to the organization by motivating the people who work with you. You should motivate the people below you in a positive manner. Ask for the lab staff's input and opinions. Take seriously any suggestions for improving the lab. Do not overwork your employees unless absolutely necessary, and even then be generous with the overtime and thankful for their work. Be generous to the rank and file employees. Buy them lunches and dinners. Eat lunch with the lab staff on a regular basis and listen to their input. Don't say or do anything to another person that you wouldn't want said or done to you.

From my discussion with other pathologists, many pathology groups have issues within the group and issues with their hospital's administration. Many groups will not survive and will instead dissolve due to these conflicts. There is no magic solution here, nor in any other Pathology books. The above advice is the best I can give.

Chapter 30 – How to chair a meeting

According to most hospital's bylaws, the Lab Directorship comes with automatic membership on some hospital committees and also typically comes with automatic chairmanship of the Blood Utilization and Transfusion Review (BUTR) Committee and the lab departmental meetings.

Blood utilization review is mandated by TJC and all hospitals will have such a committee. In my experience it is most commonly called the Blood Utilization and Transfusion Review (BUTR) Committee, but I have also seen it called the Tissue and Transfusion (T&T) Committee. In almost all hospitals, the Lab Director chairs this committee.

Before I started my first Lab Directorship, I had been the member of several hospital committees, but had never been the chair. At the time, I was overloaded with slides to look at, and my committee membership was quite slack. I would pick a seat toward the back or behind someone else, so as not to be clearly visible to the people at the head of the table. I only spoke when asked to, completed all assignments in a timely manner, but never volunteered for additional work.

When I was promoted to Lab Director, the table was turned, in a literal as well as a figurative sense. I was assigned the chairmanship of two committees, and went from hiding at the back of these committees to sitting in the driver's seat. I quickly learned how to chair a meeting.

Your committee chair work will be assisted by a secretary, typically a secretary from the Medical Staff Office. The secretary will reserve meeting room space for the date and time of the meeting.

The work of chairing a committee begins well in advance of the meeting. You should prepare the agenda at least one week in advance of the meeting. The secretary will then E-mail the agenda to all members of the committee along with a reminder of the time, date and place of the meeting. An additional reminder E-mail should be sent to all committee members about 24 hours before the meeting.

The day of the meeting you should arrive early. Lead by example. The secretary will lay out multiple copies of the agenda, last month's meeting minutes and an attendance sign-in sheet in the meeting room. The secretary will take notes for this meeting and later type the minutes. Breakfast may or may not be served.

As people come in, remind them to sign the attendance sheet. This is important, since you need to document a quorum. Also, the physicians present typically have meeting attendance requirements needed for renewal of privileges every two years. If anyone comes but forgets to sign in, it counts as an absence for attendance purposes.

Count the number of members present, and call the meeting to order when you have reached a quorum. Typically a quorum is 50% plus one of the members. With the BUTR Committee, there was little attendance, and most months we didn't reach quorum. If quorum is not met, the session in the meeting room is called a "working session" instead of a meeting. You can still do most of the work of a committee, but anything requiring a vote has to be put off until there is a quorum.

Go down the agenda one item at a time. Start with the approval of last month's minutes. Looking over last month's minutes can jog your memory as to unfinished items that need to be discussed again at the current meeting. Then go over the old business, new business, etc.

Most of the committee work will be unobjectionable. The statistics for blood usage will be presented. The blood utilization fall-out cases will be reviewed. For example Patient XYZ was transfused with a hemoglobin of 16 g/dL. This patient's chart has been pulled for the meeting. Review of the chart indicates a substantial gastrointestinal bleed. Everyone agrees that the transfusion is indicated. The case is closed.

If there is a case that is still seen as a fallout after chart review, it is referred to the department of the physician that ordered the transfusion. For example Patient Z got transfused with a hemoglobin of 12 g/dL and the indication on the chart and requisition form is "anemia". The physician that ordered the transfusion is a Family Practitioner so the case is referred to the Family Practice Department to review.

If the Family Practice Department feels the transfusion is indicted, the case is closed. If the Family Practice Department has a problem with the transfusion, they may mandate continuing medical education, or other remediation on the physician involved. The Family Practice Department may punt the case back to the BUTR Committee to do the investigation and remediation.

This is where the situation starts to get tricky. You will have a clinician coming into the BUTR Committee trying to explain why he or she ordered this particular transfusion. Usually, they will stick to their story - the patient was symptomatic, the patient needed oxygen carrying capacity, etc. I have only rarely seen a patient in person since finishing medical school 29 years ago and I was not present during that patient's physical exam, so I have no way of knowing if this physician is telling the truth or not. In this circumstance, you have to give the benefit of the doubt. The committee determines that the transfusion was indicated and the case is closed.

Even before the meeting starts I know that the case will likely be closed in that clinician's favor, just like virtually every other case in the history of the committee. While the clinician is there for the committee meeting I make sure the clinician is very clear on the indications for red blood cell transfusion. This is presented as an educational "oh, by the way, did you hear about our committee's transfusion criteria" and not presented as a corrective action.

While I have this clinician as a captive audience in my committee meeting, I am going to remind him or her of all the criteria for red blood cell transfusion at that hospital - bleeding with hypotension, bleeding more than 750ml or more than 15% of the patient's blood volume, hemoglobin less than 8 g/dL with symptoms of anemia, hemoglobin less than 10 g/dL in a preoperative patient, etc. In my experience, the combination of calling that clinician in front of a committee and informing that clinician of the transfusion criteria at that hospital almost always prevents recurrence of inappropriate transfusion.

The committee then moves on to other business, routine matters such as presenting statistics and approving the biennial renewal of the contract with the regional Blood Bank. Award letters are passed around for signatures thanking the champion blood donors who just completed their 30th, 40th, 50th donations, etc.

After finishing all the business, make a double check of the agenda to see that all items on the agenda were brought up at the meeting. Ask the members if there is any business that is not on the agenda but needs to be brought up. If there is no further business the meeting is adjourned with an announcement that the next meeting will be held the same day next month.

Immediately after the meeting is over, look at the attendance sheet and make a note of the absent physicians. Towards the close of the same working day, call these physicians one-by-one, informing them of the events that transpired at the meeting and reminding them that there is a meeting attendance requirement. Most will tell you that they were too busy to come, had a conflicting clinic schedule, etc. Any clinicians with less than 50% attendance over the past several months should be asked to send proxies, or turn their committee seats over to other physicians.

In my experience, the main job of the chairman is to keep the meeting flowing smoothly, and prevent the meeting from getting bogged down in one or more unimportant details. You don't need to be an expert in parliamentary rules of debate.

I bought a copy of Robert's Rules of Order, and found that at most meetings it was of little help. Even though there are few meetings where you will need a copy of Robert's Rules, make sure to keep a copy with you at all meetings. As detailed below, the need could come up at any time.

As the committee chair you are tasked with handling all procedural issues that come up in the meeting. If a procedural matter came up, and you didn't have a copy of Robert's Rules with you, you might not know how to proceed. In this situation you should table (i.e. postpone) that one item to the next meeting and research how to handle the procedural issue. Avoid making up the rules as you go along.

The most important point is that you have to be fair and impartial. If there is debate, allow both sides of the debate equal time. Make it clear to everyone that each side is allowed the same amount of time to present their case. That is more important than knowing all the intricacies of the parliamentary rules of debate.

In every meeting there is likely to be one or more person that likes to talk too much and/or likes to be the center of attention. If one person is talking for more than 5 minutes and not allowing anyone else to speak, interject as politely as possible that debate for this topic will be limited to another 2 minutes in order to discuss all topics at this meeting. Let the person talk another 2 minutes then politely but firmly tell him or her the meeting has to go on to other topics in order for the meeting to accomplish its agenda in the time allotted.

Not many issues needed to be voted on, and few of these issues were contentious. There were only a few instances where the debate seemed to trail on and on. When this happens, interject that you are setting a limit of 10 minutes for the debate. After the 10 minutes are up, close the debate and bring the matter to a vote.

In my many years experience as a chairman, there was only one instance where a clinician was called into a meeting and became very defensive. This was a case of red blood cell transfusion fallout. Transfusion was given to a patient with a hemoglobin around 9.5 g/dL. The clinician must have known he did something wrong. Instead of trying to justifying the transfusion, he attempted all sorts of parliamentary maneuvers such as quorum call, points of order, question of privilege, motion to table discussion, etc.

Luckily, I had brought my copy of Robert's Rules with me. As each motion and point of order was made, I'd look in Robert's Rules to see how to handle it. This slowed the committee meeting to a snail-pace but the work did eventually get done. The committee determined that the case did not require a corrective action. The case was closed in the clinician's favor, in spite of the parliamentary maneuvering and in spite of the fact he never tried to justify the transfusion.

If the case had been of a serious nature, I would have called in the hospital Medical Director to take over chairmanship of that particular meeting. The hospital Medical Director chaired multiple committees that routinely dealt with physician discipline. Thus, the Medical Director was much more experienced with parliamentary maneuvering and much more proficient at dealing with it than I was. Always know your limits, and be prepared to call in an expert if necessary.

In my experience significant problems in lab are dealt with on-the-fly and do not usually require committee meetings to work on the problem. In my experience when trying to solve significant problems in lab the best course of action is to analyze the problem, determine the causes of the problem, determine the possible solutions, pick the best possible solution, implement the solution chosen and evaluate the effectiveness of the solution. Most of this work should be done independently of committee meetings. If the plan of action requires approval by any committee, the plan of action is presented to that committee for a vote of approval.

At most hospitals, the Lab Director position comes with an automatic seat on the hospital's Medical Executive Committee (MEC), but not the chairmanship. In the hospitals where I have worked, the MEC is the most important and powerful of the medical staff committees. The MEC is the main steering committee of the hospital tasked with hearing appeals of disciplinary decisions made at the departmental level, grievances, and matters related to physician privileging among other issues.

You need to know the basics of physician privileging in order to sit on this committee, so I will provide a brief overview of the topic. The CMS regulations state that all physicians are required to be privileged at every hospital they practice at. If they practice telemedicine, they must be privileged at the hospital where they are physically located, but not necessarily at the hospital where the patient is located. The hospital where the patient is located must have a contract with the hospital where the physician is privileged.

The medical staff must be accountable to the hospital's governing body for the quality of care provided to patients. The medical staff must ensure the criteria for privileging are individual character, competence, training, experience, and judgment. The granting of privileges cannot be dependent solely upon certification, fellowship, or membership in a specialty body or society. The reference is 42 CFR § 482.12(a).

The CMS's interpretive guidelines for 42 CFR §482.22(a)(2) state there must be a mechanism established to examine credentials of individual prospective members (new appointments or reappointments) by the medical staff. The individual's credentials to be examined must include at least a request for clinical privileges, evidence of current licensure, evidence of training, professional education, documented experience and supporting references of competence.

The CMS considers its medical staff regulations to be a Condition of Participation, and any violations are taken particularly seriously. In the typical hospital-wide inspection, the CMS will review the credentialing folders of many providers. If the CMS inspectors catch even one unqualified practitioner on your hospital's medical staff, they could give the hospital an Immediate Jeopardy citation, the most severe citation CMS can give. Hence, it is very important for the medical staff to properly verify the credentials of anyone applying for privileges.

Credentialing is a subset of the privileging process and involves the review of the applicant's credentials. Privileging is the evaluation of the applicant using the information gathered in the credentialing process. In order to become privileged, a physician must fill out an application form and provide primary source verification of credentials. Primary source verification means that the applicant's transcripts, proof of residency training, proof of board certification and other documentation have come directly from the source to the hospital without passing through the hands of the physician being privileged. If primary source verification is not possible, documents coming from a Credentials Verifying Organization (CVO) or reliable secondary sources are allowed. All hospitals are required to have bylaws, and the bylaws must stipulate the pathway to privileging. The hospital bylaws must be followed to the letter. The reference is TJC Standard MS.06.01.03.

Every hospital bylaws I have ever seen state that the burden is on the physician to prove that he or she is qualified. There is no obligation on the hospital to track down this physician's transcripts, proof of training, etc.

The hospital is required to query the National Practitioner Data Bank (NPDB). The reference is TJC Standard MS.06.01.05. Although the hospital is required to make this query, there are no specific requirements as to how much derogatory information disqualifies an applicant. I once sat on an MEC that approved privileging for a physician with multiple malpractice settlements recorded in NPDB. In another instance the same MEC approved privileging for someone whose NPDB profile showed medical licenses revoked in two distant states. This hospital was desperately short of doctors, and willing to take anyone. In both these cases, the derogatory NPDB information was noted in passing, and the physician was privileged. Noting that the MEC is aware of the derogatory NPDB information is sufficient to meet regulatory requirements.

The physician cannot be privileged until every last document has been received. The privileging process typically does not start until all documents are present. After all the documents are received, the usually pathway to privileging involves review by the department where the practitioner applied for privileges followed by the Credentials Committee review.

If there are no problems the relevant committees will recommend approval. The MEC then votes a rubber stamp approval and the application for privileges is signed off by the Medical Staff President, hospital Medical Director, hospital Board and/or Hospital Administrator. The new privileges are valid after the required chain of signatories is complete. The newly privileged physician is assigned a proctor to review his or her work.

Some of the most contentious meetings I have ever attended have been MEC meetings in regard to physicians with spotty track records applying for privileges. In one instance a Pediatrician had applied for privileges that as one person put it "He repeated PGY2 maybe four or five times, did not get to PGY3 and he wants to count this as a residency". The department involved was badly short of staff, desperate to hire, and obviously willing to take anybody.

The Pediatrics Department signed off on the privileging, but the Credentials Committee objected. This resulted in a huge argument at an MEC meeting. As with any difficult cases brought before the MEC it resulted in multiple MEC members loudly quoting from the hospital bylaws during the meeting. I am not really familiar with Pediatrics training, so I sat this battle out without saying anything. The MEC then voted not to allow privileging for this Pediatrician.

The Pediatrician would have an appeals process spelled out in the hospital bylaws, appealing the unfavorable Credentials Committee and MEC decisions to the Hospital's Administrator and/or Board. The CMS regulations give the final say to the hospital's Governing Body. The reference is 42 CFR § 482.12(a)(2). At most hospitals the committee referred to by the CMS as the hospital's "Governing Body" is called the Board of Trustees, Advisory Board, or something similar. In theory, the Board has the authority to overrule the Hospital Administrator, overrule the MEC, overrule the Credentials Committee and approve a doctor for privileging against the advice of all others concerned. In my experience this has never happened. No hospital administrator or board would ever overturn an MEC decision made under these circumstances. The Pediatrician referenced above was not credentialed at that hospital and found work elsewhere.

Another sticky situation at MEC meetings results from expired privileges. Privileges cannot last longer than 2 years from the date of issue. The CMS regulations state that a physician needs privileges to practice at any given hospital. Implied but not outright stated is that a physician cannot practice at a hospital where the privileges have expired. Otherwise CMS is silent on how to deal with expired privileges. Each hospital's bylaws should state how to deal with expired privileges. The MEC will hear all sorts of appeals from physicians that forgot to renew their privileges on time. This is a very common problem, particularly among older physicians who are becoming forgetful.

My advice is to always keep track of the expiration date of your privileges at every hospital where you work and begin the renewal process at least 3 to 6 months in advance. Do not wait for a letter to arrive reminding you of the need to renew. If you do not keep track of the expiration date, and the medical staff secretary forgets to send you the renewal reminder letter, you will be in deep trouble. The same applies for all your state licensures, BLS certification and Board Certification as applicable. Keep track of the expiration dates and start the renewal process as early as possible.

When dealing with expired privileges the MEC will usually grant as much leniency as possible, allowing physicians to renew expired privileges. If possible, avoid making the physician apply for new privileges (i.e. start the application process over from the beginning). The new application will require submission of primary source verification documents, which is time consuming and could take months. In the meantime that physician cannot practice at that hospital because his or her privileges are expired.

One important caveat is that the MEC hears very sensitive cases. These discussions should be treated as top secret, and never discussed or disclosed outside of the closed doors of the meeting. Anyone divulging confidential information from an MEC meeting could be accused of being a disruptive practitioner.

One hospital I worked at had several instances in which a pair of physicians would ask to come before the MEC, air out their petty grievances in front of the MEC, and then accuse each other of disruptive practitioner. This involved physicians who were either competitors in a tight market, or hated each other or both. The problem is how to adjudicate this at the level of the MEC.

I have seen "disruptive practitioner" defined in many different ways such as violating rules of civil behavior, unprofessional etiquette, disrupting the efficient and orderly operation of the hospital or interfering with patient care. The AMA in one of its opinions states "personal conduct, whether verbal or physical, that negatively affects or that potentially may negatively affect patient care constitutes 'disruptive behavior.' This includes but is not limited to conduct that interferes with one's ability to work with other members of the health care team."

The problem is that "disruptive practitioner" is defined extremely broadly, such that saying something someone else doesn't want to hear could be counted as "disruptive practitioner".

In each case, the MEC would tell both physicians involved to settle their disputes at the departmental level, and that disruptive practitioner involves serious behavioral problems on the part of a physician. A finding of "disruptive practitioner" is NPDB reportable and that is anathema to most hospital MECs. The above described situation, in which multiple pairs of physicians asked to come before the MEC to air out their petty grievances, is a sign the physicians at that hospital were cliquish and did not get along with each other very well.

As pointed out above, the MEC will hear disputes that cannot be solved at the departmental level. As a general principle of management, all disputes should be settled at the lowest level possible. For a dispute between two physicians of the same specialty, this would involve mediation by their departmental chair. For two physicians of different specialties, the mediation should involve both their departmental chairs. The dispute should only be "run up the chain of command" to the MEC if the dispute cannot be solved at this level. Depending on how well your hospital's medical staff get along with each other, you may never see a case like this at your MEC, or you could spend hours every month dealing with these cases at the monthly MEC meeting.

Chapter 31 – Lab Director hiring, orientation, competency testing, promotion, retention and retirement

The CLIA requirements for a high complexity testing Lab Director are given in 42 CFR § 493.1443. The requirements for a moderate complexity testing Lab Director are lower. However, in the typical hospital lab there is a mix of waived, moderate and high complexity testing. The Lab Director needs to meet the criteria for a for high complexity testing Lab Director or the lab will be cited for doing testing that the Lab Director is not qualified to direct. Thus, the criteria given in 42 CFR § 493.1443 serve as the minimum hiring criteria for the Lab Director of the typical hospital lab.

There are several permutations that would meet CLIA requirements. The most common situation requires that the Lab Director must be an MD, DO, or DPM and must possess a current medical license issued by the State in which the laboratory is located, and must be certified in anatomic or clinical pathology, or both, by the American Board of Pathology or the American Osteopathic Board of Pathology. The other permutations involve qualifications that CLIA considers equivalent.

CLIA allows an MD, DO, or DPM that is not a Pathologist to be a high complexity testing Lab Director if the practitioner meets the following criteria: must possess a current medical license issued by the State in which the laboratory is located, must have at least one year of laboratory training during medical residency (for example, physicians certified either in hematology or hematology and medical oncology) or have at least 2 years of experience directing or supervising high complexity testing. In my experience, this is limited to Lab Directors of labs doing subspecialty hematology/oncology testing. I do not know of a general hospital Lab Director meeting these criteria.

CLIA allows the Lab Director to have an earned doctoral degree in a chemical, physical, biological, or clinical laboratory science if certified by a board approved by HHS. Although CLIA allows this, it is generally only done in subspecialty laboratories. For example, a person with a PhD in Microbiology and Board Certified by the American Board of Medical Microbiology could serve as Lab Director for a microbiology laboratory or public health laboratory, but not for the typical hospital lab.

The Lab Director at a hospital lab also doubles as the Clinical Consultant. There typically isn't enough work to justify one person for each position so one person typically carries out the work of both positions. In all States, medical consultations require an MD, DO or possibly a DPM degree and medical licensure by the State.

Thus the combination of the CLIA requirements and the State's requirements for medical licensure preclude anyone other than an MD, DO or possibly a DPM from acting as a simultaneous Lab Director and Clinical Consultant at a hospital lab.

There are unusual permutations that would be acceptable under CLIA. For example separating the Lab Director and Clinical Consultant positions, allowing someone with an earned doctoral degree in science and certified by a board to serve as Lab Director. The Clinical Consultant duties could then be delegated to any physician licensed in the same State as the Laboratory.

This permutation was attempted at the hospital mentioned in a prior chapter that could not find a Lab Director for more than a year. It was basically a desperation maneuver; the CMS was threatening regulatory closure if that hospital did not find a Lab Director immediately. The CMS allowed this permutation of PhD Lab Director plus MD Clinical Consultant temporarily on the understanding that the hospital was making a good faith effort to hire an MD or DO board certified Pathologist into the Lab Director position.

In my 29 years experience in Pathology and Lab Medicine, this is the only instance I know of where the Lab Director position was split from the Clinical Consultant position, with each position occupied by a different person. Since it was a desperation maneuver on the part of a lab facing regulatory closure, I assume this is not the normal state of affairs, even though it is allowed under the CLIA regulations.

The requirements for a moderate complexity testing Lab Director are lower and are given at 42 CFR § 493.1405. If your lab is only doing moderate complexity testing (i.e. most respiratory labs since arterial blood gas testing is typically moderate complexity) the qualifications for the Lab Director could be as low as an earned Bachelor's degree plus 2 years of laboratory training or experience plus 2 years of supervisory laboratory experience in non-waived testing.

In my experience Lab Directors tend to be older Pathologists that are cutting back on their work as they age. I am not much different than the average. When I graduated from training in 1996, I took a Pathologist position at a small municipal hospital. As the Lab Director of that hospital slowly aged and cut back on work I was assigned more and more of the Lab Director duties. He retired in 2005 at which time I was promoted to the Lab Director position vacated by his retirement.

Sometime around 2004 the pharmacist-businessman referenced in chapter 27 started his lab for which I was hired as Lab Director. By 2007 that lab had grown to be a large, full service outpatient lab.

Thus over the course of many years I went from being only a Pathologist to both Lab Director and Pathologist. In 2013 I would cut back on the Pathology, and end up predominantly to exclusively a Lab Director. This is the typical pathway to being a Lab Director, with the exception that I am retiring to Lab Director work a little early in life compared to most others.

CLIA lists the Lab Director's duties at 42 CFR § 493.1445. To summarize this list, the duties of the Lab Director are:

1. responsible for the overall operation and administration of the laboratory, including the employment of sufficient number of personnel with appropriate education who are competent to perform test procedures, record and report test results promptly, accurately and proficiently, and for assuring compliance with the applicable regulations. Ensures all testing personnel have the appropriate education, experience, orientation, competency testing and when necessary remedial training to improve skills.
2. must be accessible to the laboratory to provide on-site, telephone or electronic consultation as needed.
3. ensures that testing systems developed and used for each of the tests performed in the laboratory provide quality laboratory services for all aspects of test performance.
4. ensures that the physical plant and environmental conditions of the laboratory are appropriate for the testing performed and provide a safe environment in which employees are protected from physical, chemical, and biological hazards.
5. ensures that the test methodologies selected have the capability of providing quality lab results, that verification procedures used are adequate and laboratory personnel are performing the test methods as required for accurate and reliable results.
6. ensures that the laboratory is enrolled in proficiency testing and that the proficiency testing samples are tested as required, the results are returned by the due date, all proficiency testing reports received are reviewed to evaluate the laboratory's performance and to identify any problems that require corrective action and a corrective action plan is followed when any proficiency testing result is found to be unacceptable.
7. ensures quality control and quality assessment programs are established and maintained to assure the quality of laboratory services provided and to identify failures in quality as they occur.
8. ensures the establishment and maintenance of acceptable levels of analytical performance for each test system.
9. ensures that all necessary remedial actions are taken and documented whenever significant deviations from the laboratory's established performance characteristics are identified, and that patient test results are reported only when the system is functioning properly.
10. ensures that reports of test results include pertinent information required for interpretation.
11. ensures that policies and procedures are established and an approved procedure manual is

available to the testing personnel.
12. specifies in writing the responsibilities and duties of each consultant and each supervisor, as well as each person engaged in the performance of the testing stating what each individual is authorized to perform, whether supervision is required for testing or reporting and whether supervisory or director review is required prior to reporting test results.

The following responsibilities are not CLIA requirements but I have seen these commonly in many hospital Lab Director job descriptions:

13. must participate as a member of the various quality improvement committees of the institution. Typically 50% meeting attendance is required as a minimum.
14. performs planning, setting goals, developing and allocating resources.
15. laboratory budget planning with responsible financial management and selection of equipment and supplies. Responsible for laboratory cost effectiveness.
16. provides educational programs for the medical and laboratory staff, and participates in educational programs of the institution.
17. selects and monitors all reference laboratories for quality of service.
18. must have leadership skills and must maintain a working relationship with the lab staff, medical staff, hospital administration and accrediting and/or regulatory agencies.

The Lab Director typically doubles as the clinical consultant. CLIA lists the clinical consultant's responsibilities at 42 CFR § 493.1457 as:

1. provides consultation regarding the appropriateness of the testing ordered and interpretation of test results.
2. must be available to provide consultation to the laboratory's clients.
3. must be available to assist the laboratory's clients in ensuring that appropriate tests are ordered to meet the clinical expectations.
4. ensures that reports of test results include pertinent information required for specific patient interpretation.
5. ensures that consultation is available and communicated to the laboratory's clients on matters related to the quality of the test results reported and their interpretation concerning specific patient conditions.

In terms of staffing, the Lab Director position is considered essential. Under CLIA, it can only be left vacant for 30 days. Leaving it vacant for longer than 30 days will result in the citations referenced in prior chapters.

In terms of recruitment, good luck. Lab Directors are harder to find than Pathologists, Pathologists are harder to find than lab techs, and a good lab tech is hard to find. If your lab is essential to its municipality, and having regulatory problems, give me a call. I might try my hand at fixing it up. Otherwise you will be placing advertisements on the internet and in pathology publications such as CAP Today, AJCP, Laboratory Medicine, etc.

When I took my current Lab Director position in a small municipal hospital lab, my orientation lasted maybe two weeks and occurred coincident with the preparation for a CMS inspection. Thus I was signing the procedure manuals in preparation for a CMS inspection at the same time I was reading them for orientation. Reviewing the remainder of the lab's paperwork, such as QA manuals, competency evaluations, preventive maintenance logs, etc. took another three weeks. I have never seen another person start work as a Lab Director, so can't speak as to how long someone else might need for orientation.

Under CLIA the Lab Supervisor is charged with all competency evaluations in Lab. This includes the Lab Director position. This arrangement for the Lab Director's competency testing is problematic. The Lab Supervisor does not have an MD, but is being called upon to evaluate the work done by an MD. This evaluation is beyond the training and experience of a Lab Supervisor.

This arrangement also is conflicted, since the Lab Supervisor is subordinate to the Lab Director. The conflict of interest arises from the Lab Supervisor's temptation to write his or her immediate supervisor a good evaluation, and suppress any derogatory information.

In my 29 years in Pathology and Lab Medicine, I have only had one instance in which the Lab Supervisor wrote a less than stellar evaluation of me as Lab Director. In the preceding CMS inspection, there were a number of problems in the chemistry section in which the Lab Director position was cited along with the chemistry section. These types of citation on the Lab Director position are common, and do not reflect the job performance of the Lab Director per se but occur secondarily to a citation occurring elsewhere in Lab. The Lab Supervisor was new on the job, and carried the CMS citations onto my evaluation.

When I received this evaluation, I thanked the Lab Supervisor for taking the time to write the evaluation, and politely said that the CMS citations on the Lab Director position were unrelated to the job performance. I was as polite and tactful as possible. I did not suggest any changes to the evaluation, and that evaluation is probably still present buried in a file folder somewhere.

Keep in mind that other people are entitled to their opinions. Their opinion of you may not be the same as your opinion of yourself; but still they are entitled to their opinion. It is very difficult to evaluate the job performance of an administrative position such as a Lab Director position. Hence, all evaluations are an opinion, and the Lab Supervisor is entitled to any opinion at all.

As Lab Director your job turns not on the Lab Supervisor's evaluations, but on the opinion of the medical staff at the hospital where you work. If the other doctors think highly of you, you will be able to stay in that job forever, well into old age. If the other doctors think poorly of you, your days on that job may be numbered.

As a Lab Director you are subject to Ongoing Professional Practice Evaluation (OPPE) at least every 6 months if you work in an institution accredited by TJC. You will be evaluated by your immediate supervisor the hospital Medical Director. The hospital Medical Director is likely to be of a different specialty, and have little knowledge of Pathology. Furthermore, you are in an administrative position, and evaluation for such positions is difficult.

In some instances the Medical Director has evaluated me based on meeting attendance, personality, appearance, absence of complaints, and overall lab turnaround time. In other instances, the hospital Medical Director did not know what to put down, and asked me what he should put down on my OPPE. In those circumstances, try to be modest while writing your own evaluation.

Lab Directors are also subject to Focused Professional Practice Evaluation (FPPE). Triggering events include your hiring to a new hospital, you apply for increased privileges, and/or you have made one or more mistakes significant enough to trigger an FPPE. I have changed jobs twice in my 29 year career in Pathology and Lab Medicine. Each move presumably triggered an FPPE. I never received a copy of any FPPE forms that resulted. Since Lab Director positions are administrative, it would be hard to imagine a need to increase privileges. I am not aware of any Lab Director ever receiving an FPPE due to performance issues.

In terms of promotion, the Lab Director position is the highest position in Lab. The next higher administrative position in a hospital is the Medical Director position. Many years ago, I had been offered a hospital Medical Director position, but turned it down. It would have involved slightly more pay, but I would not have felt comfortable with the territory.

The hospital Medical Director must maintain discipline among the Medical Staff. At most hospitals the Medical Staff is composed of strong personalities such that the Medical Director must have a very assertive or aggressive personality in order to be effective. This type of personality is uncommon among Pathologists and Lab Directors. I have only known one Pathologist to occupy a hospital Medical Director position.

Retention of Lab Directors is not usually a problem. Most Lab Directors are older, set in their ways, and have roots in the community they live in. They will not usually move to a new community for the remainder of their career. In my experience most Lab Directors including myself are financially secure, and not really working for the money. The other benefits are more important, such as giving back to the community, self-actualization, accomplishment, close friends with coworkers, and/or having too much time on your hands if fully retired. Thus, most Lab Directors will remain in the same position indefinitely. On the other hand, rapid turnover of the Lab Director position is a warning sign of a troubled clinical lab.

I have seen numerous voluntary retirements of Lab Directors. In most instances the medical staff and administration was begging the retiree to stay, and felt that it would be impossible to find a replacement. I have only seen Lab Directors removed for cause six times:

1. Story #1 – major shift in INR. This happened in a small municipality about 125 miles from where I worked at the time. A lab tech receives a new lot of INR reagent and began using the reagent without recalibrating the analyzer or resetting the analyzer to use the ISI of the new lot. The tech continued using the controls from the old lot. The tech apparently did not realize that he was using a new lot of INR reagent. This resulted in a major shift in INR, the results were far too low. The shift persisted for weeks before it was discovered. In this time, one patient died of intracerebral bleeding and a dozen others had major bleeding episodes. The lab tech and Lab Director of that lab were fired.

2. Story #2 – Inappropriate relationship. A male Lab Director in his late-60s had an ongoing inappropriate relationship with a much younger female lab tech working in the same lab. The Lab Director and lab tech were married to other people, not married to each other. The Lab Director and lab tech did not try to hide the relationship from the other people in Lab. The hospital administration found out and forced the Lab Director to retire.

3. Story #3 – Lab Director not in touch with the modern day world. The Lab Director in this story is around age 75. He has been working at the same hospital for over 40 years. He is living in the past and likes to talk about his glorious accomplishments in the 1960s. He hates computers, hates Ipads, doesn't like cellphones, and can't figure out most modern technology. More than 20 years ago, he allowed an AS400 computer into his lab. This computer is now outdated, but he

has been refusing to allow a new computer system into lab. The hospital is getting a new computer system. The Hospital Administrator calls in the Lab Director and tells the Lab Director that the existing computer system in lab is hopelessly outdated. The hospital has paid millions to get a new computer system and Lab is part of the deal. Since the hospital has already paid millions, the computer will go into lab. The Lab Director digs in his heels and refuses to allow this computer system into lab. The Lab Director is forced to retire involuntarily and the new computer system goes into Lab.

4. Story #4 – Lab Director disability. This same story was referenced in the chapter above on Pathologist retirement. In this story an 86 year old Lab Director with Parkinson's disease becomes wheelchair-bound. He is forced to retire involuntarily.

5. Story #5 – Lab regulatory closure. This same story was referenced in the chapter on regulatory scrutiny syndrome. This unfortunate Lab Director headed up a small private lab that was caught sink testing. Sink testing involves disposing of patient specimens and turning out fraudulent test results. The Lab Director in question almost certainly must have known what was going on in his own lab. When the CMS found out about it, they performed a regulatory shutdown on his lab immediately on the spot. This Lab Director lost his business, and was banned for a time from re-entering the business. He tried to re-enter the business after the banning period ended, but no one would hire him. This was a heavy price to pay, but on the other hand his lab had committed the greatest sin in the laboratory world.

6. Story #6 – Mutiny on the laboratory. This is the story referenced in the chapter on lab conflict. This elderly Lab Director was unseated by his 10 employee Pathologists in a disagreement over workload and layoffs. This Lab Director was in his early 80s at the time, and retired after being forced out from his job.

Of these stories above #2, #5 and #6 were avoidable, #4 was unavoidable while #1 and #3 might have been avoidable. In any event, Lab Directors #1 to #4 would have had an appeals process spelled out in the hospital bylaws. Lab Director #5 would have had a CMS appeals process available. Lab Director #6 could sue for breach of contract.

Every hospital is obligated to follow its bylaws. In any ensuing lawsuit the plaintiff's attorney will look for ways in which the hospital did not follow its own bylaws. If the hospital deviates even one iota from its bylaws in a physician employee removal process, the physician employee will likely get reinstatement with back pay.

The Lab Director who became disabled would additionally have protections from the Americans with Disabilities Act (ADA) which requires a series of hearings before one can be removed from a job position. If the hospital deviates one iota from these requirements, the physician employee will likely get reinstated with back pay.

In my 29 years experience in Pathology and Lab Medicine I have changed jobs twice. The first time was related to salary, I took a higher paying job. The second time I moved was basically a retirement. I took a job with slightly less pay, but with much less workload.

Retiring from Pathology to Lab Director work is nice. I have plenty of spare time to do the things I like, such as writing this book. As mentioned above, I am up for any challenge involving fixing up a lab. If your lab is essential to its municipality, and having regulatory problems, give me a call. I might try my hand at fixing it up.

Chapter 32 – Advanced topics in Lab Directorship

Topic #1 - How to handle certificates and PT when patient testing is spread across multiple sites

CLIA allows multiple laboratories on one certificate only in limited circumstances. If a hospital system has multiple laboratories in non-contiguous buildings these will all need their own Certificate of Compliance, Certificate of Accreditation, Certificate of PPM, etc. as applicable. The exceptions to this rule include multiple laboratories in contiguous buildings under common direction, mobile satellite labs, and public health testing limited to 15 or less analytes. In most cases the decision to apply for one or multiple certificates is straightforward. Generally speaking it simplifies things if you put as much as possible on one certificate, as opposed to splitting your labs onto multiple certificates.

However, there are some situations where you would want some of the testing split onto a separate certificate. For example, one of the hospitals I previously worked at had the respiratory lab physically separate from the main lab on different floors of the same building. I was Lab Director of the main lab and someone else was Lab Director of the respiratory lab. The CMS inspector said we could combine both labs onto one certificate if we wanted to because they are in the same building. The CMS inspector said this would save money on certificate fees. I said an emphatic "no thanks" to this offer, since the respiratory lab was having major problems. I had been asked to help with the respiratory lab's most recent inspection responses and was surprised by the number and severity of the citations they had received.

If the labs were combined it would become my responsibility to fix all the citations of both labs, and I had my hands full with the main lab. Furthermore the respiratory lab was under different leadership such that if they were on the same CMS certificate as main lab, I would be responsible for fixing the citations but would not have any authority in the lab generating the citations. You do not want to find yourself in the situation where you have citations but cannot fix them.

Under CLIA all proficiency testing (PT) specimens must be treated the same as patient specimens. CLIA also prohibits referral of PT specimens to an outside laboratory. The reference is 42 CFR § 493.801.

This creates a catch 22 when patient testing is spread across multiple sites with different CMS Certificate of Compliance numbers. In this situation, you must break one rule (treat PT specimens the same as patient specimens) or break the other rule (no referral). In all circumstances the "no referral" rule supersedes the "same treatment" rule.

As an example, I will use the typical state Public Health system. If you walk into a Public Health facility in any state and ask for HIV testing, you will likely get a point of care test for HIV. The typical protocol is to sign out any negative test in-house and refer out any specimen that tests positive to that State's Central Public Health Lab for confirmatory testing.

Although PT is not required for a waived test, let's say they do PT for their point of care HIV test. If the point of care test is negative, they would sign the specimen out as negative in-house. For all negative PT specimens put "negative" down on the PT result form.

If a patient specimen is positive, they would refer the specimen to the State Central Public Health Lab.

Thus, positive results are not reported to the PT provider. Instead "test not performed" is put down on the PT result form, since the specimen would have been referred to a different lab with a different CLIA number.

As another example, let's say a small clinic is doing point of care hemoglobin under a Certificate of Waiver. All specimens are subsequently sent to the municipal hospital lab for a Complete Blood Count (CBC).

Point of care hemoglobin is a waived test and does not require PT testing. If a PT event was ever attempted for the point of care hemoglobin test, all the PT specimens would have to be reported as "test not performed" since all specimens would have been referred to the municipal hospital lab for a subsequent CBC. Thus, in this setting where all specimens are referred after testing, ordering a PT event is a futile maneuver, since the results could not be reported.

Topic #2 - How to perform verification for a non-waived qualitative analyzer

The typical lab analyzer is FDA cleared or approved, non-waived and produces quantitative results, in other words the results are expressed in numbers. Chapter 7 lists the steps for setting this type of lab analyzer into service.

Some analyzers give qualitative results. Qualitative results by definition cannot be numbers, but instead describe a quality of the specimen. This is typically limited to microbiology. Organism identification is a qualitative test. When testing for a single infectious organism results are typically either "positive" or "negative". For antibiotic sensitivity testing the results are usually expressed as "sensitive", "intermediate", or "resistant".

CLIA requires verification of an FDA cleared or approved, non-waived qualitative analyzer. The rules given in 42 CFR § 493.1253 apply to all non-waived analyzers. However, the guidelines given refer to reportable range and other parameters that are not applicable to qualitative testing. There are no guidelines for qualitative analyzer verification, in effect leaving the entire process to the lab's discretion. Thus, my recommendations in this section are suggestions and not regulatory requirements.

Setting an FDA cleared or approved, non-waived qualitative analyzer into service is easier than setting the typical lab analyzer into service. Linearity, AMR, reportable range, calibration and calibration verification are not applicable for analyzers that return qualitative results.

I will begin by discussing verification for tests that can only return a positive or negative test result (i.e. positive or negative for gonorrhea, positive or negative for chlamydia, etc.). The verification is different for organism identification and antibiotic sensitivity testing, since these return more complicated results as compared to a test that can only return positive or negative results. I will discuss verification of organism identification and antibiotic sensitivity testing at the end of this section.

For a test that can only return a result of positive or negative, precision consists of testing the same specimens over and over to see if you get the same result each time. My recommendation is to make 10 repeats of the positive control and 10 repeats of the negative control. I have never seen failure of precision (positive control tests negative and/or negative control tests positive) on this type of analyzer.

Accept the manufacturer's reference range and critical values. For infectious agent testing, the reference range is "negative", and the critical value is "positive".

Correlation is performed by splitting 20 or more patient specimens, running a split in your new analyzer and testing the other split by a reference method (old analyzer or send-out testing). The minimum of 20 is recommended, but not a regulatory requirement. If you don't have enough patient specimens, you are allowed to use controls and/or proficiency testing (PT) specimens to reach the minimum number needed for a correlation. Even so, there should be some patient specimens included, not all controls and PT specimens. For some specimen types you will virtually never see a positive in real life (smallpox, rabies, etc.) in which case the correlation will have to be done with negative patient specimens, controls and PT specimens.

Here is an example of a passing correlation:

Specimen number	In-house test result	Send-out test result	Concordance
Patient #1	Negative	Negative	Concordant
Patient #2	Negative	Negative	Concordant
Patient #3	Positive	Positive	Concordant
Patient #4	Negative	Negative	Concordant
Patient #5	Negative	Negative	Concordant
Patient #6	Negative	Negative	Concordant
Patient #7	Positive	Positive	Concordant
Patient #8	Negative	Negative	Concordant
Patient #9	Negative	Negative	Concordant
Patient #10	Negative	Negative	Concordant
Pos control repeat #1	Positive	Positive	Concordant
Pos control repeat #2	Positive	Positive	Concordant
Pos control repeat #3	Positive	Positive	Concordant
Pos control repeat #4	Positive	Positive	Concordant
Pos control repeat #5	Positive	Positive	Concordant
Neg control repeat #1	Negative	Negative	Concordant
Neg control repeat #2	Negative	Negative	Concordant
Neg control repeat #3	Negative	Negative	Concordant
Neg control repeat #4	Negative	Negative	Concordant
Neg control repeat #5	Negative	Negative	Concordant

This is how a correlation should appear for a qualitative analyzer that can only return positive or negative results. All test results are concordant when comparing the in-house to the send-out testing. There are no discordant results to resolve, and the analyzer can be considered to be verified.

Here is an example of a correlation with discordant results:

Specimen number	In-house test result	Send-out test result	Concordance
Patient #1	Negative	Negative	Concordant
Patient #2	Negative	Negative	Concordant
Patient #3	Positive	Negative	**DISCORDANT**
Patient #4	Negative	Negative	Concordant
Patient #5	Negative	Negative	Concordant
Patient #6	Negative	Negative	Concordant
Patient #7	Positive	Positive	Concordant
Patient #8	Negative	Negative	Concordant
Patient #9	Positive	Negative	**DISCORDANT**
Patient #10	Negative	Negative	Concordant
Pos control repeat #1	Positive	Positive	Concordant
Pos control repeat #2	Positive	Positive	Concordant
Pos control repeat #3	Positive	Positive	Concordant
Pos control repeat #4	Positive	Positive	Concordant
Pos control repeat #5	Positive	Positive	Concordant
Neg control repeat #1	Negative	Negative	Concordant
Neg control repeat #2	Negative	Negative	Concordant
Neg control repeat #3	Negative	Negative	Concordant
Neg control repeat #4	Negative	Negative	Concordant
Neg control repeat #5	Negative	Negative	Concordant

According to the literature, all discordant results must be resolved before the analyzer can be considered to be verified. This implies that if any discordant results cannot be resolved, you have to reject the analyzer and tell the manufacturer to take it back and replace it with a new one.

I have not seen any discordant results when performing verification on analyzers of this type. If ever there were discordant results you could try to resolve the problem by re-testing the specimen, or sending a split of the specimen to a different outside lab for testing.

If the in-house test uses different methodology compared to the send-out test (e.g. your analyzer uses DNA amplification and the send-out lab uses culture) discordant results can be attributed to the differing methodology. In order to prove this, retest a split of the specimen (if any remains) at any outside lab using the same methodology that you are trying to verify.

An "easy out" would be attributing any discordant results to sampling error in which low numbers of the organism were present in one split of the sample but not the other. This would be grasping at straws, and it would be unlikely for a CMS inspector to accept this.

After any discordant results are resolved, the test is considered to be verified. The remainder of setting the analyzer into service follows the same steps as outlined in Chapter 7 - make a procedure manual, make standing orders for reagents, supplies, controls and proficiency testing specimens, train the staff on how to use the instrument, document this training, connect the instrument to the hospital's information system, and go live with testing.

Next I will discuss the verification of an analyzer that performs organism identification and/or antibiotic sensitivity testing. This is more complex than verifying a test that can only return positive or negative results. In this situation, the analyzer is capable of returning multiple possible results (S. aureus identified, E. coli identified, sensitive to 1 mg/l, sensitive to 2mg/l, sensitive to 4mg/l, etc.). In this regard the verification is similar for any analyzer that returns graded or titered results.

For organism identification, test at least five QC organisms once each for 20 days on both the new analyzer and the old analyzer. If the new analyzer and the old analyzer give the same results for the QC organisms at least 95% of the time the new analyzer can be considered to be verified. If not, a corrective action is needed before repeating the verification studies. The typical hospital lab has little experience with verification of a microbiology analyzer, and will be quick to call the manufacturer for help if any problems occur in verification. The new analyzer must pass verification before it can be put into service for patient testing.

For antibiotic sensitivity testing, run at least five isolates of known sensitive and known resistant organisms once each on the new analyzer and old analyzer for at least five days. Avoid using organisms with sensitivity near the breakpoint as this will complicate things. Use isolates representative of the problem organisms at your hospital (MRSA, VRE, etc.).

In this setting a major error is when one analyzer reports sensitive and the other reports resistant on the same isolate. A minor error is when one analyzer reports intermediate and the other analyzer reports sensitive or resistant for the same isolate. In order to pass verification the major error rate should be less than 5% and the sum of major error plus minor error should be less than 10%. If the new analyzer does not pass verification a corrective action is needed before repeating the verification studies. The typical hospital lab has little experience with verification of a microbiology analyzer, and will be quick to call the manufacturer for help if any problems occur in verification. The new analyzer must pass verification before it can be put into service for patient testing.

Here is an example of a correlation for antibiotic sensitivity testing:

Isolate and day number	New analyzer result	Old analyzer result	Concordance
Isolate #1 Day #1	Sensitive	Sensitive	Concordant
Isolate #2 Day #1	Resistant	Resistant	Concordant
Isolate #3 Day #1	Sensitive	Sensitive	Concordant
Isolate #4 Day #1	Intermediate	Intermediate	Concordant
Isolate #5 Day #1	Resistant	Sensitive	**MAJOR ERROR**
Isolate #1 Day #2	Sensitive	Sensitive	Concordant
Isolate #2 Day #2	Resistant	Resistant	Concordant
Isolate #3 Day #2	Sensitive	Sensitive	Concordant
Isolate #4 Day #2	Intermediate	Intermediate	Concordant
Isolate #5 Day #2	Resistant	Resistant	Concordant
Isolate #1 Day #3	Sensitive	Sensitive	Concordant
Isolate #2 Day #3	Resistant	Resistant	Concordant
Isolate #3 Day #3	Sensitive	Sensitive	Concordant
Isolate #4 Day #3	Intermediate	Intermediate	Concordant
Isolate #5 Day #3	Resistant	Resistant	Concordant
Isolate #1 Day #4	Sensitive	Sensitive	Concordant
Isolate #2 Day #4	Resistant	Resistant	Concordant
Isolate #3 Day #4	Sensitive	Sensitive	Concordant
Isolate #4 Day #4	Intermediate	Intermediate	Concordant
Isolate #5 Day #4	Resistant	Resistant	Concordant
Isolate #1 Day #5	Sensitive	Sensitive	Concordant
Isolate #2 Day #5	Resistant	Resistant	Concordant
Isolate #3 Day #5	Sensitive	Sensitive	Concordant
Isolate #4 Day #5	Intermediate	Sensitive	**MINOR ERROR**
Isolate #5 Day #5	Resistant	Resistant	Concordant

For the above correlation, the major error rate is $1 \div 25 = 4.0\%$, the minor error rate is $1 \div 25 = 4.0\%$ and the sum of major error plus minor error is 8.0%. This is a passing correlation given the rules presented on the previous page.

The old analyzer should not be considered the gold standard. Neither the new analyzer nor the old analyzer are a gold standard. Notice that in the above correlation both the minor error and the major error occurred because the old analyzer is giving different results for the same isolate on different days. The sensitivity for an organism should not change from day to day indicating that the problem is likely with the old analyzer, not the new analyzer.

After completing verification, the remainder of setting the analyzer into service follows the same steps as outlined in Chapter 7 - make a procedure manual, make standing orders for reagents, supplies, controls and proficiency testing specimens, train the staff on how to use the instrument, document this training, connect the instrument to the hospital's information system, and go live with testing.

Topic #3 - How to perform "off label" test verification

In this section I will go through the steps of verifying a test that is not FDA cleared or approved. These same steps of verification are required for any test that is modified from the manufacturer's instructions. If you modify a test, you have in effect become the manufacturer of the new test you have created. This is in contradistinction to Chapter 7 which discusses verifying an unmodified, FDA cleared or approved, non-waived quantitative analyzer.

A test that is not FDA cleared or approved is referred to as a laboratory developed test (LDT) or "off label" test. Such a test can only be performed in-house. The testing equipment cannot be sold to or used in another lab without FDA clearance or approval. However, other labs can send you specimens for "off label" testing.

In 2014, the FDA notified the US Congress that it plans to change the way it regulates LDT's, stratifying them into low risk, medium risk and high risk. These proposed changes will take several years to fully implement. As a Lab Director, your approach to LDT's is likely to change considerably as the new regulations are implemented. At the time of this writing, all LDT's are treated the same by the FDA, and the information given below is current as of late 2019.

If a test is not FDA cleared or approved it is automatically high complexity. Even if it uses a methodology that is waived under other circumstances (e.g. latex agglutination on a card) it is automatically high complexity because it is not FDA cleared or approved.

Let's review the regulations. Per CLIA each laboratory that introduces an unmodified, FDA-cleared or approved test system before reporting patient test results must demonstrate that it can obtain performance specifications comparable to those established by the manufacturer for the following performance characteristics: accuracy, precision and reportable range of test results. The lab must verify that the manufacturer's reference intervals (normal values) are appropriate for the laboratory's patient population. The laboratory must determine the test system's calibration procedures and control procedures based upon the performance specifications it has established. The laboratory must document all these activities.

If the test is not FDA cleared or approved you would additionally need to establish the following: analytical sensitivity, analytical specificity to include interfering substances, reference intervals (normal values) and any other performance characteristic required for test performance. The reference for the above is 42 CFR § 493.1253.

My assessment: The added requirements placed on tests that are not FDA cleared or approved make verification extremely difficult such that it typically exceeds the ability of most small hospital labs. Thus, this is typically only done at reference labs and university hospital labs.

Before you start, you have to decide what is passing for each of the criteria listed (accuracy, precision, etc.). Under CLIA the requirement for passing each of these criteria are left up to the discretion of the

Lab Director. In theory, it would be possible to set the bar so low that you are bound to pass. In actual practice, your CMS inspector would object if you did this.

It is permissible to use scientific literature to establish the analytical sensitivity and specificity.

When validating "off label" testing, you are required to test the effects of possible interfering substances. This can be done by spiking positive and negative controls with known concentrations of possible interfering substances to determine the effects of these substances on the test being verified.

There is typically a long list of possible interfering substances. You must evaluate the effects of all possible interfering substances at varying concentrations of each possible interfering substance. You could end up doing hundreds or thousands of individual tests to get past this step. Thus, this step will be costly and time consuming.

The Limit of Detection (LoD) can be determined by repeatedly testing blank specimens. This is another costly and time consuming step due to the number of repeats necessary to establish the mean of blanks and standard deviation of the blanks. The LoD is typically set higher than the 95th percentile of the blanks. With the LoD set above this level you can be at least 95% sure that a positive test really is positive.

The Limit of Quantitation (LoQ) and the Analytical Measurement Range (AMR) can be derived from a linearity proficiency test. The LoQ is the lower limit of linearity, and the AMR runs from the lower limit of linearity to the upper limit of linearity.

The reference range and critical values can be derived from the literature.

Accuracy can be measured by splitting patient samples, testing one split using the method being verified and testing the other split by a different method. The results obtained from using the new method are correlated to the results obtained from using the different method. A correlation coefficient of at least 0.95 is preferred but not required. See Chapter 7 for extensive discussion regarding correlation.

Precision is tested by repeatedly running the same specimens over and over. I would recommend using three levels of controls run seven times each for a total of 21 repeats. Calculate the Coefficient of Variation (CV) for each of these 3 levels. The CV is calculated as Standard Deviation ÷ mean x 100%. CV is a measure of imprecision. The higher the CV the more imprecise the test, the lower the CV the more precise the test. You typically want the CV for each level of control to be less than 10%, and preferably less than 5%, unless you are testing near zero, where a larger CV is allowed.

CLIA mandates that you determine "any other performance characteristic required for test performance". This is so broad that it could include just about anything - carryover, trueness, robustness, etc. Robustness refers to a test's ability to remain unaffected by small variations in test methods and test conditions.

There are nearly infinite possibilities to "small variations in test methods and test conditions". Add one minute to incubation time, add 2 minutes to incubation time, incubate at 30°C, incubate at 31°C, add/remove extraction steps, increase/decrease each of the reagents slightly, etc. You must run one test for each of these nearly infinite possibilities and permutations. As a result, this will be the step that defeats most attempts at "off label" test verification. At the minimum, this will make "off label" test verification prohibitively expensive and time consuming for a small hospital lab.

After you have exhausted the nearly infinite resources and time needed to get past this step, the next step is to determine the test system's calibration and control procedures. If you are modifying an existing test you may still be able to adopt the manufacturer's calibration and control procedures. If you are making the new test from nothing, you could buy calibrators and controls and adopt the calibration and control procedures used on any other analyzer in your lab. The controls should be run at least once each day of testing unless you have an IQCP in place. The calibration is done at least every 6 months, after changing reagent lots, after major repairs to the analyzer, etc. If the analyte you are measuring is unstable, you should run controls and calibration more frequently.

After you pass all the above steps, the remainder of setting the analyzer into service follows the same steps as outlined in Chapter 7 - make a procedure manual, make standing orders for reagents, supplies, controls and proficiency testing specimens, train the staff on how to use the instrument, document this training, connect the instrument to the hospital's information system, and go live with testing.

Topic #4 - How to make an Individualized Quality Control Plan (IQCP)

CLIA has two exceptions to the rule regarding daily use of controls. These exceptions are the Equivalent Quality Control (EQC) procedure and the Individualized Quality Control Plan (IQCP).

The Equivalent Quality Control (EQC) plan has been phased out. Any lab using this plan should have discontinued it by January 1, 2016. The replacement is the Individualized Quality Control Plan (IQCP). There are a few differences between these two plans, and many similarities.

The main difference is that the IQCP takes risk into consideration while EQC does not. Otherwise they are similar. Both programs are voluntary. In other words, if you want to continue doing daily QC you are free to do so. These programs can only be used when the manufacturer's instructions specify less frequent quality controls than CLIA does or when the manufacturer's instructions are silent on the frequency of QC.

With EQC, the frequency of external QC was determined by whether the test had internal monitoring that checked all, some or none of the test parameters. You then had to do monitoring of the test for a specified number of days using external controls to make sure the system was stable. After doing this, if the results were acceptable, you could drop the external QC to weekly or monthly provided that the results are acceptable during the evaluation period.

IQCP is much more complex. It involves calculating the risk associated with a large series of possible problems. Risk assessment must include the 5 required components of environment, test system, reagents, testing personnel, and specimen. It must also cover the preanalytical, analytical and postanalytical phases of testing. If the data shows that the system is stable you can then drop the external QC to the manufacturer's minimum requirement, or to monthly QC, whichever is more frequent.

To make an IQCP, you need to examine each of the steps in the testing process to determine the possible problems at each step. Next you determine the likelihood of these potential problems occurring, the degree of risk to patient care and determine if there is any way to prevent these potential problems from occurring. This should specify ways to immediately detect problems when they occur.

Next you make a Quality Control Plan (QCP). This could be as simple as stating that you will run QC weekly (as opposed to daily) and specify the acceptable QC results. The IQCP is then signed by the Lab Director and put in place. There must be an ongoing monitoring of the IQCP. These reviews of the IQCP should occur at least annually. This could be as simple as an additional review of the QC at the end of each month to ensure the QC is acceptable. The documentation from these periodic reviews should be stored in the same binder as the IQCP.

The easy option is to buy a computer program that can make IQCP's. There is already a computer program being sold by COLA which does this risk assessment. My advice is that there is no need to reinvent the wheel. All you have to do is buy the COLA program or any equivalent computer program sold by any other vendor, answer a series of questions, and print out an IQCP Summary Report detailing your risk.

The COLA computer program will grade you as a low, intermediate or high risk of having problems if you use IQCP. I have only seen this computer program used twice at a hospital where I worked. It gave a GeneXpert analyzer a "low risk" for IQCP on TB testing and combined chlamydia/gonorrhea testing. Regardless of the risk that is reported, the decision to use or not use IQCP is left to you as Lab Director. There are no statutory requirements as to how much risk is too much.

If the computer program assesses a "low risk", all you have to do is print out the IQCP Summary Report detailing your risk, sign as Lab Director the statement that the risk is acceptable and file this at the back of the procedure manual. Then reduce the external QC to the manufacturer's minimum requirement or to weekly or to once every 30 days or on opening a new lot, whichever comes first, etc.

If the computer program assesses you a "moderate risk" or "high risk" my advice is that you should look over the data entered into the program to make sure it is correct and there are no transcription errors.

If the entered information is correct and the computer program assesses you a "moderate risk" or "high risk" this would indicate you are not doing things optimally in your laboratory. Go down the list of questions and determine what can be optimized. Are two identifiers checked before drawing all patients? Does the test have internal positive and negative controls? Do the clinicians have adequate instructions on how to collect the specimen?

After doing this, re-run the program. If it now returns "low risk" implement the IQCP as above. If the risk is still "moderate risk" or "high risk", go through the list of questions again to see what is wrong, and try to correct it. Repeat this process until such time as the computer program reports "low risk". Since many of the questions on this list involve laboratory best practices, anything other than "low risk" on this assessment implies that you are not following laboratory best practices.

Repeat the above process for each analyte you want to have an IQCP. If you have two or more of the same analyzer, you only need to make one IQCP per analyte for each set of identical analyzers.

If you don't have access to any computer programs that can make an IQCP, you can make the IQCP yourself. The only situation where I had to make an IQCP myself was for Microbiology Petri plate testing and for a Vitek at a small hospital I worked at. An IQCP does not need to be lengthy. The one I made for Microbiology Petri plate testing fits onto a single page. The risk assessment in this document is a "best guess". The risk assessment does not need to be perfect and can be a best guess. The example IQCP on page 223 passed a CMS inspection for the small hospital I work at. Since Microbiology Petri plate testing is essentially the same everywhere, you should be able to copy verbatim this example IQCP as your own Microbiology Petri plate IQCP.

If you are using IQCP, it could take up to 30 days to find out if your test goes out of control and begins to fail external controls. In that time, it would be possible to turn out a large number of erroneous test results. If you find your test is out of control and you have to bring it back into control, you would have to re-test any remaining specimens examined since the last external QC thirty days ago. Thus IQCP is a two edged sword, you could lower your costs by using less QC materials, but there are risks to doing this.

Laboratory Name: MY LABORATORY

Test System Name: Microbiology Petri plates

Tests: Organism Identification

MY PROCEDURE MANUAL
example IQCP

CMS Component	Risk Assessment		Risk Evaluation				Development of an Individualized Quality Control plan is indicated for non-waived testing only.		Risk Mitigation	
	Risk Identification									
	Risk Identification	Failure detectable by the petri plates?	Failure Impact on Patient Care	Probability	Severity	Acceptable?	test system features that mitigate failure risk	educational resources that mitigate failure risk	Manufacturer Mitigation of Risk Effective?	Laboratory action or plans to mitigate failure risk	Supporting Documentation
Specimen	Specimen labelled as to wrong specimen type	No	False Negative or False Positive Results	Very Low	Minor	Yes	1. Competency testing on the phlebotomy and nursing staff 2. Specimen handling procedures	Training and orientation on the phlebotomy and nursing staff	No	Training and competency testing on the phlebotomy staff	Training and annual competency testing documentation on the phlebotomists
	Samples frozen or otherwise subjected to conditions that would kill bacteria (i.e. addition of bleach or antibiotics to the sample)	No	False Negative Results	Very Low	Minor	Yes	1. Competency testing on the phlebotomy and nursing staff 2. Specimen handling procedures	Training and orientation on the phlebotomy and nursing staff	No	Training and competency testing on the phlebotomy staff	Training and annual competency testing documentation on the phlebotomists
	Specimen left for extended periods before testing	No	False Negative Results	Low	Minor	Yes	Staffing of lab 24/7/365	Training and orientation on the lab staff	No	Training and competency testing on the lab staff	Training and annual competency testing documentation on the lab staff
	Sample labelled as to wrong patient	No	False Negative or False Positive Results	Very Low	Serious	Yes	1. Competency testing on the phlebotomy and nursing staff 2. Specimen handling procedures	Training and orientation on the phlebotomy and nursing staff	No	Training and competency testing on the phlebotomy staff	Training and annual competency testing documentation on the lab staff
Environment	Testing area or storage areas are not at appropriate temperature.	No	False Negative Results	Low	Minor	Yes	Temperature monitoring of lab's storerooms and testing area	Lab staff record the temperatures on the storeroom and call maintenance if acceptable range exceeded	No	Lab staff record the temperatures in lab every 8 hours and call maintenance if acceptable range exceeded	Temperature monitoring logs in lab
	Test specifications for temperature are not followed.	No	False Negative Results	Low	Minor	Yes	Temperature monitoring of lab's storerooms and testing area	Training of lab staff on acceptable temperatures in lab	No	Lab staff record the temperatures in lab every day and call maintenance if acceptable range exceeded	Temperature monitoring logs for storeroom and incubators
Reagents	Plates accidentally contaminated	No	False Positive Results	Low	Serious	Yes	Micro petri plate QC	Training of lab staff on handling Petri plates	No	Training of lab staff on handling Petri plates	Training and annual competency testing documentation on the lab staff
	Use of expired Petri plates	No	Unknown	Very Low	Minor	Yes	Lab staff trained to never use expired Petri plates	Training of lab staff to check expiration dates	No	Training of lab staff to check expiration dates	Training and annual competency testing documentation on the lab staff
	QC organisms deteriorate and/or fail to grow	Yes	False Negative Results on QC testing	Low	Minor	Yes	Degradation of QC organisms should be detectable by failure to grow QC organisms	Training of lab staff on corrective actions	No	Training of lab staff on corrective actions	Training and annual competency testing documentation on the lab staff
	Petri plates arrive contaminated	Yes	False Positive Results	Very Low	Minor	Yes	External QC is run with each new lot of plates. External QC will fail if plates contaminated.	Lab staff are trained to run external QC with each new lot of Petri plates.	No	Lab staff are trained to run external QC with each new lot of petri plates.	Training and annual competency testing documentation on the lab staff
	Petri plates degrade during storage	Yes	False Negative Results	Low	Minor	Yes	None	Weekly QC done on the Petri plates	No	Weekly QC on the Petri plates	QC logs for the Petri plates
Test System	Incorrect interpretation of color change reactions on the Petri plates	No	False Negative or False Positive Results	Very Low	Serious	Yes	None	Training and competency testing on the lab staff	No	Training and competency testing on the lab staff	Training and annual competency testing on the lab staff
	Cross contamination of organisms from one Petri plate to another	No	False Positive Results	Very Low	Serious	Yes	None	Training and competency testing on the lab staff	No	Training and competency testing on the lab staff	Training and annual competency testing on the lab staff
Testing Personnel	Results interpreted incorrectly	No	False Negative or False Positive Result	Very Low	Serious	Yes	None	Training and competency testing on the lab staff	No	Training and competency testing on the lab staff	Training and annual competency testing documentation on the lab staff
	Results transcribed incorrectly	No	False Negative or False Positive Results	Very Low	Serious	Yes	None	Training and competency testing on the lab staff	No	Training and competency testing on the lab staff	Training and annual competency testing documentation on the lab staff

Quality Control Plan: Run QC once per week or with each new lot of Petri plates whichever comes first. Acceptable QC is 95% concordance or better.

Lab Director approval: _____ Date: _____

Review 2020 Q1	Review 2020 Q2	Review 2020 Q3	Review 2020 Q4	Review 2021 Q1	Review 2021 Q2	Review 2021 Q3	Review 2021 Q4	Review 2022 Q1	Review 2022 Q2	Review 2022 Q3

Topic #5 - Public relations. Lab Director as Public Information Officer (PIO)

In a freestanding lab the Lab Director acts as the Public Information Officer (PIO) for the Laboratory. This means that all information released to the news media must go through you or at least needs your approval for release. My advice is to only release positive information. If any negative information regarding lab surfaces, refute the information if you can. If you can't refute the information, remain tight-lipped and refer all calls to the lab's attorney.

In most hospitals, the Hospital Administrator acts as PIO for the entire hospital. In a hospital lab, the Lab Director needs permission from the Hospital Administrator for public release of information and that release of information is usually made by the Hospital Administrator. Generally speaking, the hospital's leadership will want to claim the limelight for all positive news regarding the lab.

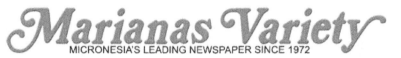
MICRONESIA'S LEADING NEWSPAPER SINCE 1972

| CNMI | REGIONAL NEWS | COMMUNITY BULLETINS | VARIETY FEATURES | ADVERTISING | CONTACT US | GUÅHAN NEWS |

CHC laboratory receives compliance certificate

Published on Monday, March 24, 2014 00:00 By Emmanuel T. Erediano - @mvariety.com - Variety News Staff

THE Commonwealth Healthcare Corp. has received from the federal government a compliance certificate for the laboratory.

CHC Chief Executive Officer Esther L. Muna and hospital administrator Jesse Tudela joined laboratory director Dr. Philip Dauterman and his staff for lunch on Friday to celebrate.

The certificate of compliance was issued by the Centers for Medicare & Medicaid Services' Clinical Laboratory Improvement Amendments.

Muna said it is a very important certification that assures the hospital has adequate equipment, supplies and staff to provide diagnostic tests for patients.

She said CHC almost lost its certification two years ago when CMS found a number of areas in the laboratory that required "correction."

"It is very important to have the laboratory services," she added. "Without them, we will be missing out on finding the true causes of our patients' health problems. So this is really important."

Aside from stressful days over the last couple of years, the CEO said it also cost the corporation close to $1 million "to get everything back up to standard."

"But we needed to comply. We needed to spend that money in order to get our laboratory fully equipped. So it was all worth it for the community's health and safety," Muna said.

COMMONWEALTH HEALTHCARE CORP. LABORATORY DIRECTOR DR. PHILIP DAUTERMAN, CENTER, HOLDS THE CERTIFICATE OF COMPLIANCE AS HE POSES WITH LABORATORY STAFFERS, CHC CHIEF EXECUTIVE OFFICER ESTHER L.MUNA, PARTLY HIDDEN AT THE BACK, AND HOSPITAL ADMINISTRATOR JESS TUDELA, FIFTH FROM RIGHT. PHOTO BY EMMANUEL T. EREDIANO

Tudela applauded the CEO and the laboratory staff for "an awesome job of following up on the plan of correction."

He said without Muna's efforts to find and procure the necessary equipment, staff and supplies to ensure that we can provide the diagnostic tools "the hospital would be pretty much handicapped."

Lab Director positions tend to be quiet, behind the scenes positions. Media limelight such as that depicted above is extremely rare in my experience. My advice is to avoid publicity seeking and that excessive publicity could limit one's ability to work behind the scenes.

My advice is that if you receive a call from a journalist asking to interview you, always ask what the news story pertains to. In general, journalists will give honest answers or at least you can tell from their answer if the story will be favorable or unfavorable to your lab. If the story is unfavorable to your lab, remain tight-lipped and refer the call to the Hospital Administrator. If the story will be favorable to your lab, ask the Hospital Administrator for permission to step in front of the media spotlight.

In the above news article, the reporter has made a minor factual error - Certificates of Compliance are issued by CMS not by CLIA. This mistake is insignificant; however, it indicates there was miscommunication during the interview. In my experience, most reporters do not have much medical knowledge and misunderstandings such as this are common. My advice is that at the end of any interview always ask the reporter to read back his or her notes. This will help ensure the reporter understands the information you have given.

The above recommendations should be sufficient to get you through an interview with local news media. Local news interviews tend to be more informal and unstructured compared to interviews by national level news media. In my experience local news reporters do not have a political agenda. The biggest risk in this situation is that they will get the message mixed up or garbled.

It is my understanding that when being interviewed by national level news media there is a significant risk the reporter will have a political agenda and/or try to lead you astray. In this situation, the reporter will want to discuss topics unrelated to the intended topic of the interview. If this occurs, you should try to return the interview to the intended topic immediately.

For example, in the above news article the topic is the recent CMS inspection on the local laboratory. During the interview a reporter with a political agenda might ask you "What do you think about the recent tweet messages coming from the US President?". In this situation I would respond "That is unrelated to the topic of this interview. This interview is about the recent CMS inspection of our local laboratory. Our lab did very well in this inspection. I would like to thank the lab staff and hospital personnel who all worked very hard to help our lab pass this inspection."

A national level news interview will require much more preparation than a local level news interview. The news organization will contact your lab or hospital and ask for the interview. Both sides must agree to the date, time, venue, topic of the interview, which topics are off limits, etc. If there is no agreement on these specifics the interview will not occur. You should prepare in advance of the interview by reviewing as much information as you can on the topic that will be discussed. You should have a general idea of the questions that are likely to be asked, and be prepared to answer them. It is helpful to have practice interviews in advance of the real interview.

The reporter may ask you to make "off the record" comments. In this setting, there is no such thing as "off the record". Everything you say could appear in the news media. Try to keep your answers short and to the point. If you have an important message to present, be prepared to summarize it as a "sound bite" of 10 seconds or less.

Do not provide any information that is not needed to answer the question. Avoid using technical jargon or lab terminology that would not be understood outside of laboratory. If you do not know the answer to a question, state that you do not know. Do not lie, speculate or guess in an interview. Be polite in the interview. The reporter may ask questions intended to upset or anger you, but you should remain calm and friendly. Do not get into an argument with the reporter.

The interviewer may try to pressure you by asking questions rapid-fire. In this case, try to slow things down. It helps to repeat the question, as this will give you some time to think of an answer. Try to talk at a slow to moderate pace, even if the interviewer is speaking rapidly when asking questions.

I have never been interviewed by national level media, only by local media. My knowledge of national level interviews comes from classroom and training sessions at an APHL Biosafety Leadership Workshop.

> Topic #6 - Lab Director liability (malpractice) insurance

Liability insurance, also known as malpractice insurance, protects the purchaser (the "insured") from the risk of lawsuits. Every hospital I have ever worked at covered me under its umbrella plan for liability insurance. At one time, I applied to work at a hospital that required liability insurance for all physicians working there and required that the insurance must be bought from one particular insurance company. I did not take the position at that hospital, for other reasons. Although I never worked there, I saved the relevant application correspondence including the price list for liability insurance.

Looking over the price list for liability insurance, the highest rates are for the operative specialties. OB/GYN will pay the most at $47,520/yr. followed by orthopedic surgery at $30,103/yr. At the bottom of the list is "Other Low Risk Specialties" at $4,300/yr. and "General Medical Practitioner" at $2,310/yr. Pathology and Lab Directorship are not on the list. I asked for the "General Medical Practitioner" pricing, but they told me I'd get the "Other Low Risk Specialties" pricing.

Keep in mind that the insurance industry stratifies the specialties by risk. OB/GYN has the highest risk of getting sued so they pay the most per year. Lab Directors are very unlikely to be sued so we pay less.

In my experience, I am not aware of any Lab Director anywhere being sued for malpractice. This is in distinction to Pathology (i.e. reading slides) where there is significant risk. Pathology is included in most studies of litigation risk across all medical specialties. Pathologists face about a 7% to 9% per year risk of being sued, depending on which study you look at. Given these numbers, the average Pathologist is sued once every 11 to 14 years.

However, there is little literature summarizing the risk for Lab Directors. Lab Directors are not listed in the studies of litigation risk across all medical specialties. From reading the literature, the high risk areas (FNA, Cytopath, breast biopsy, etc.) all fall under anatomic pathology, not clinical pathology. However, the literature does indicate a small number of liability cases almost all related to Blood Bank. These studies were searches of legal databases containing many year's worth of data for the entire US and found only a few dozen cases. This averaged to maybe 2 or 3 Lab Director lawsuits per year for the entire US. In my opinion, this confirms that lawsuits naming Lab Directors are vanishingly rare.

My advice is that if you are looking at a position, and they require you to buy malpractice insurance, add the cost in to your salary requirements. Let me use the hospital above as an example. If I had been hired there, it would have been locum tenans coverage for 2 weeks per year while their pathologist is on vacation. Let's say I am willing to work for $100/hr. For 2 weeks at 40 hours per week that comes out to 80 hours or $8,000 per year. Add in the $4,300/yr. for the liability insurance and that comes to $12,300 for working there 80 hours per year. Divide by the 80 hours and that comes out to $153/hr. When negotiating for this position, I upped my salary request from $100/hr. to $153/hr. to compensate for the malpractice insurance, and asked for the contract to stipulate that they would reimburse me for the cost of the insurance if they didn't call me up for locum tenans work at least 2 weeks per year. The negotiations fell apart for other reasons, and I never worked at that hospital.

Most outpatient labs will either cover you under their umbrella plan or not require you to have malpractice insurance. All outpatient labs I have ever worked at have covered me under their umbrella plan. As Lab Director of an outpatient lab with no Blood Bank, I would not have been uncomfortable "flying blind" without malpractice insurance. In my opinion, the risk in this setting (outpatient lab with no Blood Bank) is so low that malpractice insurance wouldn't be worthwhile.

Topic #7 - Laboratory Information Technology (IT) and Laboratory Information Systems (LIS)

There is a great deal written in the laboratory literature on Laboratory Information Technology (IT) and Laboratory Information Systems (LIS). This stresses the need for maximum interoperability, upgrade-ability, interfacing with other departments (billing, purchasing, accounts payable, etc.), confidentiality of information, ease of use, etc. In this literature, there is a nearly universal assumption that lab will select the LIS without input from other areas of the hospital. In my experience, this is completely unrealistic.

In my experience in the typical hospital lab the LIS is a part of the entire Hospital Information System (HIS). The hospital will only get a new HIS very rarely, in my experience less than once per decade. The LIS will typically only be changed when the HIS changes. Every time the lab gets a new LIS, it would need to be interfaced to the HIS. This type of interface is very expensive and time consuming, hence the HIS and LIS typically are only changed in unison. In my experience, they are only changed when there is some impetus, such as newly added federal regulations on HIS/LIS systems.

There is a vast multitude of potential HIS/LIS systems to choose from. When selecting a new HIS/LIS the purchase decision is made by the Hospital's administration and Information Technology (IT) department based on the needs of the hospital as a whole, not just lab. When selecting a new HIS/LIS the hospital will typically start by making a tentative selection and informing all departments. At this stage of the game, it is imperative to check that the proposed new system can be easily interfaced with all of lab's instruments and can interface with the lab's reference lab. You will typically be allowed to veto the tentatively selected HIS/LIS. You should use this veto power on any proposed HIS/LIS that is not capable of interfacing with all instruments in lab or the lab's reference lab. I will go into more detail on this below.

All other areas of the hospital should be checking that the proposed HIS/LIS will work for them, and they are allowed veto power as well. The hospital's billing department should ensure that the billing for lab tests will work in the proposed new HIS/LIS. This should not be lab's responsibility, although in some situations the billing department may ask lab for information and/or input. The same applies for the hospital's other departments - procurement department, accounts payable department, etc. They should ensure that the new computer system will work for their departments, and not make it lab's responsibility to ensure that the lab's procurement, accounts payable, etc. are compatible with the proposed new HIS/LIS.

There are a multitude of HIS/LIS systems to choose from. If one is vetoed another will be tentatively selected. Be prepared that there may be multiple cycles of tentative selection followed by veto as one after another various departments determine that the proposed new HIS/LIS will not work for them.

This process continues until a HIS/LIS is selected that the entire hospital can agree to. Then the purchase documents are completed and the new HIS/LIS is put in place. The installation of cables, computer interfacing, training on use of the new system, etc. should not be lab's responsibility and should be the responsibility of the HIS/LIS vendor or the hospital's IT department.

The typical hospital lab has one or two lab techs trained as "super-users" able to change some details in the computer system such as reference ranges, critical values, etc. The other lab techs are able to result tests, but can't change reference ranges, critical values, etc. Anything requiring substantial changes to the computer system is referred to the hospital's IT department.

The LIS is very complicated and tends to be a problem area in most labs. For example, I am familiar with a small hospital that got a new HIS/LIS in 2013. The impetus for the purchase was newly enacted federal regulations on Meaningful Use (MU). The hospital's old HIS/LIS did not meet the new regulations at the time the regulations were enacted. This hospital was cash-strapped and obtained an HIS/LIS that was already an older model when it was installed. At about the same time in 2013, the hematology analyzers were replaced on an expedited basis due to problems with the analyzers. Technical issues delayed the interfacing of the hematology analyzers to the new HIS/LIS computer system. For at least a month's time the hematology results had to be typed into the HIS/LIS manually until the interface could be set up. During this time the hematology techs were very upset because the manual entry of test results is time consuming, laborious and carries the risk of transcription error.

This same HIS/LIS was not set up to interface with the lab's reference lab. As a result, all send out testing was reported as printout on a dedicated printer in lab. The phlebotomists had to manually transcribe the send-out results into the lab's HIS/LIS. Technical issues resulted in a protracted delay before the interface could be set up. This was very upsetting to the phlebotomists because the manual entry of test results is time consuming, laborious and carries the risk of transcription error.

This points out the need for lab to ensure any proposed new computer system can easily interface with all instruments in lab and with the lab's reference lab. Try as best you can to veto any proposed HIS/LIS that cannot do this. In this setting, I would further recommend that acquisition of new instruments should be delayed until the new HIS/LIS is in place, unless the acquisition is an emergency. In my case, this was not possible as the new HIS/LIS was a free gift from an outside organization, the existing HIS/LIS was outdated and could not meet newly enacted regulatory requirements, the hospital could not afford a better HIS/LIS and the hematology analyzers had unexpected breakdowns requiring expedited replacement.

If you find that your new computer system is not able to interface with lab's instruments and/or reference lab be prepared that the lab staff will be very upset with the manual entry of data; since it is slow, time consuming, and carries the risk of transcription error.

In my experience the most common Laboratory IT problem you will have to deal with is protracted downtime of the LIS and/or HIS. Always have a backup plan in case the computer system goes down and can't be brought back up quickly. In my experience, most labs revert to paper ordering and resulting if the computer system is going to be down for 2 hours or more. After the computer system comes back up the test results that were initially paper-reported are then entered into the computer via instrument interface.

Do your best to ensure that there are adequate backups of patient test results. As mentioned in a previous chapter, record retention is a CLIA requirement. Loss of recent lab test records is a CLIA violation, and should be avoided. However, the safekeeping of lab's records is typically entrusted to the hospital's IT department. Lab typically has little control over how the hospital's IT department handles backups. My advice is to query the IT department as to how it is handling the backups of lab's data. If you don't like the answer you get, ask the head of the IT department to add layers of backups and/or discuss with the Hospital Administrator that you would like better backups of lab's data.

Topic #8 - The End. How to perform voluntary closure of a laboratory

There are a number of situations where voluntary closure of a laboratory may become necessary:

1. The hospital as a whole is closing down.
2. The hospital is consolidating, merging and/or reorganizing and feels your lab is no longer necessary.
3. Your lab has failed so many PT that one more failed PT will result in regulatory closure.
4. Your lab is facing imminent regulatory closure for reasons other than failed PT.
5. Your lab has been consistently losing money, and is no longer financially viable.

In my 29 years experience in Pathology and Lab Medicine I have never had to perform voluntary closure of a laboratory. I have dodged this bullet so far. Therefore, the entirety of this information is based on my knowledge of distant lab closings and not speaking from personal experience.

My assumption is that voluntary closure of a lab is more or less the reverse of starting a new lab. The date of closure should be known well in advance. If the hospital as a whole is closing down, merging, or reorganizing, etc., you should have at least 6 months advance notice. If you are closing the lab due to failed PT, you will know the date of the next PT shipment. PT is sent three times per year, so you should have a few months advance notice to close your lab before the next PT is due to be sent.

As soon as the decision is made to close your lab you should notify your regulator (CMS, CAP, etc.) of the pending closure and the planned closing date. You will need to submit the relevant forms to your regulator notifying them of the pending closure.

All standing orders for reagents and supplies are discontinued in advance of the closure date such that there will be minimal inventory remaining on the closure date. If you time the discontinuation of shipments correctly, you should have just barely enough inventory left to get you through to the closure date.

The lab staff should be given notice that the lab is closing. The Federal government mandates a minimum 60 days notice if you have more than 100 employees. Some states mandate a minimum notice period (typically 60 days notice) for all layoffs regardless of the number of employees. The employees may have a longer notice period (e.g. 90 days notice) or severance packages stipulated in their employment documents. Given the time frame of the typical lab closure, you should have enough advance notice of the lab closing to meet the minimum notice periods.

The layoffs will be the most onerous part of the lab closure to carry out. As a Lab Director, you are responsible in many ways for the well-being of your lab staff. If you have been working with the lab staff for many years these layoffs will make you feel like you are Judas, the betrayer.

If the hospital as a whole is closing, you don't need to make arrangements to hand off testing to anther lab. There will be no patients left to test after the hospital closes.

If you are heading an outpatient lab that is closing, inform all hospitals, clinics and doctors in your municipality well in advance of the closure date that your lab will no longer accept patients as of the closure date. The hospitals, clinics and doctors will then refer their patients to any other available lab in that municipality.

If the hospital remains open, but the lab is closing, there must be some way of handing off the patient testing to a new lab, or an outside lab. The new or outside lab should be able to do all STAT testing on-site. The routine testing could be referred to the main testing site for that lab. In other words, the new or outside lab must set up at least a STAT lab on-site but could otherwise be a draw station with the testing referred out.

If there is a new lab taking the place of your lab, ask that lab to accept as many of your lab staff as possible to work in that lab. This will decrease the dislocation on your lab staff. The other labs in your municipality will likely have at least a few vacant job positions and will likely gladly accept new hires coming from your lab.

At the close of the last business day there is usually a very sad going away party, and a notice of closure is placed on the front door of the lab. No one will be present in the lab and valuable equipment will still be left in the lab until such time as the equipment can be disposed. This situation invites theft. Be careful to have sufficient security, at least an alarm or monitored cameras, and not just a lock on the front door. After the equipment has been disposed and removed from your lab you can drop the security. It is the laboratory's responsibility to dispose of all hazardous materials (hazardous chemicals, bacterial cultures, etc.) in a manner meeting regulations.

After the closure date passes, the lab will no longer be doing any testing. There will be essentially no reagents or supplies left. The lab needs to dispose of all remaining items in its possession, the most valuable of which is the equipment. For any equipment that is leased or rented, ask the owner to take the equipment back. Any equipment owned by the lab will need to be sold. Each piece of equipment is removed from your lab after its disposition is determined.

The lab will likely have ongoing financial obligations after the closure date (rent, equipment lease expenses, etc.) and no way to pay the bills. The testing has ceased so there is no income. The sale of equipment may raise some cash, but this is not likely to meet expenses for long. Hence, liquidation is time sensitive and should be completed as expeditiously as possible. The lab as a corporation will likely have to file bankruptcy to eliminate its obligations.

Make sure you pick a reputable legal office to handle the bankruptcy. This legal office will typically handle all affairs for your defunct lab after the bankruptcy is completed. Make arrangements that all correspondence addressed to your lab should be forwarded to this legal office. After the bankruptcy is completed, the lab no longer exists as a going entity.

The records of patient testing must be retained for the length of time specified under CLIA. For an outpatient lab, this is usually accomplished by leaving the testing records with the same legal office that handled the bankruptcy. This legal office will handle any release of patient test results for your defunct lab. For an inpatient lab, these records are left with the hospital's medical records department.

Other records, such as PT, preventive maintenance, etc. are usually given over to the lab that acquires the relevant equipment. Any lab that acquires your equipment will need to produce 2 years worth of PT, preventive maintenance records, etc. at their next CMS or CAP inspection. Thus, the acquiring lab will not likely accept your equipment without the relevant records.

After the last remaining items are disposed from your lab, the rented space can be turned back over to the landlord. Immediately before this handover, make one last pass through this now empty rented space which used to be your lab to make sure that nothing of value remains. The landlord will dispose of anything you leave behind, clean the space, remove all your company's logos, and rent the space to the next tenant.

MY LABORATORY   MY PROCEDURE MANUAL
INDEX
page 1 of 4

Topic	Page
Accuracy	9
Analyte Specific Reagent (ASR)	42-43
Analytic Measurement Range (AMR)	52-54, 70, 74
Analyzer breakdowns	62-65
Causes	62
Diagnosing	62-63
Repairing	63-65
Antibiotic sensitivity testing, verif. of	216-218
Application for certification	61, 183-184, 188
Timing of application	184, 188
As Soon As Possible (ASAP) test ordering	7
Calibration	51
Calibration verification	51-52
CAP	27, 37, 54-55, 78, 121, 123, 131-132, 151
Additional requirements under CAP as compared to CLIA	27, 46, 78, 151
CAP deemed status from CMS	150-151
CAP critical value policy requirements	54-55
CAP lab director duties	121, 131-132
CAP lack of unscheduled PT events	37
CAP procedure manual requirements	78
CAP requirement for a lab disaster plan	123
CAP requirements for test verification	46
CAP requiring PT of waived analytes	27
Chain of command	3-4
CLIA	3
CMS Certificates	151, 183-184, 185-186, 188
Certificate of Compliance	151
Certificate of PPM	185-186
Certificate of Registration	188
Certificate of Waiver	183-184
CMS form 116 App. for Certification	61, 183, 188
CMS form 209 Lab personnel report	4-7
CMS form 2567 Inspection deficiencies	156-169
Coefficient of Variation (CV)	219
College of American Pathologists – see CAP	
Color of drawing tube tops	7-8
Complaints involving lab	86, 90-91
Conflict and conflict resolution	195-199

Topic	Page
Controls	56-57
Assayed controls	56
In control defined	57
Out of control defined	57
Requirement to verify all controls	57
Unassayed controls	56
Corrective action	22-41, 50, 86-90, 156-169
for correlation	50
for inspection citations	156-169
for out of control tests	22-23
for PT, multiple failed	36-41
for PT, single failed	33-36
for QA	86-90
Correlation	47-51
Credentialing	203
Credible Allegation of Compliance	163
Critical values	54-55, 59, 61-62
Current Procedural Terminology (CPT) codes	59
Daily maintenance	60
Disaster planning	123-130
Disaster with loss of infrastructure	125-130
Disaster with mass casualties	123-125
Disruptive practitioner	205
Equivalent Quality Control (EQC)	58, 220
Error, in measurement	9
Bias, in measurement	9
Random error	9
Systematic error	9
Ethics	191-195
Expert witness	175-182
Expert witness scheduling	177, 180-181
Expert witness bill of rights	180-181
Expired reagents and supplies, use of	140
False negative	10-12
False positive	10-12
Fire Drills	123
Food and Drug Administration (FDA)	41-43
Clearance or approval of lab tests	42-43
Regulatory authority over all lab tests	41-42

MY LABORATORY — MY PROCEDURE MANUAL
INDEX
page 2 of 4

Topic	Page
FPPE	146, 209-210
Function checks	59-60
HIPAA	172-175
Authorization to disclose PHI form	174
Protected Health Information (PHI)	172
Incident reports involving lab	91-93
Individualized Quality Control Plan (IQCP)	58, 220-223
Example IQCP	223
Infection Control in lab	140
Inspections of lab	150-169
Choosing inspection agency	151
Credible Allegation of Compliance	163
Day of the inspection	155-157
Deemed status inspecting agencies	150-151
Plan of correction	156-169
Preparing for the inspection	151-155
Re-inspections	157
Responding to citations	156-169
Inventory control	136-140
Minimum Operating Inventory	137, 139
Par level - see Minimum Operat. Inventory	
ISO nomenclature and regulations	9
Job descriptions	130-131
Lab Directors	205-211
Competency testing	209-210
Duties and responsibilities	207-208
Staffing & recruitment	208
Orientation	208-209
Promotion	210
Qualifications	205-206
Retention	210
Retirement	210-211
Laboratory Information System (LIS)	227-228
Lab mutinies	196-198
Lab planning	121-122
Deciding on in-house testing	121-122
Lab Supervisors	133-140
Competency testing	135
Delegation of duties	136
Duties and responsibilities	134-135
Promotion	135
Qualifications	134
Retention	135
Lab techs	108-120
Competency testing	112-117
Competency testing form	114-115
Discipline and termination	118-120
Staffing and recruitment	109-112
Orientation	112
Promotion	117
Qualifications	108-109
Retention	117-118
Retirement	117
Lab workflow	122
Lab work shifts	4
Leadership skills	198-199
Legal considerations	175-182
Court testimony	177-182
Expert witness scheduling	177, 180-181
Expert witness bill of rights	180-181
Deposition	177, 182
Subpoena	175-176, 182
Levels of complexity of lab tests	3
Levey-Jennings charts	13-14
Liability insurance	226-227
Limit of detection (LoD)	11-12
Limit of quantitation (LoQ)	11
Linearity	52-53, 66-77
Malpractice insurance	226-227
Medicare Exclusion Database (MED)	171
Meetings	199-205
Chairing a meeting	199-202
Medical Executive Committee	202-205

MY LABORATORY   MY PROCEDURE MANUAL
INDEX
page 3 of 4

Topic	Page
Memorandum	77
MSDS – see Safety Data Sheets	
New analyzer, setting into service	41-60, 213-220
Correlation	47-51
Deciding to buy, rent or lease	45-46
Imprecision allowable	52
Maintenance, routine and preventive	59-60
"Off label" test verification	218-220
Qualitative analyzer verification	213-218
Quantitative analyzer verification	41-60
Regulatory requirements	41-43, 213, 218
Selecting new analyzer	43-45
Validation, definition of	42
Verification, definition of	42
New test, setting into service	60-62
Normal values – see Reference range	
OPPE	146-147, 209
OPPE form	147
Ordering of Lab tests	7
Organism identification, verification of	216-218
OSHA regulations covering lab	79-80, 92, 123
Panic values – see Critical values	
Pathologists	143-150
Pathologist competency testing	145-148
Pathologist hiring	143-144
Pathologist orientation	144
Pathologist promotion	144
Pathologist qualifications	143
Pathologist retention	144
Pathologist retirement	148-150
Personnel problems	93-102
Behavioral issues	100-101
Disagreements between employees	96-99
Late to work employees	99-100
Performance issues	101-102
Potentially homicidal employee	94-95
Potentially suicidal employee	95-96
Physician demands on lab	102-103
Physician ordering practices	102
Physician privileging	202-204
Plan of correction	156-169
Plasma	8
Policy	77
Precision	9, 52, 213, 219
Preventive maintenance (PM)	59-60
Problem solving	202
Procedures	56, 77-84
CLIA requirements	79-84
OSHA requirements	79-80
Professional relations	103-108
Proficiency testing (PT)	27-41, 56, 58, 61, 68, 212
CLIA requirements	27-30, 36
Educational challenge and no consensus	32
Example of failing PT	33, 36
Example of passing PT	31
Initial unsuccessful participation in PT	36-40
Passing defined	27-28, 36
Peer group	31, 68
PT failure mitigation – see Corrective Action	
Repeat unsuccessful participation in PT	40-41
Ordering	56, 58, 61
When testing is done at multiple sites	212-213
Provider Performed Microscopy (PPM)	185-186
Public Information Officer (PIO)	224-226
Public release of information	224-226
Quality Assurance (QA)	84-93
Analytical phases of lab testing	85
CLIA and CMS requirements	85
QA, definition of	84
QA form, monthly	87
QA indicators	84
Quality Control (QC)	15, 22, 23, 84
QC, definition of	84

MY LABORATORY — MY PROCEDURE MANUAL
INDEX
page 4 of 4

Topic	Page
Record retention	60, 80, 84
Changed procedures	84
Daily controls	60
Employee training and competency testing	60
Patient test reports	60
Preventive Maintenance	60
Proficiency testing	60
Quality control records	60
Retired procedures	80
Test requisitions	60
Reference laboratories	131-133
Monitoring the performance of	132-133
Requirement for contract with	132
Selection of	131
Reference range	54, 59, 61-62
Regulatory closure	163-164, 170-172
Reportable range	53
Definition of reportable range	53
Expanded reportable range	53
Robustness of a test	42, 219
Root Cause Analysis (RCA)	92-93
Routine test ordering	7
Ruggedness of a test	42
Safety Data Sheets (SDS)	79-80, 123
Section Supervisors	141-142
Competency testing	142
Duties and responsibilities	141
Promotion	142
Qualifications	141
Retention	142
Selection of reference laboratory	131
Sensitivity	10-12
Serum	8
Service pin, example	125
Shift	21, 25, 27

Topic	Page
Sop	58-59, 79
Specificity	10-12
Starting a new lab	186-191
STAT test ordering	7
Test modification	43, 185, 218
The Joint Commission - see TJC	
Timed test ordering	7
TJC	54-55, 123, 139, 146-148, 150-151, 203
Blood Utilization Review Requirement	139
TJC deemed status from CMS	150-151
TJC critical values policy requirements	54-55
TJC requirement for a lab disaster plan	123
TJC requirement for FPPE	146
TJC requirement for OPPE	146-148
TJC requirements for privileging	203
Trend	21, 25, 27
True positive	10-11
True negative	10
Turnaround time of lab tests	7
Validation	42
Definition of validation	42
Verification	41-60, 213-220
Definition of verification	42
Qualitative analyzer verification	213-218
Quantitative analyzer verification	41-60
Verif. of organism identification	216-218
Verif. of antibiotic sensitivity testing	216-218
"Off label" test verification	218-220
Voluntary closure of a laboratory	229-230
Waived testing	182-185
Westgard rules	15-27
Passing QC defined	22
Rule failure corrective action	22, 23
Rule failure defined	22

Pictures of me having a bad year in 2015

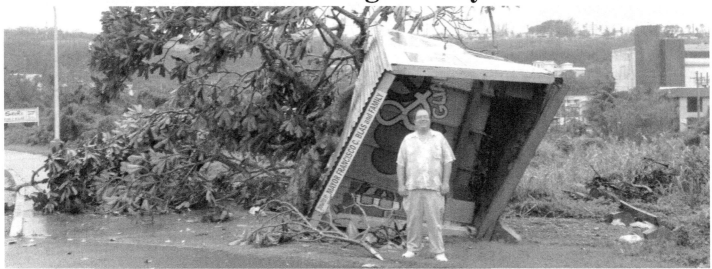

Picture of me on Guam the day after Typhoon Dolphin. I was on a temporary 2 week assignment to Guam in May, 2015 when Typhoon Dolphin hit. This photo shows typical Category 1 Hurricane damage – flimsy wooden structure overturned but not completely disintegrated. The tree trunk is still standing with large branches down on the sidewalk. There is no damage to any concrete structure in this photo.

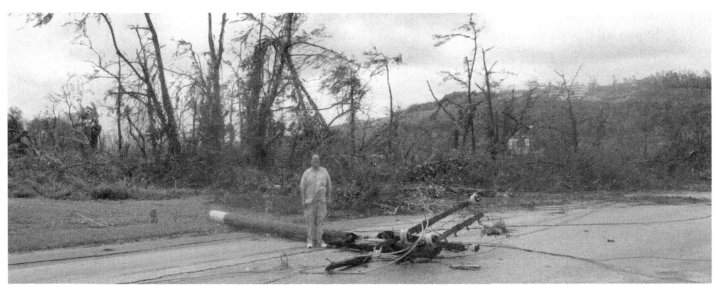

Picture of me on Saipan the day after Typhoon Soudelor. I work full time on Saipan where Typhoon Soudelor hit August 2, 2015. This photo shows hurricane damage typical of Category 3 or higher – a downed telephone pole with multiple large trees broken at the trunk or entirely uprooted. An entire forest has been felled, such that structures are visible on the distant hillside that would not ordinarily be visible through a forest. Disintegrated structures and debris from disintegrated structures can be seen on the hillside.

I lost 23 pounds on the Hurricane Diet Plan

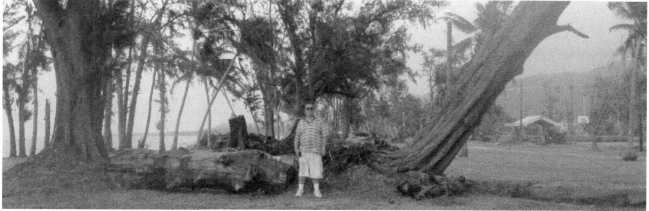

Picture of me on Saipan taken October 24, 2015 about two and a half months after Typhoon Soudelor hit August 2. The debris has been largely removed but a few downed trees remain. In the background, both concrete and wooden phone poles can be seen. Each concrete phone pole replaces a downed wooden phone pole. At the time of this photo, my apartment still did not have electric power restored after the storm. In that time I lost 23 pounds, down from 248 pounds at the time of the storm to 225 pounds in this photo. If you don't have electric power you can't cook your food and your refrigerator doesn't work either. After a major hurricane, the food supply will be so disrupted you literally won't know where your next meal is coming from. I refer to this as the Hurricane Diet Plan.

About the author

Dr. Dauterman received his M.D. Degree from Ross University followed by residency training in anatomical and clinical pathology at Eastern Virginia Medical School in Norfolk, Virginia. He completed his pathology training with a surgical pathology fellowship at SUNY Health Science Center, Brooklyn, New York. He spent the next 16 years practicing pathology at Guam Memorial Hospital, initially as a staff pathologist and eventually Laboratory Director. During his time on Guam, he served as a pathology consultant for the U.S. Navy. Dr. Dauterman accepted a Pathologist position at Jack C. Montgomery VAMC, Muskogee, OK for one year.

Dr. Dauterman returned to the Mariana Islands where he is currently serving as a Laboratory Director and Consultant for Saipan and Guam as well as the American Samoa Department of Public Health.

Dr. Dauterman is board certified in Anatomic and Clinical Pathology and a Fellow of the College of American Pathologists.

This book is a practical guide designed for physicians, medical technologists and doctoral level scientists involved in Laboratory Medicine. Pathologists and pathology residents may find it especially useful as these topics are rarely covered in-depth during the rigorous training of pathology. Dr. Dauterman's practical advice covers many complicated topics such as quality control, laboratory administration and accreditation, hospital and peer relations as well as employee relations. He covers these topics with humorous stories from real life events teaching us how to be a Laboratory Director.

About the Author is written by Timothy Sorrells, MD

Made in the USA
Middletown, DE
20 November 2020